Baillière's
CLINICAL
OBSTETRICS
AND
GYNAECOLOGY
INTERNATIONAL PRACTICE AND RESEARCH

Baillière's
CLINICAL OBSTETRICS AND GYNAECOLOGY
INTERNATIONAL PRACTICE AND RESEARCH

Volume 5/Number 1
March 1991

Factors of Importance for Implantation

M. SEPPÄLÄ MD, FRCOG
Guest Editor

Baillière Tindall
London Philadelphia Sydney Tokyo Toronto

This book is printed on acid-free paper.

Baillière Tindall   24–28 Oval Road,
W.B. Saunders   London NW1 7DX

The Curtis Center, Independence Square West,
Philadelphia, PA 19106–3399, USA

55 Horner Avenue
Toronto, Ontario M8Z 4X6, Canada

Harcourt Brace Jovanovich Group (Australia) Pty Ltd,
30–52 Smidmore Street, Marrickville, NSW 2204, Australia

Harcourt Brace Jovanovich Japan, Inc,
Ichibancho Central Building,
22-1 Ichibancho, Chiyoda-ku, Tokyo 102, Japan

ISSN 0950–3552

ISBN 0–7020–1533–4 (single copy)

Baillière's Clinical Obstetrics and Gynaecology is published four times each year by
Baillière Tindall. Annual subscription prices are:

TERRITORY	ANNUAL SUBSCRIPTION	SINGLE ISSUE
1. UK	£55.00 post free	£27.50 post free
2. Europe	£61.00 post free	£27.50 post free
3. All other countries	Consult your local Harcourt Brace Jovanovich office for dollar price	

The editor of this publication is Margaret Macdonald, Baillière Tindall,
24–28 Oval Road, London NW1 7DX.

Baillière's Clinical Obstetrics and Gynaecology was published from 1983 to 1986 as
Clinics in Obstetrics and Gynaecology.

Typeset by Phoenix Photosetting, Chatham.
Printed and bound in Great Britain by Mackays of Chatham PLC, Chatham, Kent.

Contributors to this issue

MATS ÅKERLUND MD, PhD, Associate Professor and Consultant, Department of Obstetrics and Gynaecology, University Hospital, S-22185 Lund, Sweden.

MAARIT ANGERVO MD, Department I of Obstetrics and Gynaecology, Helsinki University Central Hospital, SF-00290 Helsinki, Finland.

CHRISTINE BERGERON MD, Institut de Pathologie Cellulaire, 53 rue des Belles Feuilles, 755116 Paris, France.

PHILIPPE BOUCHARD MD, Professor of Medicine, Service d'Endocrinologie et des Maladies de la Reproduction, Hôpital Bicêtre, 78, rue du Général Leclerc, 94270 Le Kremlin-Bicêtre, Paris, France.

TIM CHARD MD, FRCOG, Professor, Reproductive Physiology, St. Bartholomews Hospital, London EC1A 7BE, UK.

DAVID A. CLARK MD, PhD, FRCPC, Professor, Departments of Medicine/Obstetrics-Gynaecology, McMaster University, 1200 Main Street West, Hamilton, Ontario, Canada L8N 3Z5.

ROBERT G. EDWARDS CBE, DSc, FRCOG, Hon MRCP, FRS, Scientific Director, Bourn Hall Clinic, Courn, Cambridge CB3 7TR, UK.

J. K. FINDLAY BAgSc, PhD, Prince Henry's Institute of Medical Research, PO Box 118, South Melbourne, Victoria 3205, Australia.

RENE FRYDMAN MD, Chief, Department of Obstetrics & Gynaecology, Hôpital Antoine Béclère, 157 avenue de la Porte de Trivaux, 92141 Clamart, France.

GERALDINE M. HARTSHORNE BSc, PhD, Bourn Hall Clinic, Courn, Cambridge, CB3 7TR, UK.

DAVID L. HEALY BMedSci, MBBS, PhD, FRACOG, Professor in Obstetrics and Gynaecology, Monash University and Chief, Reproductive Biology Unit, Monash Medical Centre, Melbourne, Australia.

ELISABETH JOHANNISSON MD, PhD, Consulting Professor, Clinic of Sterility, Department of Obstetrics and Gynaecology, Faculty of Medicine, University of Geneva, Switzerland.

MERVI JULKUNEN MD, Department I of Obstetrics and Gynaecology, Helsinki University Central Hospital, SF-00290 Helsinki, Finland.

RIITTA KOISTINEN PhD, Hormone Laboratory, Department I of Obstetrics and Gynaecology, Helsinki University Central Hospital, SF-00290 Helsinki, Finland.

RICHARD G. LEA BSc(Hons), PhD, McMaster University, Room 4H13, 1200 Main Street West, Hamilton, Ontario, L8N 3Z5, Canada.

SVEND LINDENBERG MD, Research Fellow, Department of Obstetrics and Gynaecology, Chromosome Laboratorium, 4051, Rigshospitalet, University of Copenhagen, Blegdamsvej 9, Denmark 2100.

ADRIAN LOWER BMedSci, BMBS, MRCOG, Research Fellow, Academic Unit of Obstetrics and Gynaecology, The Royal London Hospital; PIVET Medical Centre, 166–168 Cambridge St, Perth, Western Australia.

JULIA MARRAOUI MD, Post-Doctoral Fellow, Service d'Endocrinologie et des Maladies de la Reproduction, Hôpital Bicêtre, 78 rue du Général Leclerc, 94270 Le Kremlin-Bicêtre, Paris, France.

MARIA-REBECCA MASSAI MD, Post-Doctoral Fellow, Service d'Endocrinologie et des Maladies de la Reproduction, Hopital Bicêtre, 78, rue du Général Leclerc, 94270 Le Kremlin-Bicêtre, Paris, France.

DANIEL MEDALIE, Graduate Student, Serive d'Endocrinologie et des Maladies de la Reproduction, Hôpital Bicêtre, 78, rue du Général Leclerc, 94270 Le Kremlin-Bicêtre, Paris, France.

CHRIS O'NEILL BSc, PhD, Director, Human Reproduction Unit, Royal North Shore Hospital of Sydney, St. Leonards, New South Wales 2065, Australia.

MARTINE PERROT-APPLANAT MD, Directeur de Recherche, INSERM U 135, Hôpital Bicêtre, 78, rue du Général Leclerc, 94270 Le Kremlin-Bicêtre, Paris, France.

LEENA RIITTINEN MSc, Hormone Laboratory, Department I of Obstetrics and Gynaecology, Helsinki University Central Hospital, SF-00290 Helsinki, Finland.

LOIS A. SALAMONSEN PhD, Research Officer, Prince Henry's Institute of Medical Research, PO Box 118, South Melbourne 3025, Australia.

MARKKU SEPPÄLÄ MD, FRCOG, Professor, Department I of Obstetrics and Gynaecology, Helsinki University Central Hospital, SF-00290 Helsinki, Finland.

STEPHEN K. SMITH MBBS, MD, MRCOG, Professor, Department of Obstetrics and Gynaecology, University of Cambridge, Rosie Maternity Hospital, Cambridge CB2 2SW, UK.

JOHN YOVICH MBBS, MD, FRACOG, FRCOG, previously: Medical Director, Pivet Medical Centre, Perth, Western Australia; currently: Medical Director, Hallam Medical Centre, 112 Harley Street, London W1N 1AF, UK.

DOMINIQUE DE ZIEGLER MD, Associate Professor of Medicine, Department of Obstetrics & Gynaecology, Hôpital Antoine Béclère, 157 avenue de la Porte de Trivaux, 92141 Clamart, France.

Table of contents

PREVIOUS ISSUES

FORTHCOMING ISSUES

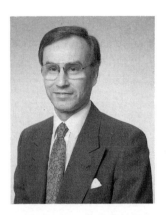

Foreword

Implantation is a sequence of events whereby the fertilized ovum, having hatched from the zona pellucida and reached the blastocyst stage, attaches into the uterine wall. Implantation remains the most difficult single part of assisted reproduction, and an understanding of its mechanisms is the key for any advance to be made in this field. Much of our current knowledge is based on studies in laboratory animals because ethical restraints prevent reproductive experimentations in the human.

From epidemiological data, it has been estimated that as many as 80% of human conceptions are lost before term. Evidence for this is reviewed in the chapter by Tim Chard. Not all implantation failures can be attributed to anatomical and chromosomal defects. The role of embryonic factors is presented in a comprehensive overview by pioneers in the field from Cambridge, UK. Many biologically active substances have been identified in the embryo; they include chorionic gonadotrophin and growth factors. Vasoactive products, such as platelet-activating factor, histamine and prostaglandins, and other embryonic factors, such as polyamines, are dealt with in the articles by Chris O'Neill, Stephen Smith and Richard Lea and David Clark.

As to maternal factors, cyclical changes in the uterus in response to hormonal stimuli can also be studied in the absence of an embryo. Elisabeth Johannisson, Svend Lindenberg and Mats Åkerlund have contributed chapters on microscopic and ultrastructural changes in the endometrium and implantation, and on the function of blood vessels relative to implantation. The role of adaptive and para-immune systems is extensively reassessed by Richard Lea and David Clark, while the interactions of prolactin with white blood cells in the decidual reaction, and paracrine factors relative to implantation are reviewed by Jock Findlay and Lois Salamonsen. Chapters on endometrial steroid receptors and protein secretion are also included. Finally, the results of current clinical practice to improve the implantation rate are evaluated by John Yovich and Adrian Lower.

Besides writing the chapters the authors themselves have contributed greatly to the new information presented. It has been a privilege to edit this volume for them. I wish to thank the authors for their devoted work and

hope the volume will be a worthwhile account of the current state of the art
in implantation research and clinical practice.

MARKKU SEPPÄLÄ

1

Ultrastructure in human implantation: transmission and scanning electron microscopy

SVEND LINDENBERG

After normal fertilization and development of the mammalian ovum to the blastocyst stage, implantation takes place in the uterus. Implantation is the process by which the embryo becomes intimately connected with the maternal tissue of the uterus. As mammalian implantation involves embryonic and maternal processes, it is useful to separate the events of implantation into a series of developmental phases: apposition, adhesion and penetration (Figure 1).

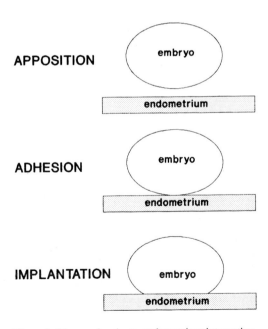

Figure 1. Phases of embryo–endometrium interaction.

Baillière's Clinical Obstetrics and Gynaecology—
Vol. 5, No. 1, March 1991
ISBN 0–7020–1533–4

Apposition and adhesion of the trophoblast cells to the uterine surface

Little is known about the molecular basis of the acquisition of adhesiveness by the trophoblast and uterine surface, but both the plasmalemma of the trophoblast and the uterine epithelium contain molecules which have been associated with specific fundamental processes. Chavez (1986) found a molecular modification of the trophoblast surface at the time of attachment using lectins, indicating a change in the complex carbohydrate moieties of the glycopeptides, glycolipids or glycosaminoglycans located on the surface of the attaching trophoblast. The carbohydrate complexes of the luminal uterine surface have also been shown to change during the adhesive phase (Chavez and Anderson, 1985; Anderson et al, 1986). This carbohydrate-rich domain is termed the glycocalyx.

In recent studies by Lindenberg et al (1989, 1990) and Kimber et al (1990), a specific oligosaccharide determinant on the surface of the uterus in mice appears at the time of implantation due to hormonal induction. This determinant corresponds to a lectin receptor on the trophoblast at the time of attachment of the embryo, thus facilitating the initial attachment and implantation. There is evidence that corresponding glycoconjugate–receptor interactions are involved in human implantation (S. Lindenberg and S. J. Kimber, unpublished data).

Penetration of the trophoblast into the uterine epithelium

Penetration of the trophoblast into the epithelium has been extensively studied in vivo in different mammalian species. These studies have revealed three primary types of penetration: (1) a fusional type, such as observed in the rabbit (Larsen, 1961; Schlafke and Enders, 1975), where the trophoblast fuses with the epithelial cells of the endometrium; (2) an intrusive type, as in the ferret (Enders and Schlafke, 1972), where trophoblast cells extend cytoplasmic protrusions between individual epithelial cells; and (3) a displacement type, such as that observed in the rat and mouse (Tachi et al, 1970; Finn, 1982), where trophoblast cells simply displace the epithelial cells, i.e. lift them away from the stroma.

All these mechanisms for penetration of the uterine epithelium represent the initial process in the development of the placental organ, which is in direct contact with the maternal blood circulation (and is therefore named haemochorial placentation), securing intimate contact and nutrients for the embryo. However, a fourth mechanism, not primarily involving a phase of penetration of the uterine epithelium by the trophoblast, can be observed in the cow (Wathes and Wooding, 1980) and pig (Dantzer, 1985). Here, the trophoblast grows on the uterine epithelium without penetration. Thus the placental organ in these animals is organized on the uterine epithelial lining (and is therefore called epitheliochorial placentation), in contrast to the aforementioned, where the placental organ is located within the uterine tissue.

Interestingly, all these different types of placentation have at least one element in common, namely a specialized close cell–cell interaction between the trophoblast and the surface epithelium of the uterus.

REGULATION OF IMPLANTATION

The concept of mammalian implantation described above has been based upon morphological criteria from observations of histological specimens of implantation sites in vivo. Until the early 1960s implantation was considered to start at the stage when invasion of the endometrium by the embryonic cells, or the uterine response to this invasion, as evidenced by morphological criteria. Now it is known that this implantation process is preceded by a series of embryo–maternal interactions (Heald, 1976; Bazer and Roberts, 1983; Heap et al, 1986; Hearn, 1986; Nieder et al, 1987).

The mammalian implantation involves extensive modifications of the embryo and endometrium. As well as cell–cell contact between the embryo and the uterus, extracellular signals of a specific nature pass both ways between the blastocyst and the uterine epithelium (Surani, 1977; Heap et al, 1979; Nieder and Macon, 1987).

Furthermore, an exact synchrony between embryonic development and the state of the uterus (also named the receptive phase) seems to be essential for successful implantation, at least in the mouse (McLaren and Michie, 1956; Psychoyos, 1976; Heap et al, 1979; Vanderhyden and Armstrong, 1988). In the human the receptive phase may be longer, and a less exact synchrony may be necessary (Cecco et al, 1984). However, significant asynchrony might have an impact on success following in vitro fertilization and embryo transfer in the human (Edwards et al, 1981).

Observations on pig embryos by Samuel and Perry (1972) also stress the importance of specific regulation between the trophoblast and the uterine organ. The pig embryo normally forms a chorioepithelial placentation without syncytium formation and penetration of the uterine epithelial cells in utero, but when Samuel and Perry transferred these embryos to ectopic sites, a syncytium was observed in addition to invasive trophoblast activity. In rodents, a similar phenomenon is seen when embryos are transferred to an ectopic site (Kirby, 1962). This led to the hypothesis that the uterus might be the most hostile place for the embryo, except at the time for implantation.

HUMAN STUDIES

To gain specific information about development of the human peri-implantation embryo, considerable efforts have been made to sample human embryos and implantation sites in vivo (Hertig et al, 1956, 1958; Larsen and Knoth, 1971; Knoth and Larsen, 1972; Croxatto et al, 1978, 1979; Buster et al, 1985). This work has enabled us to estimate the time taken for transport of the embryo through the fallopian tubes and for the development of the embryo to various stages in the early post-implantation period. However, no information on the time and mode of attachment and initial penetration has been obtained. Attempts to extrapolate animal data to explain human implantation mechanisms have failed and it is clear that comparisons can only be made with caution, even between closely related species (Ramsey et al, 1976). An alternative approach has been to investigate the potential of an in vitro implantation model.

Results of studying human implantation in vitro

With the introduction of human in vitro fertilization (IVF) and embryo transfer (ET) techniques (Edwards et al, 1970, 1981; Trounson and Conti, 1981) human embryos have become accessible on a large scale. Holmes and Lindenberg (1988) observed human trophoblastic outgrowth in vitro from blastocysts cultured on plastic. This study could only demonstrate that human blastocysts can develop to the hatched blastocyst stage in vitro.

By using techniques specifically developed for culturing human endometrial epithelial monolayer cells (Lindenberg et al, 1984), it was possible to produce a system for studying attachment of the human blastocyst to these epithelial cells in vitro (Lindenberg et al, 1985).

Admittedly, development of human embryos in vitro does not exactly reflect the situation in vivo, for the following reasons: (1) the endometrial stromal and maternal hormonal influences are lacking; (2) no decidualization can take place; and (3) the growth potential is limited. Nevertheless, it seems reasonable to believe that some aspects of the development of embryos in vitro reflect what happens in vivo (Sherman and Wudl, 1976), including the attachment mechanism (Jenkinson, 1977), and in endometrial monolayer cultures (Fay et al, 1990a, 1990b).

The study of attachment in vitro (Lindenberg et al, 1986, 1989) initially revealed a considerable embryonic loss during development from oocytes to hatched blastocysts. Only 10% (4/42) of mature oocyte–cumulus complexes reached the hatched blastocyst stage. These data are in accordance with Fishel et al (1985), who reported that 5% (10/192) of human ova developed to hatched blastocysts.

Morphological changes in the blastocyst

When the in vitro developed blastocysts were fully hatched, only the polar

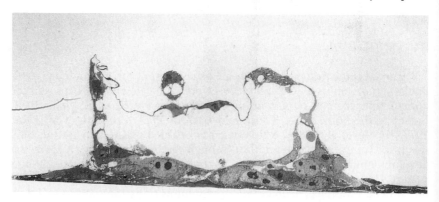

Figure 2. Implanting blastocyst with an expanded blastocoele displacing the endometrial epithelial monolayer cells.

trophoblast cells were involved in the primary adhesion to the endometrial cells (Lindenberg et al, 1986, 1989) (Figure 2), confirming that polarity of the human blastocyst has already developed by the attachment phase, as is also the case in the mouse. This orientation of the implanting blastocyst during culture seems to be consistent with the few reports on human implantation sites in vivo (Hertig et al, 1956; Knoth and Larsen, 1972) that comprise later stages of implantation. This conclusion should be made with caution, however, because, in the mouse, initial attachment takes place at the abembryonic pole of the blastocyst, but later the polar trophectoderm forms the embryonic side of the placenta, both in vivo and in vitro (Rossant, 1977, 1979; Gardner, 1978; Lindenberg et al, 1989).

The morphological changes involved in inner cell mass (ICM) differentiation, trophoblast differentiation, and outgrowth and initial contact between the trophoblast and endometrium are of particular significance for the understanding of the implantation mechanism. Only the trophoblast cells covering the ICM were involved in the initial contact and subsequent outgrowth. It is possible that an interaction between the ICM and the trophoblast influences the polarity of the human blastocyst. In a human in vitro attachment study, the human trophoblast had long microvilli projecting into the ICM cells (Lindenberg et al, 1986) (Figure 3). Furthermore, failure of human blastocyst development might be due to the anomalous formation of the ICM (Lindenberg et al, 1986, 1989), which regulates the continuous differentiation of trophectoderm in mouse embryos (Gardner,

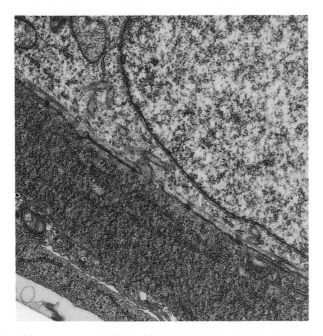

Figure 3. Detail from a cytotrophoblast with a long slender projection which invaginates the plasmalemma of an embryonic cell at a position close to its nucleus.

1978). Some human blastocysts in culture possess a widely diffuse and thin ICM and this might lead to failure of the critical ICM–trophectoderm interaction (Copp, 1979) regulating the development of the trophectoderm. A major defect in ICM function might result in the formation of trophoblast vesicles which would secrete human chorionic gonadotrophin (hCG) and be recognized as biochemical pregnancies in IVF–ET treatments, preclinical abortions or blighted ova (Lindenberg et al, 1984).

Concerning the development of the human trophoblast in vitro, early syncytial formation was observed in the central part of the implantation site. This observation is in accordance with the suggestion by Enders (1976) that a correlation exists between early syncytial formation and invasiveness of the trophoblast, which according to our findings (Lindenberg, 1986, 1989) takes place less than 24 h after adhesion.

Trophoblast–endometrial cell interaction

The initial penetration of the epithelium by the trophoblast involves two separate components: the trophoblastic outgrowth and the endometrial epithelial response.

At the time of adhesion the surfaces of both the endometrial cells and the trophoblastic cells are already changing. The endometrial cells surrounding the attachment site lose their microvilli and the surface facing the blastocyst becomes smoother, as viewed by scanning electron microscopy (Figure 4).

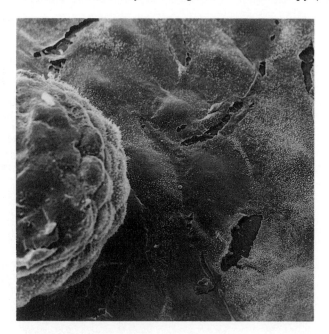

Figure 4. Scanning electron micrograph showing a human blastocyst (left) attaching to the uterine epithelial monolayer. The monolayer cells close to the attaching blastocyst exhibit remarkably fewer microvilli than more distant cells.

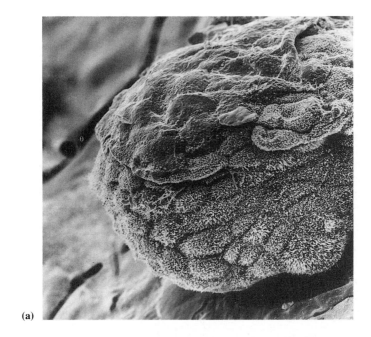

(a)

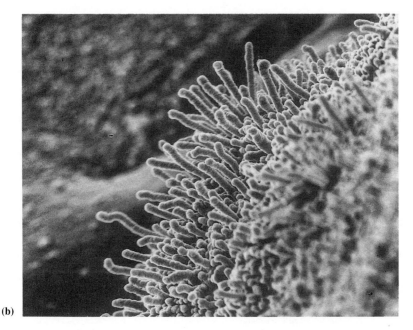

(b)

Figure 5. (a) Scanning electron micrograph of a human blastocyst attaching to a human endometrial monolayer culture. Note the abundance of microvilli on the surface of the mural trophoblast. (b) Microvilli on the surface of a human implanting blastocyst.

This observation is in accordance with in vivo findings by Nilsson (1974) in rodents. The opposite changes take place on the surface of the blastocyst. Here the mural trophoblast, besides being covered by mucin-like material, also exhibits long microvilli in abundance (Figure 5).

An intriguing feature of human in vitro implantation was the finding that the polar trophoblast had displaced the endometrial cells in the central part of the implantation site (see Figure 2). Furthermore, in the contact zone between endometrial and trophoblast cells the endometrial cells were stacked into a multilayer of 2–3 cells (Figure 6). Whether this is a result of 'pushing' by the invading trophoblastic cells (Larsen and Knoth, 1971; Knoth and Larsen, 1972), or a local redistribution of the endometrial cells themselves, as seen in the rat (Enders, 1976), is not clear.

The endometrial cells respond by a remarkable membrane activity, i.e. numerous invaginations of the plasmalemma in the areas facing the cyto-trophoblast (Figure 7). Whether this reflects endocytosis or exocytosis remains to be settled, but in cyclic cows (Hyttel, 1985) and in the peri-implantational phase in rats (Enders and Nielson, 1973; Parr and Parr, 1974) and in mice (Parr and Parr, 1977) a similar membrane activity of the epithelial cells in vivo was shown to be endocytotic. Furthermore, the trophoblasts were not cytolytic in these initial phases of in vitro implan-tation, as no degenerating epithelial cells were seen next to the outgrowing trophoblast cells.

The cytotrophoblast penetrates the endometrial monolayer by long,

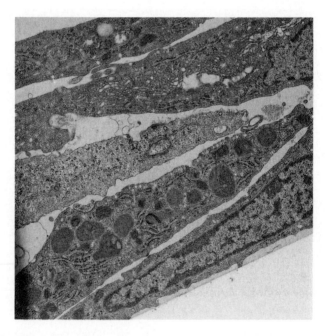

Figure 6. Detail from the periphery of an attachment site. The trophoblastic cells are insinuated between the stacked monolayer cells (darker cells).

slender, ectoplasmic protrusions which insinuate themselves between the endometrial cells and disrupt their desmosomes. These observations of human in vitro implantation are in accordance with the intrusive type of implantation seen in vivo (Enders and Schlafke, 1972).

Although the implantation sites collected by Hertig and Rock (now in the Carnegie Collection) (Section 8020, 6-5-1, × 300; studied from photographs kindly provided of Professor J. F. Larsen, University of Copenhagen, Denmark) represent day 7 of gestation, careful observation, especially of one implantation (a blastocyst half nidated into the endometrium in vivo), reveals several features supporting our findings from embryos implanting in vitro (Figures 8 and 9):

1. The polar trophoblast penetrates deep into the maternal tissue.
2. Syncytiotrophoblastic multinucleate cells are located in the polar trophoblast area.
3. The 'stacking' of the endometrial epithelial cells is also found in the periphery of the implantation site.

Thus from the author's own work on human implantation in vitro and the study of a human implantation site in vivo the following sequence of attachment and early penetration can be seen:

1. In the appositional and adhesional phases the human blastocyst attaches primarily at the embryonic pole.

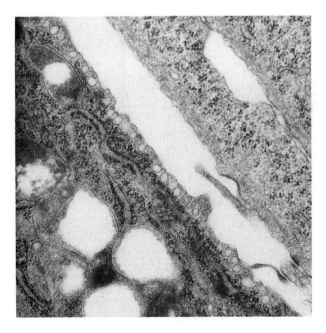

Figure 7. Trophoblastic cells and endometrial cells (darker) in close apposition. Note the remarkable number of membrane invaginations in the endometrial cell plasma membrane.

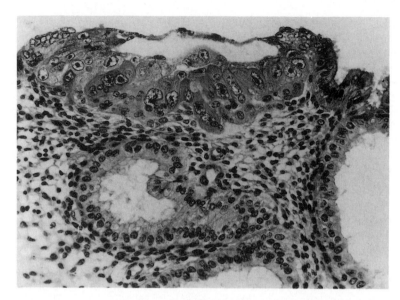

Figure 8. Micrograph of the human implantation site in vivo. Note the stacking of the endometrial cells in the periphery of the implantation.
(Section 8020, 6-5-1, × 300; Carnegie Collection studied by Professor J. F. Larsen)

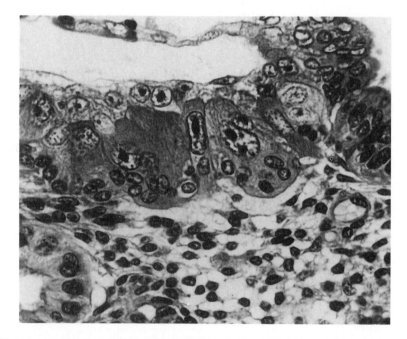

Figure 9. Magnification of Figure 8, illustrating the stacking of the human endometrial cells and possible intrusive behaviour of the trophoblast.

2. Less than 24 h after attachment the trophoblast has initiated an intrusive type of epithelial monolayer penetration.

DISCUSSION

Several practical issues are raised as a result of our research on in vitro implantations of the human blastocyst:

1. The fast development of a complex placentation comprising several cell–cell interaction phenomena.
2. The considerable embryonic loss which leads to the question: how far can take-home-baby rates go with conventional in vitro fertilization?
3. In vitro co-cultures of human embryos and endometrial cells.

From our in vitro studies on human embryo attachment to endometrial epithelial cells it is evident that at a very early stage in implantation/adhesion several complex cell–cell interaction mechanisms are of importance.

First, the orientation of the ICM and organization of the trophoblast in the polar and mural trophoblastic areas takes place. This change in embryonic morphology always precedes the attachment proper. At the stage of attachment, transformation of trophoblast into syncytiotrophoblastic cells and organization of specialized cells, which in the periphery grow out in between the endometrial cells, takes place. This initial trophoblast–endometrial epithelial cell interaction has been shown in rodents to be highly dependent on the glycoconjugate–receptor interactions on the cell membrane. Furthermore, the expression of such glycoreceptor interactions are hormone dependent (Kimber et al, 1990).

Thus from these data it is possible to explain some of the failures in practical clinical IVF treatments, such as a rise in hCG without any fetal echoes on ultrasound, or the development of blighted ova. Both these findings might be dependent on insufficient ICM rotation or development (Gardner, 1978). In addition, the very early embryonic loss after implantation might be due to either low expression or no expression of glycoconjugates of importance for trophoblast–endometrium interaction, which might be a hormone dependent failure.

Concerning the embryonic loss during in vitro culture, several authors following both in vivo and in vitro observations report an embryonic loss of 60–90% after fertilization. This is also of importance when one is measuring the success following routine IVF treatment in humans. Here almost 90% of all ova retrieved after ovarian hyperstimulation will not give rise to a healthy offspring.

What is more interesting is the fact that both in vivo and in vitro studies indicate the same magnitude of embryonic wastage. This might imply a fundamental defect in most human ova and raises the question of how successful conventional routine IVF–ET can be. The author's views about IVF results reaching a barrier are based on the fact that calculating the outcome of infertility therapy, as shown by Cramer et al (1979), and using data from other published papers (Wilkes et al, 1985; Guzick et al, 1986;

Sharma et al, 1988; Padilla and Garcia, 1989) provide us with a cumulative pregnancy rate no different from that of natural fertilization.

Another practical feature in the future development of in vitro cultures for human embryos might be the co-culture system. Here, different types of cells are co-cultured with embryos. In our work this has led to advanced development of human embryos. Several reports on human and bovine embryos have shown the benefits of such a culture strategy for embryos in an IVF programme. Whether these co-culture systems simply detoxify the medium, supply the medium with growth factors or metabolize wastage from the embryos remains to be determined.

REFERENCES

Anderson TL, Olsen GE & Hoffman LH (1986) Stage specific alterations in the apical membrane glycoproteins on endometrial epithelial cells related to implantation in rabbits. *Biology of Reproduction* **34:** 701–720.

Bazer FW & Roberts RM (1983) Biochemical aspects of conceptus–endometrial interactions. *Journal of Experimental Zoology* **228:** 373–383.

Buster JE, Bustillo M, Rodi IA et al (1985) Biologic and morphologic development of donated human ova recovered by nonsurgical uterine lavage. *American Journal of Obstetrics and Gynecology* **153:** 211–217.

Cecco L, Capitanio GL, Croce S, Forcucci M, Gerbaldo D & Rissone R (1984) Biology of nidation and ectopic implantation. *Acta Europaea Fertilitatis* **15:** 347–355.

Chavez DJ (1986) Cell surface of mouse blastocysts at the trophectoderm–uterine interface during the adhesive stage of implantation. *American Journal of Anatomy* **176:** 153–158.

Chavez DJ & Anderson TL (1985) The glycocalyx of the mouse uterine luminal epithelium during estrus, early pregnancy, the peri-implantation period, and delayed implantation. I. Acquisition of *Ricinus communis* I binding sites during pregnancy. *Biology of Reproduction* **32:** 1135–1142.

Copp AJ (1979) Interaction between innercell mass and the trophectoderm of the mouse blastocyst. II. The fate of the polar trophectoderm. *Journal of Embryology and Experimental Morphology* **51:** 109–120.

Croxatto HB, Ortiz ME, Diaz S, Hess R, Balmeceda J & Croxatto HD (1978) Studies on the duration of egg transport by human oviduct. *American Journal of Obstetrics and Gynecology* **132:** 629–634.

Croxatto HB, Ortiz ME, Diaz S & Hess R (1979) Attempts to modify ovum transport in women. *Journal of Reproduction and Fertility* **55:** 231–237.

Dantzer V (1985) Electron microscopy of the initial stages of placentation in the pig. *Anat Embryol* **172:** 281–293.

Edwards RG, Steptoe PC & Purdy JM (1970) Fertilization and cleavage in vitro of preovulator human oocytes. *Nature* **227:** 1307–1309.

Edwards RG, Purdy JM, Steptoe PC & Walters DE (1981) The growth of human pre-implantation embryos in vitro. *American Journal of Obstetrics and Gynecology* **141:** 408–416.

Enders AC (1976) Anatomical aspects of implantation. *Journal of Reproduction and Fertility (Supplement)* **25:** 1–15.

Enders AC & Nielson DM (1973) Pinocytotic activity of the uterus of the rat. *American Journal of Anatomy* **138:** 277–300.

Enders AC & Schlafke S (1972) Implantation in the ferret: epithelial penetration. *American Journal of Anatomy* **133:** 291–316.

Fay TN, Lindenberg S, Teisner B, Westergaard LG, Westergaard JG & Grudzinskas JG (1990a) De novo synthesis of placental protein-14 (PP14) and nor PP12 by monolayer cultures of glandular epithelium of gestational endometrium. *Journal of Clinical Endocrinology and Metabolism* **70:** 515–518.

Fay T, Lindenberg S, Teisner B, Westergaard LG & Grudzinskas JG (1990b) Identification of specific serum proteins synthesized de novo by monolayer cultures of glandular cells of gestational endometrium. *Human Reproduction* **5:** 14–18.

Finn CA (1982) Cellular changes in the uterus during the establishment of pregnancy in rodents. *Journal of Reproduction and Fertility (Supplement)* **31:** 105–111.

Gardner RL (1978) The relationship between cell lineage and differentiation in the early mammalian embryo. In Gehring WJ (ed.) *Genetic Mosaics and Cell Differentiation*, pp 205–241. Heidelberg: Springer-Verlag.

Guzick DS, Wilkes C & Jones HW (1986) Cumulative pregnancy rates after in vitro fertilization. *Fertility and Sterility* **46:** 663–667.

Heald PJ (1976) Biochemical aspects of implantation. *Journal of Reproduction and Fertility* **25:** 29–52.

Heap RB, Flint AP & Gadsby JE (1979) Role of embryonic signals in the establishment of pregnancy. *British Medical Bulletin* **3:** 129–135.

Heap PB, Rider V, Wooding FBP & Flint APF (1986) Molecular and cellular signalling and embryo survival. In Sreenan JM & Diskin MG (eds) *Embryonic Mortality in Farm Animals*, pp 46–73. Boston: Martinus Nijhoff.

Hearn JP (1986) The embryo–maternal dialogue during early pregnancy in primates. *Journal of Reproduction and Fertility* **76:** 809–819.

Hertig AT, Rock J & Adams EC (1956) A description of 34 human ova within the first 17 days of development. *American Journal of Anatomy* **98:** 435–491.

Hertig AT, Rock J, Adams EC & Mulligan WJ (1958) On the preimplantation stage of the human ovum: a description of four normal and four abnormal specimens ranging from the second to the fifth day of development. *Embryology* **240:** 201–220.

Holmes PV & Lindenberg S (1988) Behaviour of mouse and human trophoblast cells during adhesion to and penetration of the endometrial epithelium. In Chapman GP, Ainsworth CC & Chatham CJ (eds) *Eukaryote Cell Recognition: Concepts and Model Systems*, pp 225–237. Cambridge: Cambridge University Press.

Hyttel P (1985) The epithelium of uterine biopsies from cyclic cattle: ultrastructure and endocytotic activity. *Acta Anatomica* **123:** 93–100.

Jenkinson EJ (1977) The in vitro blastocyst outgrowth system as a model for the analysis of peri-implantation development. In Johnson MH (ed.) *Development in Mammals*, vol. 2, pp 151–172. North-Holland Publishing.

Kimber SJ & Lindenberg S (1990) Hormonal control of a carbohydrate epitope involved in implantation in mice. *Journal of Reproduction and Fertility* **89:** 13–21.

Kimber SJ, Lindenberg S & Lundblad A (1988) Distribution of some Gal-β-1-3-(4)GlcNAc related carbohydrate antigens on the mouse uterine epithelium in relation to the peri-implantational period. *Journal of Reproduction and Immunology* **12:** 297–313.

Kirby DRS (1962) The influence of the uterine environment on the development of mouse eggs. *Journal of Embryology and Experimental Morphology* **10:** 496–506.

Knoth M & Larsen JF (1972) Ultrastructure of a human implantation site. *Acta Obstetricia et Gynecologica Scandinavica* **51:** 385–393.

Larsen JF (1961) Electronmicroscopy of the implantation site in the rabbit. *American Journal of Anatomy* **109:** 319–334.

Larsen JF & Knoth M (1971) Ultrastructure of the anchoring villi and trophoblastic shell in the second week of placentation. *Acta Obstetricia et Gynecologica Scandinavica* **50:** 117–128.

Lindenberg S, Lauritsen JG, Nielsen MH & Larsen JF (1984) Isolation and culture of human endometrial epithelial cells. *Fertility and Sterility* **41:** 650–652.

Lindenberg S, Nielsen MH & Lenz S (1985) In vitro studies of human blastocyst implantation. *Annals of the New York Academy of Sciences* **442:** 368–374.

Lindenberg S, Hyttel P, Lenz S & Holmes PV (1986) Ultrastructure of the early human implantation in vitro. *Human Reproduction* **1:** 533–538.

Lindenberg S, Sundberg K, Kimber SJ & Lundblad A (1988) The milk oligosaccharide, lacto-*N*-fucopentaose I, inhibits attachment of mouse blastocysts on endometrial monolayers. *Journal of Reproduction and Fertility* **83:** 149–158.

Lindenberg S, Hyttel P, Sjögren A & Greve T (1989) A comparative study of attachment of human, bovine and mouse blastocysts to uterine epithelial monolayer. *Human Reproduction* **4:** 446–456.

Lindenberg S, Kimber SJ & Kallin E (1990) Carbohydrate binding properties of mouse embryos. *Journal of Reproduction and Fertility* (in press).

McLaren A & Michie D (1956) Studies on the transfer of fertilized mouse eggs to uterine foster-mothers. I. Factors affecting the implantation and survival of native and transferred eggs. *Journal of Experimental Biology* 33: 394–416.

Nieder GL & Macon GR (1987) Uterine and oviducal protein secretion during early pregnancy in the mouse. *Journal of Reproduction and Fertility* 81: 287–294.

Nieder GL, Weitlauf HM & Suda-Hartman M (1987) Synthesis and secretion of stage-specific proteins by peri-implantation mouse embryos. *Biology of Reproduction* 36: 687–699.

Nielsson O (1974) The morphology of blastocyst implantation. *Journal of Reproduction and Fertility* 39: 187–194.

Padilla S & Garcia JE (1989) Effect of maternal age and number of in vitro fertilization procedures on pregnancy outcome. *Fertility and Sterility* 52: 270–273.

Parr MB & Parr EL (1974) Uterine luminal epithelium: protrusions mediated endocytosis, not apocrine secretion, in the rat. *Biology of Reproduction* 11: 220–233.

Parr MB & Parr EL (1977) Endocytosis in the uterine epithelium of the mouse. *Journal of Reproduction and Fertility* 50: 151–153.

Psychoyos A (1977) Hormonal control of uterine receptivity for nidation. *Journal of Reproduction and Fertility (Supplement)* 25: 17–28.

Ramsey EM, Houston ML & Harris JWS (1976) Interaction of the trophoblast and maternal tissue in three closely related primate species. *American Journal of Obstetrics and Gynecology* 124: 647–652.

Rossant J & Ofer L (1977) Properties of extra-embryonic ectoderm isolated from post implantation mouse embryos. *Journal of Embryology and Experimental Morphology* 39: 183–194.

Rossant J & Tamura LW (1979) The possible dual origin of the ectoderm of the chorion in the mouse embryo. *Developmental Biology* 70: 249–254.

Samuel CA & Perry JS (1972) The ultrastructure of pig trophoblast transplanted to an ectopic site in the uterine wall. *Journal of Anatomy* 113: 139–149.

Schlafke S & Enders AC (1975) Cellular basis of interaction between trophoblast and uterus at implantation. *Biology of Reproduction* 12: 41–65.

Sharma V, Riddle A, Mason BA, Pampiglione J & Campbell S (1988) An analysis of factors influencing the establishment of a clinical pregnancy in an ultrasound-based ambulatory in vitro fertilization program. *Fertility and Sterility* 43: 468–478.

Sherman MI & Wudl LR (1976) The implanting mouse blastocyst. In Poste G & Nicholson GL (eds) *The Cell Surface in Animal Embryogenesis and Development*, pp 81–125. Amsterdam: Elsevier.

Surani MAH (1977) Radiolabelled rat uterine luminal proteins and their regulation by estradiol and progesterone. *Journal of Reproduction and Fertility* 50: 289–296.

Tachi S, Tachi C & Lindner HR (1970) Ultrastructural features of blastocyst attachment and trophoblastic invasion in the rat. *Journal of Reproduction and Fertility* 21: 37–56.

Trounson A & Conti A (1982) Research in human in-vitro fertilisation and embryo transfer. *British Medical Journal* 285: 244–248.

Vanderhyden BC & Armstrong DT (1988) Decreased embryonic survival of in-vitro fertilized oocytes in rats is due to retardation of preimplantation development. *Journal of Reproduction and Fertility* 83: 851–857.

Wathes DC & Wooding FBP (1980) An electronmicroscopic study of implantation in the cow. *American Journal of Anatomy* 159: 285–306.

Wilkes CA, Rosenwaks Z, Jones DL & Jones H (1985) Pregnancy related to infertility diagnosis, number of attempts, and age in a program of in vitro fertilization. *Obstetrics and Gynecology* 66: 350–352.

2

Function of blood vessels relative to implantation

MATS ÅKERLUND

The coiled arterioles of the endometrium in humans possess unique properties in that each month they develop in a specific and complex way in order to provide for the nutrition of a newly nidated ovum. Not only is the anatomy of the vascular tree repeatedly changing with the variations in hormonal state, but the motor responses of the smooth muscle of vessels and myometrium to different vasoactive substances are also often modified. The purpose of this chapter is to give an overview of present knowledge about the circulation of the human uterus, particularly of the endometrium, and to put this information into perspective with respect to the process of implantation.

ANATOMY OF UTERINE BLOOD VESSELS

The uterine arteries, which are the most important vessels for providing the blood supply to the human uterus, as well as to the fetoplacental unit during pregnancy, reach the uterus at the level of the upper cervix. There, a descending ramification, the vaginal artery, is given off, while the ascending main branch follows the lateral part of the uterus between the folds of the broad uterine ligament. Numerous branches are given off to the myometrium and, after further ramifications, the vessels eventually reach the endometrium (Figure 1). They connect with the coiled arterioles, which are well developed at the time of ovulation, and finally ramify into capillaries. At the lateral, upper part of the uterus, below the isthmic part of the fallopian tube, the uterine artery splits into the ovarian and tubal branches, both of which anastomose with branches of the ovarian artery, which also contributes to the uterine circulation. In principle, the venous circulation follows a corresponding pattern.

CHANGES IN ANATOMY OF ENDOMETRIAL BLOOD VESSELS RELATIVE TO IMPLANTATION

The anatomical changes in endometrial vessels of primates relative to implantation have recently been studied (Kaiserman-Abramof and

Baillière's Clinical Obstetrics and Gynaecology—
Vol. 5, No. 1, March 1991
ISBN 0–7020–1533–4

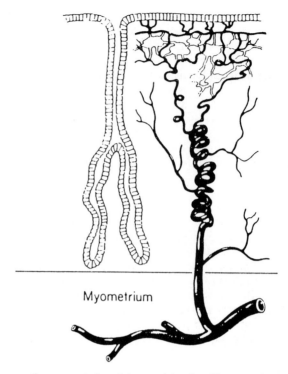

Myometrium

Figure 1. Diagrammatic representation of the arterial and capillary vasculature of the primate endometrium.

Padykula, 1989). The postovulatory period of the menstrual cycle is characterized by rapid growth of the coiled arterioles and development of capillaries and venules. Definitive coiled arterioles consist of interlinked endothelial and smooth muscle cells which provide flexibility for rapid changes in shape. Progressive differentiation continues up to the premenstrual stage. This abundant angiogenesis may reflect preparation and maintenance of a suitable uterine environment for possible implantation and pregnancy during each menstrual cycle.

The anatomical changes during the menstrual cycle in humans have also been confirmed in vivo by microhysteroscopic studies (Van Herendael et al, 1987). These allowed a definition of five different and typical phases of the menstrual cycle, i.e. early proliferative, late proliferative, early secretory, late secretory and premenstrual–menstrual phases.

INNERVATION OF HUMAN UTERINE ARTERIES

The presence of an adrenergic and cholinergic nerve supply to the uterine arteries has been known for many years (see Owman and Stjernquist, 1988). Recent in vitro studies demonstrated that the postjunctional contractile adrenoceptors are primarily of the α_1-type (Stjernquist and Owman, 1990).

This agrees with results of previous studies in the guinea-pig, which also demonstrated that relaxant adrenoceptor effects and neuronal and extra-neuronal uptake are of minor importance in the main branch of the uterine artery (Fallgren and Edvinsson, 1986).

Recent immunohistochemical studies of peptide-containing nerves in the smooth muscle of vascular walls in human uterine arteries also revealed the presence of separate fibres with vasoactive intestinal peptide, peptide histidine methionine, neuropeptide Y or, to some extent, leu-enkephalin (Ekesbo et al, 1990). In guinea-pig uterine arteries, fibres with substance P together with calcitonin gene related peptide and vasoactive intestinal peptide together with neuropeptide Y were demonstrated (Fallgren et al, 1989).

OVARIAN STEROIDS AND ENDOMETRIAL CIRCULATION

Immunohistochemical studies demonstrated oestrogen and progesterone receptors in the muscle cells of human uterine arteries (Perrot-Applanat et al, 1988). Specific binding of oestradiol appears to be mainly to the nucleus of cells from these arteries (Batra and Iosif, 1987). These results suggest that sex steroids may regulate uterine blood flow through a direct effect on uterine arterial walls.

During the menstrual cycle there are variations in the endometrial blood flow; these variations were described in the classic reports by Markee (1950) and Prill and Götz (1961). Markee studied endometrial transplants in the eye chamber of monkeys, and Prill and Götz, although studying humans, used a primitive thermodilution technique. The more recent quantitative estimations by Fraser et al (1987), using the ^{123}Xe technique, gave similar but not identical results, probably due to discrepancies in the techniques employed.

Endometrial blood flow studies using the ^{123}Xe technique showed blood flows ranging from 10 to 70 ml/100 g tissue/min in healthy women of fertile age (Fraser et al, 1987). When results obtained at different days of the menstrual cycle were compared, a significant correlation between plasma oestradiol levels and endometrial blood flow was seen in the follicular phase, with an elevation of flow in the days preceding ovulation. This is in agreement with previous studies indicating a potent vasodilatory effect of oestrogens on uterine arteries (Makowski, 1977). In the luteal phase there was no correlation between blood flow and oestradiol levels (Fraser et al, 1987) but a gradual increase until the onset of menstruation, when a fall was observed. Women with non-ovulatory dysfunctional bleeding had exceedingly variable flow rates.

SPONTANEOUS BLOOD FLOW OF ENDOMETRIAL VESSELS: INFLUENCE OF THE MYOMETRIUM AND VASCULAR SMOOTH MUSCLE

With the thermoconduction–thermistor technique (Hansson et al, 1987; Hauksson et al, 1988), pulsed synchronous variations in flow of the endometrial arteries were recorded. During spontaneous, well-demarcated

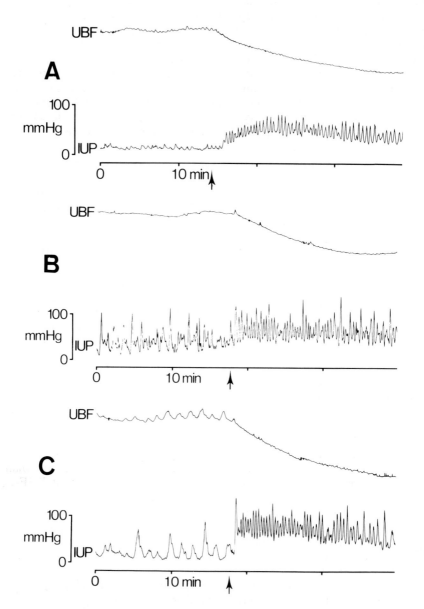

Figure 2. The effect of intravenous lysin vasopressin (0.8 μg; injections indicated by arrows) on local endometrial blood flow (UBF) and intrauterine pressure (IUP) in a woman **(A)** 7 days after, **(B)** 7 days before and **(C)** 2 days before a menstruation.

uterine contractions, which occur around the onset of menstruation (Figure 2C), blood flow generally decreases, presumably as a result of a compressing effect of the increased intrauterine pressure on uterine vessels (Hauksson et al, 1988). In primary dysmenorrhoea, myometrial hyperactivity causes uterine ischaemia and pain by compressing uterine vessels, but blood flow recordings also indicated that a vasoconstrictive agent acts directly on the vessel walls (Åkerlund et al, 1976). One important such factor has been demonstrated to be vasopressin (Åkerlund et al, 1979). During the time period from mid-follicular phase until a few days before the onset of menstruation the uterine activity is not co-ordinated throughout the uterus, contractions being only local in the myometrium, and the effects of these on the endometrial blood flow are limited (Figure 2A,B) (Åkerlund and Andersson, 1976a, 1976b).

The relative influence of uterine contractions compared with the effect of the smooth muscle of uterine vessels on endometrial blood flow in non-pregnant women is difficult to assess in the light of available data. However, it might be anticipated that the effects of myometrial activity on blood flow is more important in the non-pregnant than in the pregnant condition because of the differences in diameter of the uterine cavity. Much higher intrauterine pressures can occur in non-pregnant women.

EFFECTS OF VASOACTIVE SUBSTANCES ON HUMAN UTERINE BLOOD FLOW

In vitro findings

In studies of the contractile potency of some neuropeptides and of other important humoral factors on the small branches of the human uterine arteries (Figure 3), it was found that arginine vasopressin was the most potent, followed by oxytocin, noradrenaline together with neuropeptide Y, noradrenaline alone, and dopamine (Ekesbo et al, 1990). No effect was seen with acetylcholine or tyrosine; vasoactive intestinal peptide caused relaxation of contractile activity induced by prostaglandin $(PG)F_{2\alpha}$. In small human intracervical arteries, noradrenaline, and to some extent $PGF_{2\alpha}$, caused contraction, whereas PGE_2, vasoactive intestinal peptide and substance P induced relaxation of precontracted vessels (Allen et al, 1988).

The important role of the different prostaglandins in the regulation of menstrual bleeding has been known for some time and has been extensively reviewed (Christiaens et al, 1981; Granström et al, 1983). With respect to the function of endometrial blood vessels, an interesting recent finding (Meigaard et al, 1985) was the difference in response to $PGF_{2\alpha}$ and PGE_2 of extramyometrial and intramyometrial arteries. Both prostaglandins, particularly $PGF_{2\alpha}$ in higher dose, stimulated contractions of extra-myometrial arteries. By contrast, both compounds caused relaxation of intramyometrial arteries of smaller diameter. Changes in response between extramyometrial and intramyometrial vessels were also seen with other vasoactive substances (M. Åkerlund et al, unpublished data).

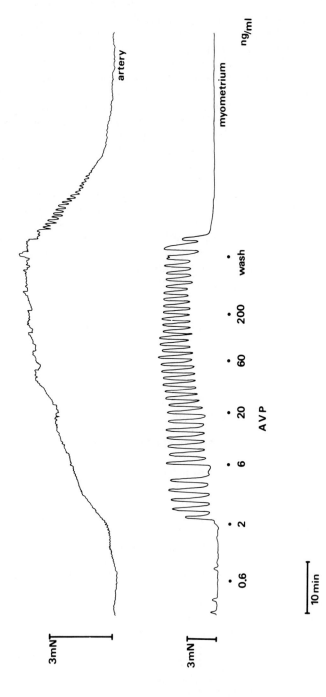

Figure 3. Cumulative dose–response curves from isolated artery and myometrium of a human after administration of increasing amounts of arginine vasopressin (AVP).

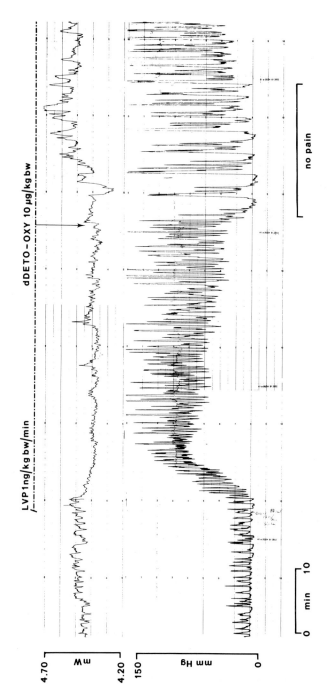

Figure 4. Recording of intrauterine pressure and added power reflecting uterine blood flow in a non-pregnant woman at the onset of menstruation. Infusion of lysin vasopressin (LVP) induced uterine hyperactivity, reduction of blood flow and dysmenorrhoea-like pain, which was counteracted by injection of the oxytocin and vasopressin antagonist, 1-deamino-2-D-Tyr(OEt)-4-Thr-8-Orn-oxytocin (dDETO-OXY).

In vivo results

Vasopressin has a potent effect on endometrial blood flow, particularly during early menstruation (Figures 2 and 4), as shown by thermistor technique recordings during intrauterine pressure studies (Åkerlund and Andersson, 1976a; Hansson et al, 1987; Hauksson et al, 1988). When the vasopressin effect was inhibited by a newly developed oxytocin and vasopressin receptor blocking agent, the blood flow rose markedly and the uterus relaxed (Figure 4). In vitro studies confirmed that this analogue also has an inhibitory effect on the smooth muscle of the uterine arteries; a therapeutic effect in primary dysmenorrhoea was also demonstrated (Åkerlund, 1987).

There is little in vivo data about the effect of physiological and pharmacological factors on endometrial blood flow at the times of ovulation and nidation. The effects of vasopressin on myometrial activity and endometrial blood flow in healthy women at these times of the cycle were less pronounced than at the onset of menstruation (Åkerlund and Andersson, 1976b). Correspondingly, the uterine relaxation induced by a β_2-adrenoceptor stimulating agent, with parallel increases in endometrial blood flow, was also less pronounced at these times (Åkerlund and Andersson, 1976a). For other vasoactive substances new data from in vivo studies in the human are not available.

CONCLUSION

The regulation of endometrial blood flow is complex, involving aminergic and peptidergic nerves and humoral factors. A considerable amount of in vitro data on these factors is available, but the importance in the in vivo situation of neuropeptides, prostaglandins and other vasoactive substances, circulating or locally released, for the function of endometrial blood vessels relative to implantation still remains largely to be determined. Furthermore, when considering agents which influence endometrial blood flow, the implication of myometrial effects needs to be taken into account when endometrial circulatory effects are investigated. These substances can act both via effects on myometrial activity and by directly influencing the vessel walls. The relative importance of these two mechanisms remains to be determined. Ovarian steroids have both a trophic effect on the endometrial vessels, which are repeatedly changing each menstrual cycle, and oestrogens, at least, have direct effects on the vessel walls, stimulating circulation. Disturbances in either of these factors probably influence the mechanisms of nidation and nutrition of the newly concepted ovum, but so far data concerning this are scanty. This is an area of important future research.

REFERENCES

Åkerlund M (1987) Can primary dysmenorrhoea be alleviated by a vasopressin antagonist?
    Acta Obstetricia et Gynecologica Scandinavica **66:** 459–461.
Åkerlund M & Andersson K-E (1976a) Effects of terbutaline on human myometrial activity
    and endometrial blood flow. *Obstetrics and Gynecology* **47:** 529–535.

Åkerlund M & Andersson K-E (1976b) Vasopressin response and terbutaline inhibition of the uterus. *Obstetrics and Gynecology* **48**: 528–536.

Åkerlund M, Andersson K-E & Ingemarsson I (1976) Effects of terbutaline on myometrial activity, uterine blood flow, and lower abdominal pain in women with primary dysmenorrhoea. *British Journal of Obstetrics and Gynaecology* **83**: 673–678.

Åkerlund M, Strömberg P & Forsling ML (1979) Primary dysmenorrhoea and vasopressin. *British Journal of Obstetrics and Gynaecology* **86**: 484–487.

Allen J, Hansen V, Maigaard S, Andersson K-E & Forman A (1988) Effects of some neurotransmitters and prostanoids on isolated human intracervical arteries. *American Journal of Obstetrics and Gynecology* **157**: 637–641.

Batra S & Iosif S (1987) Nuclear estrogen receptors in human uterine arteries. *Gynecological and Obstetrical Investigation* **24**: 250–255.

Christiaens GCML, Sixma JJ & Haspels AA (1981) Haemostasis in menstrual endometrium in the presence of an intrauterine device. *British Journal of Obstetrics and Gynaecology* **88**: 825–837.

Ekesbo R, Alm P, Ekström P, Lundberg L-M & Åkerlund M (1990) Innervation of the human uterine artery and motor responses to neuropeptides. *Gynecologic and Obstetric Investigation* (in press).

Fallgren B & Edvinsson L (1986) Characterization of adrenoceptor mechanisms in isolated guinea-pig uterine arteries. *European Journal of Pharmacology* **131**: 163–170.

Fallgren B, Ekblad E & Edvinsson L (1989) Co-existence of neuropeptides and differential inhibition of vasodilator responses by neuropeptide Y in guinea pig uterine arteries. *Neuroscience Letters* **100**: 71–76.

Fraser IS, McCarron G, Hutton B & Macey D (1987) Endometrial blood flow measured by xenon-133 clearance in women with normal menstruation cycles and dysfunctional uterine bleeding. *American Journal of Obstetrics and Gynecology* **156**: 158–166.

Granström E, Swann M-L & Lundström V (1983) The possible roles of prostaglandins and related compounds in endometrial bleeding. A mini-review. *Acta Obstetricia et Gynecologica Scandinavica, Supplement* **113**: 91–99.

Hansson G-Å, Hauksson A, Strömberg P & Åkerlund M (1987) An instrument for measuring endometrial blood flow in the uterus, using two thermistor probes. *Journal of Medical Engineering and Technology* **11**: 17–22.

Hauksson A, Åkerlund M & Melin P (1988) Uterine blood flow and myometrial activity at menstruation, and the action of vasopressin and a synthetic antagonist. *British Journal of Obstetrics and Gynaecology* **95**: 898–904.

Kaiserman-Abramof IR & Padykula HA (1989) Angiogenesis in the postovulatory primate endometrium: the coiled arteriolar system. *Anatomical Research* **224**: 479–489.

Maigaard S, Forman A & Andersson K-E (1985) Differences in contractile activation between human myometrium and intramyometrial arteries. *Acta Physiologica Scandinavica* **124**: 371–379.

Makowski EL (1977) Vascular physiology. In Wynn RM (ed.) *Biology of the Uterus*, pp 77–100. New York: Plenum Press.

Markee JE (1950) The relation of blood flow to endometrial growth and the inception of menstruation. In Engle ET (ed.) *Menstruation and its Disorders*, pp 165–185. Springfield, IL: CC Thomas.

Owman Ch & Stjernquist M (1988) Origin, distribution, and functional aspects of aminergic and peptidergic nerves in the male and female reproductive tracts. In Björklund A, Hökfelt T & Owman Ch (eds) *Handbook of Chemical Neuroanatomy, Vol. 6: The Peripheral Nervous System*, pp 445–544. Amsterdam: Elsevier.

Perrot-Applanat M, Groyer-Picard MT, Garcia E, Lorenzo F & Milgrom E (1988) Immunocytochemical demonstration of estrogen and progesterone receptors in muscle cells of uterine arteries in rabbits and humans. *Endocrinology* **123**: 1511–1519.

Prill HJ & Götz F (1961) Blood flow in the myometrium and endometrium of the uterus. *American Journal of Obstetrics and Gynecology* **82**: 102–108.

Stjernquist M & Owman Ch (1990) Adrenoceptors mediating contraction in the human uterine artery. *Human Reproduction* **5**: 19–24.

Van Herendael BJ, Stevens MJ, Flakiewicz-Kula A & Hansch CH (1987) Dating of the endometrium by microhysteroscopy. *Gynecologic and Obstetric Investigation* **24**: 114–118.

3

Macrophages and migratory cells in endometrium relevant to implantation

RICHARD G. LEA
DAVID A. CLARK

A substantial percentage of reproductive failure is failure to implant successfully. Evidence for this comes from comparative studies of early pregnancy loss in both normal fertile couples and in couples undergoing in vitro fertilization and embryo transfer (IVFET). A number of studies on the clinical abortion rate have shown that approximately 15% of all recognized non-IVFET pregnancies are miscarried or aborted before the 28th week of pregnancy (Alberman, 1988). From analysis of epidemiological data, it was estimated that 80% of conceptions were lost before term (Roberts and Lowe, 1975); it follows therefore that with a clinical abortion rate of 15%, 65% of conceptions may be lost before the recognition of a clinical pregnancy (i.e. 35% succeed). The number of conceptions lost before or with the onset of menses includes fertilized oocytes which fail to attach to the uterine lining, and early implanted pregnancies. Fertilization can be detected using an assay for early pregnancy factor (EPF) in blood, and an implanted pregnancy during the late luteal phase can be detected using sensitive assays for human chorionic gonadotrophin β-chain (β-hCG), which are not normally done clinically. The incidence of loss of early implants (β-hCG +), depends on the stringency of the criteria required for diagnosis (Table 1). Based on Table 1, one can divide the 65% of conceptions that become unrecognized losses into 20% of fertilized oocytes which do not attempt implantation (β-hCG never positive), 28% that fail at initial contact with uterine epithelium (and provide a single low level β-hCG spike), and 17% that fail during the first 8–9 days after initial contact (i.e. peri-implantation). For the purpose of this chapter, we shall include all of these unrecognized losses under the term 'implantation failure'.

The data in Table 2 provides some interesting insight into the relative contribution of fertilization failure and implantation failure to failure to achieve a clinical pregnancy (i.e. infertility). With normal in vivo fertilization, a positive EPF assay occurred in 61–69% of cycles, which is slightly higher than the 50% rate assumed by Roberts and Lowe (1975). Oocytes from normal fertile women or from women with mechanically blocked fallopian tubes fertilized at about the same rate in vitro, and fertilization ability was only slightly less when sperm or oocytes from patients with

25

Table 1. Frequency of occult pregnancy loss in women attempting conception.

| Investigators | β-hCG criteria | | No. positive cycles | No. aborted | | Clinical rate of pregnancy/cycle (%) |
	Methodology	+ Level		Occult (%)	Clinical	
Urine						
Edmonds et al (1982)	sb6 RIA d21,23,25*,....	56 units/litre	118	67 (57)	6	51/198 (26)
Miller et al (1980)	ortho RIA same	50 units/litre or 20×2	152	50 (33)	15	102/521 (20)
Wilcox et al (1985)	r529 IRMA daily	0.47 units/litre once >once	29 21	12 (41) 4 (19)	4 4	17/19 (89)
Sharp et al (1986)	sb6 RIA d21,23,25,....	50 units/litre once >once	32 19	21 (66) 8 (42)	2 2	Subfertiles
Blood						
Whittaker et al (1983)	Amersh, RIA last week cycle	16 units/litre	92	7 (8)	11	85/226 (38)
Smart et al (1982)	bio-RIA >d9 post-ov q2-3d	5 units/litre†	9	2 (22)	1	7/19 (37)
Chartier et al (1979)	sb6 RIA >d9 post-ov q1-3d	4 units/litre	90	19 (21)	14	71/298 (24)

Summary: High sampling frequency + low β-hCG threshold
331 + cycles
150 occult losses (45%)
27 clinical aborts (8%)

Low sampling frequency ± high β-hCG threshold ± >1 positive test required
231 + cycles
40 occult losses (17%)
32 clinical aborts (13.9%)

* Day of cycle.
† Threshold of assay.
RIA, radio-immunoassay; IMRA, immunoradiometric assay.

Table 2. Failure of fertilization.

In vivo mating	Rolfe (1982)	Smart et al (1982)	
normal fertiles	69% (26 cycles)	67% (21 cycles)	
idiopathic infertiles	?	?	
In vitro fertilization:	Edwards (1985) Eggs fertilized (%)	Yovich (1985) Eggs fertilized (%)	Hull et al (1985) 1 or more egg fertilized (%)
Normal fertiles	not done	not done	82
Infertiles			
Poor sperm/cervical mucus	53	36	28
Blocked tubes	73	80	78
Endometriosis	74	58	nd
Idiopathic	65	48	68

different types of infertility were tested. Further, it appears that sperm reaches the ampulla (and oocyte) in most patients with unexplained infertility (Ramsewak et al, 1990). If fertilization now occurs at the rate expected from in vitro studies, failure to achieve pregnancy must be explained more than half the time by failure to implant and/or to survive the initial period after implantation. In the case of IVFET, 80% of transfers of 3–4 embryos fail to establish pregnancies: a 5–7% success rate per embryo compared with an expected success rate of 35% per pre-embryo (i.e. $1 - 0.65$). If the infertility in the IVFET patients was due solely to inability to fertilize in vivo, then one would have expected pregnancy success following transfer of four in vitro fertilization (IVF) embryos to reach 82.1% ($1 - 0.35^4$). It follows that an understanding of mechanisms leading to failure to attach to the uterus, and/or failure to survive the early time period after attachment, could lead to treatments that would substantially enhance fecundity.

Implantation failure has been largely attributed to anatomical and chromosomal defects (Papadopoulos et al, 1989). Despite the higher failure rate of IVF embryos to implant, the frequency of chromosomal abnormalities in embryos selected for transfer is not increased beyond normal levels. It follows therefore that if four embryos are transferred with a 50% chance of a defect, then the probability of at least one normal embryo being transferred is $1 - (0.5)^4 = 0.94$. This suggests that the implantation success rate with IVFET should be greater than the result of normal conception. These data suggest that physiological factors represent a major cause of implantation failure in IVFET and probably contribute to delay in achieving pregnancy in many normal couples. Evidence for a key role for physiological factors in recurrent clinical abortion has also been provided by Boue et al (1975), who noted that loss of a chromosomally normal embryo doubled the risk of a recurrent failure. These data taken together imply that lethal chromosome defects are unlikely to explain recurrent implantation failure.

THE ISSUE OF SYNCHRONY

A useful analogy for the implantation of the embryo into the lining of the uterus is that of the 'seed' and the 'soil', where the seed represents an appropriately developed embryo and the soil represents a suitably conditioned uterine lining. Implantation failure may occur due to defects in the 'seed', which may be in part anatomical or chromosomal in nature, as already discussed, or due to more subtle genetic/developmental influences, as mediated by the preimplantation embryo development (*Ped*) gene (see below). Defects in the 'soil' may also occur when the hormonal conditioning of the uterus is inappropriate. Altered progesterone : oestrogen ratios have been suggested to lead to implantation failure in humans and mice (Gidley-Baird et al, 1986). Another fundamental requirement for successful implantation is that there must be a synchrony between the development of the embryo and the conditioning of the uterus. Under the influence of ovarian hormones, the uterine lining reaches a transient receptive stage at which an embryo that has reached the blastocyst stage can attach (Rogers and Murphy, 1989). The transient nature of this receptive stage has led to the concept of an 'implantation window', i.e. a limited time period when attachment is possible. Any factor interfering with the normal operation of the endocrine system before the implantation window has been reached may prevent synchronization of events in the embryo and uterus.

Altered uterine physiology is an important issue in the attempt to improve the pregnancy success rate in patients undergoing IVFET. IVF patients stimulated to ovulate with hCG develop high serum oestradiol levels which in turn may exert an adverse effect on implantation by reducing uterine receptivity (Forman et al, 1988). When implantation success in standard IVFET is compared with that in donor IVF, where eggs from one donor are fertilized in vitro and are then transferred to the patient, Paulson et al (1990) found that a woman whose uterus was not subject to the effects of fertility drugs had an implantation rate three times higher than women whose uterine environment had been adversely affected by drugs (patients in the standard IVF programme). Pre-embryos generated in both programmes were exposed to drugs and thus only the status of the uterus differed between the two groups of patients. A second problem in IVFET is that IVF embryos are transferred into the uterus only 2 days after follicular aspiration, in contrast to the in vivo fertilized egg, which arrives a little later and in a more advanced stage to implant 5–7 days after ovulation. This suggests that IVF embryos may be present in the uterus before the endometrium has reached its receptive stage, i.e. standard IVF embryo transfer may be viewed as asynchronous. As elevated progesterone levels have been equated with advanced endometrial maturity (Garcia et al, 1984), a study was carried out by Ben-Nun and his colleagues (1990) to determine if progesterone supplementation initiated before ovulation could improve the success rate of implantation of transferred IVF embryos. The pregnancy rate per embryo transfer (ET) cycle for patients given progesterone supplementation was indeed significantly higher than that of controls. A more synchronous relationship between embryo and uterus may occur in the donor IVFET programmes as compared with standard IVF. Similarly, greater synchrony between embryo and uterus can be achieved in standard IVF by freezing IVF embryos and transferring them in a subsequent, more natural cycle. This has been reported to increase the chances of obtaining a pregnancy from a single oocyte recovery procedure (Testart et al, 1986). The statistical analysis of pooled IVF clinic data suggests that 40–60% of uteri achieve receptivity and 20–40% of embryos should have the capacity to implant (Walters et al, 1985). Failure or slowing of development of the pre-embryo to the blastocyst stage after transfer is also clearly a potential major cause of uterine asynchrony.

The effects of asynchronous embryo transfer on subsequent embryo development have been investigated in the sheep and the rabbit (Chang, 1950; Wilmut and Sales, 1981; Fischer, 1989). In both species, asynchrony between embryo and uterus alters the rate of embryo development. Embryos transferred to more advanced uteri developed more rapidly than normal and embryos transferred to a less advanced uterus developed more slowly than normal. In the sheep, the stimulating effect exerted by an advanced uterus on retarded embryos was greater than the effect on advanced embryos, but there was a high incidence of postimplantation embryonic mortality of retarded embryo transfers in spite of these effects (Wilmut et al, 1985). The authors suggest that the enhanced development of the embryos may be an aberrant development rather than a functional catch-up to the more advanced uterine environment. A further interesting observation in the sheep was that the simultaneous transfer of synchronous and asynchronous embryos resulted in selective failure of the asynchronous embryo; that is the asynchronous embryo could not adapt (Wilmut and Sales, 1981). In the rabbit, the transfer of embryos more advanced with respect to uterine development achieved a better rate of implantation (Chang, 1950). In the rat, decreased embryonic survival of IVF oocytes was associated with retarded embryo development at the time of transfer (Vanderhyden and Armstrong, 1988). The authors reported that IVF morulae contained fewer cells per embryo than controls but still had the capacity to implant and develop into fetuses if they were transferred to the oviduct of the recipient. Transfer of the morulae to the uterus was not, however, conducive to implantation. Similarly, the in vitro development of mouse 1-cell embryos to the blastocyst stage is better within the oviduct of pregnant females compared with the uterine environment (Papaioannou and Ebert, 1986). These data suggest exposure to the oviduct environment is particularly important in enhancing the rate of preblastocyst development. Alternatively, factors in the uterine environment might be hostile.

What is the nature of factors affecting development of the preimplantation embryo, and, in the case where maternal influences are important, does the embryo actively induce production of this activity?

FACTORS AFFECTING THE PREIMPLANTATION EMBRYO

Intrinsic cell properties

Rapidly dividing human embryos have been shown to have a better potential to implant (Wilmut et al, 1985). Both maternal and paternal genotypes influence the timing of early murine embryo cleavage and development

(Barkley and Fitzgerald, 1990). Studies in mice have shown that associated with H-2 (major histocompatibility complex, MHC) is a *Ped* gene which influences the rate of cleavage of preimplantation murine embryos (Warner et al, 1987a). The *Ped* gene has two functional alleles, designated fast and slow with respect to embryo cleavage rates, and the gene is expressed at the time of the first cleavage division (Warner et al, 1987a). Cleavage rates in mice congenic at the H-2 complex are fast when Qa-2 antigens are expressed (Qa-2^a mice) and slow in mice lacking Qa-2 antigens (Qa-2^b mice). The *Ped* gene appears to be located in the Qa-2 subregion of the MHC and the *Ped* gene product may in fact be a class I MHC (Qa-2) molecule (Warner et al, 1987b).

Direct cell-to-cell communication via gap junctions is believed to be important in directing development of a population of cells; indeed, groups of cells cease to communicate with each other once they begin to diverge along separate developmental pathways (Wolpert, 1978). In the pre-implantation embryo, gap junction communication is first evident at the 8-cell stage when cell compaction occurs (Lee et al, 1987). At this stage, electrical coupling and the transfer of Lucifer yellow (6-carboxyfluorescein) has been shown to occur between all eight cells (Goodall and Johnson, 1984). Antibodies raised against a protein isolated from rat liver gap junctions recognize gap junctions in the 8-cell stage murine pre-embryo (Lee et al, 1987). The injection of this antibody into 8-cell murine zygotes blocks gap junction communication and interferes with compaction of the embryo at the 16-cell stage (Lee et al, 1987). Compaction of the embryo is considered important as this precedes the establishment of the trophoblast and the inner cell mass lineages. These findings suggested that there was a correlation between efficient communication, compaction and embryo viability (Lee et al, 1987).

Embryos obtained from DDK females crossed with C3H/B1 males often fail to form blastocysts and only 5–10% survive to implant and develop to term (Wakasugi, 1973). At the 8-cell stage, DDK × C3H/B1 embryos undergo compaction as normal but the spread of dye throughout the embryos was slow, indicative of defective gap junction communication (Buehr et al, 1987). In addition, blastomeres obtained from these mice underwent spontaneous decompaction and resembled gap junction antibody treated normal embryos (Lee et al, 1987). The extruded blastomeres were no longer in communication with the other cells and it was at this stage that embryo loss occurred. These findings suggest that gap junction formation and compaction are important processes in the development of the preimplantation embryo. It is possible therefore that one contributor to the low rate of implantation of human IVF embryos may be impaired gap junction formation and compaction.

Polyamines

Individual human oocytes cultured in vitro release a non-specific anti-proliferative activity into the culture supernatant (Daya and Clark, 1986). IVF embryo release of this activity has been shown to correlate with the ability to establish a pregnancy (Clark et al, 1989a). Recent work in our laboratory indicates that the inhibitory activity is due to polyamines (spermine and spermidine) in the IVF supernatant, which are oxidized by the enzyme monoamine oxidase (MAO) present in the fetal bovine serum used in the medium of our cell proliferation assays (Clark et al, 1989a; Lea et al, 1990 and unpublished data). MAO oxidizes spermine into spermine dialdehyde and acrolein which act as non-specific toxins (Allen and Roberts, 1987). Oxidized spermidine is also toxic. Although spermine is a small peptide of molecular weight 202, it forms complexes and binds to proteins, which accounts for the appearance of more than one suppressive peak on high performance liquid chromatographic (HPLC) separation of IVF supernatants (Allen et al, 1977; Williams-Ashman et al, 1980).

Murine IVF embryo supernatants also exhibit non-specific inhibitory activity, which appears to be due to the presence of one or more polyamines (Porat and Clark, 1990). The origin of the IVF polyamines is uncertain. Recent studies have shown that both murine and human sperm supernatants contain high levels of spermine and exhibit polyamine mediated inhibitory activity (Porat and Clark, 1990; Clark et al, 1989a; R. G. Lea et al, unpublished data). This suggests a possible sperm origin; however, in some human IVF embryo cultures the activity in 24–48 h growth medium (from which sperm have been removed) exceeded that in 0–24 h insemination medium, indicative of an ongoing polyamine synthesis (Clark et al, 1989a). Further evidence for this idea was obtained in the mouse IVF system where fertilized oocytes from young CBA/J fertile mice gave rise to suppressive supernatants, and fertilized oocytes from old CBA/J mice, which have reduced fertility, gave rise to non-suppressive supernatant (Porat and Clark, 1990). As all oocytes were fertilized with the same young DBA/2 sperm, it appeared that polyamines produced by fertilized and dividing young oocytes were responsible for the majority of the IVF embryo supernatant inhibitory activity.

The preceding observations suggest measurement of spermine/spermidine in IVF culture supernatants could allow selection of embryos most likely to implant. In what way might the presence of a polyamine such as spermine in the IVF culture medium be a predictor of implantation?

It is possible that polyamine production is a result of rapid cell proliferation, i.e. fast embryos. Alternatively, polyamines may have two possible active roles relevant to implantation. Firstly, the biosynthesis of polyamines, particularly spermine, is essential for the proliferation and differentiation of eukaryotic cells. The selective inhibition of spermine synthesis in the murine pre-embryo leads to arrested embryo development at the 8-cell or morula stage (Zwierzchowski et al, 1986). Human pre-embryos achieving blastocyst formation have a higher success rate of implantation, and similar findings have been reported for farm animals (Bustillo et al, 1986; Butler and Biggers, 1989). These studies suggest that a spermine/spermidine deficiency in the preimplantation embryo could prevent development beyond the 8-cell stage and thus prevent implantation. In IVFET, the polyamine-containing culture supernatant is discarded at the time of embryo transfer. This may account for the higher pregnancy rates achieved via gamete intrafallopian transfer

(GIFT), where factors such as spermine/spermidine are not lost (Asch et al, 1988). The success rates of both IVF and GIFT can also be improved by the presence of ejaculate in the reproductive tract (Bellinge et al, 1986; Marconi et al, 1989). Normal human semen contains spermine in concentrations of 5–15 mM, which is in excess of the amount needed to stimulate embryo growth (Mendez, 1989). It is possible therefore that the success rate of human IVF could be increased by increasing spermine levels in IVF culture medium, and/or in the patient, in order to enhance the growth of the pre-embryo.

The IVF oocytes from old CBA/J (infertile) mice fail to develop beyond the 2-cell stage in vitro and recent studies have shown that the cleavage arrest can be reversed in some of the embryos by adding exogenous spermine to the cultures (Porat and Clark, 1990) (the occurrence of the cleavage arrest at the 2-cell stage in the old CBA/J oocytes may in part reflect a variety of lethal, age-associated defects). Whether young oocytes have a 'reserve' of polyamines which is age depleted is under study. Age has been shown to play a role in IVFET and women over the age of 42 years receiving donated oocytes from young women had a higher pregnancy rate than those receiving their own oocytes (Serhal and Craft, 1989). The higher fertility potential of oocytes from younger women may reflect their ability to produce polyamines and/or their endogenous reserve.

A second active role for polyamines such as spermine may be to neutralize maternal anti-embryo effector cells. Most of the data at this point derive from study of postimplantation pregnancy tissue. Monoamine and diamine oxidase are both present in placental homogenates, and possibly in the decidua, so that local oxidation to the active state is possible and may be employed in locally suppressing maternal anti-embryo effector activity (Morgan, 1982). Furthermore, we have recently found that a murine trophoblast cell line (Be6) is less sensitive to polyamine toxicity than murine lymphocytes (authors' unpublished data). It is possible therefore that the inhibitory products of oxidized spermine/spermidine could selectively inactivate maternal cells potentially deleterious to embryonic tissue, such as T lymphocytes, natural killer (NK) cells or macrophages. There are also maternal lymphoid cells in the tubal wall, the activity of which would otherwise affect preimplantation development. Such maternal effectors may act directly at the time of attachment or indirectly via release of cytokines into tubal fluid. There may also be maternal cells in peritoneal or tubal fluid capable of affecting the embryo, as will be discussed in the next section. Spermine might also affect these cells.

A further function of seminal spermine on the uterine wall may be to regulate the formation of clots in seminal plasma by acting as a competitive substrate for the transglutaminases secreted by the coagulating gland (Williams-Ashman et al, 1980). Polyamines have also been shown to act as inhibitors of platelet aggregation (Joseph et al, 1987) and to enhance plasminogen activator secretion, and thus enhance fibrinolytic activity (Kuo et al, 1988). The regulation of platelet aggregation and coagulation during the early stages of the decidual reaction may therefore be another important parameter affecting pregnancy success after the embryo has attached to the uterine wall.

THE PROBLEM OF THE CONCEPTUS AS A FOREIGN BODY

In 1953, Peter Medawar stated that 'the conceptus must be regarded as an intrauterine foreign graft, owing to the inheritance of paternal genes not shared by the mother'. This prompted many investigations of antigen expression by the early embryo and, indeed, from the time of fertilization through to parturition, fetal cells express foreign antigens against which the mother can respond immunologically (Billington, 1988). For this reason, the embryo is often referred to as a graft and thus recognition of paternal/ embryonic antigens should trigger the maternal immune system to mediate rejection of the embryo as a foreign tissue. The survival of the conceptus before, during and after implantation may therefore rely upon mechanisms preventing the potential harmful effects of the maternal immune system. Possible anti-rejection mechanisms may operate by preventing the generation of harmful types of immunity, by limiting any accumulation or activity of effector cells in close proximity to the embryo, or by conferring resistance of embryonic tissues to the effects of maternal effector cells capable of causing embryonic demise.

'Immunorejection' of the conceptus, resulting in clinical pregnancy loss, may occur via the two major types of maternal antigraft effector mechanisms. Such mechanisms are mediated by the adaptive and the paraimmune or innate immune systems (Clark and Chaouat, 1989). The adaptive immune response consists of T cells, B cells and antigen presenting cells such as dendritic cells or macrophages. Antigen presenting cells present antigen (usually after processing) in association with MHC class II antigen to helper T cells (Grey and Chesnut, 1985). Under the influence of the lymphokines interleukin-1 (IL-1) and interleukin-2 (IL-2) produced by macrophages and T cells respectively, T cells can proliferate and differentiate into cytotoxic T cells and delayed hypersensitivity T cells (T_{DTH}) which constitute the cellular specific effectors of the adaptive response. T_{DTH} cells produce toxic cytokines such as tumour necrosis factor-α/β (TNF-α/β) and are also responsible for initiating the cellular infiltrate, characteristic of delayed type hypersensitivity reactions, which occurs by the release of lymphokines such as IL-2, γ-interferon (IFN-γ) and interleukin-3 (IL-3). The humoral aspect of the adaptive immune response comes about by activation of B cells by soluble antigen or by immune complexes taken up by follicular dendritic cells. Some responses are MHC independent, but most require 'help' from T cells. Antibody can bind non-specific cytotoxic cell targets to produce ADCC (antibody dependent cell mediated cytotoxicity).

The innate system is non-antigen specific and is composed of NK, lymphokine activated killer (LAK) cells, macrophages and natural cytotoxic (NC) cells, some of which bear the asialo-GM1 marker. Natural effectors essentially act as a surveillance system exerting a selective toxicity against primitive embryonic-neoplastic cells, and can act without the delay inherent in adaptive immune responses. Cells of the innate immune system do not require prior exposure to antigen to kill and do not exhibit memory typical of adaptive immune responses. Killing of cells occurs by release of hydrogen peroxide, enzymes and TNF-α, as well as a number of other factors (Clark et al, 1989a).

Of particular relevance to abortion of the implanted embryo are the recent findings that trophoblast can be killed by LAK cells (Head, 1989) and that vascular endothelium may be sensitive to cytokines such as TNF-α (Eades et al, 1988). In addition, cells of the classical immune and innate resistance system are present in uteroplacental tissue (Hunt, 1989; Clark and Daya, 1990). Cytokines produced by macrophages or the specific immunological system can activate LAK precursors. It has therefore been proposed that the survival of the embryo after it has made direct contact with the uterine lining may depend on an active suppression of both the adaptive and innate immune responses occurring locally within the uterus.

Lymphocytes and macrophages are also present in normal tubal and peritoneal fluid, as already mentioned, and could affect preimplantation embryos by production of toxins or by direct cytotoxicity. It follows that similar processes relevant to rejection of implanted embryos need to be considered with respect to negative factors leading to implantation failure.

An important aspect of the interaction between mother and conceptus has been the recent discovery that certain types of immune responses may be beneficial to pregnancy and prevent 'rejection' (i.e. abortion of the implanted embryo), by natural effectors (LAKs). Cytokines such as granulocyte–

Table 3. Maternal cell population potentially relevant to early pregnancy outcome.

Embryonic event	Phase of menstrual cycle			
	Proliferative	Secretory	Late secretory* (pre-decidual)	Missed menses and clinical pregnancy
Uterine lining				
Macrophages	++	++	++/+++	+++
T cells	+	++	+	+
eGL	+	+	+++	+++
B cells	±	±/+	?	?
Polymorphonuclear lymphocytes	−	−	?	−
IEL	+++	++	+	±
NK	±	±	±	±
Fallopian tube†				
Macrophages	(+)	(+)	?	?
T cells	?	?	?	?
Peritoneal/tubal fluid				
Macrophages	+++	+++	+++++	?
T cells	+/±	+/±	+++++	?
eGL/NK‡	±	±	?	?
B cells	±	±	?	?

eGL = Endometrial granulated lymphocytes; IEL = intraepithelial lymphocytes.
* Cell numbers during the late secretory phase reflect the physiological situation in the absence of an embryo in the human. Ethical constraints have limited pre/peri-implantation anatomical studies in the human and much of the data obtained come from extrapolation from animal models.
† Macrophages may be present in fallopian tube tissue as tubal fluid macrophages appear to be either of peritoneal or tubal origin (Haney et al, 1983).
‡ Cells were detected using the NKHI antibody which detects Leu19⁺ NK and eGLs (Hill et al, 1988).

macrophage colony stimulating factor (GM-CSF) derived from T cells or macrophages can stimulate trophoblast growth (Athanassakis et al, 1987). Antibody may also lead to protective effects (Clark et al, 1990). The possibility that maternal cells in the wall of the uterus and oviduct, and luminal fluid, might exert both positive and/or negative effects on the early embryo needs to be considered. Various cell types in the uterine lining during the normal menstrual cycle and in peritoneal fluid are summarized in Table 3.

GROWTH FACTORS AND THE PREIMPLANTATION EMBRYO

Growth factors (embryo and maternal) are clearly required during pre-implantation pregnancy and regulate growth of the pre-embryo. When fertilized eggs are placed in the reproductive tract of steroid hormone depleted mice, some develop to blastocysts but a substantial number are lost. Treatment with progesterone or oestrogen reversed the defect (Roblero and Garavagno, 1979). This suggests that in addition to autocrine embryo derived factors such as polyamines, pre-embryo development requires additional paracrine factors produced by the reproductive tract in response to progesterone and oestradiol. Preimplantation embryos can, however, develop into blastocysts in vitro in a simple medium, but the growth rate is slower and there are fewer cells in the in vitro grown blastocysts (Papaioannou and Ebert, 1986). This could be explained by the absence of reproductive tract derived growth factors and/or dilution of embryo produced factors in the culture medium. Two-cell mouse embryos cultured singly in 25 μl microdrops show an inferior rate of development into blastocysts and have fewer cells per blastocyst compared with embryos cultured in groups of five or ten (Paria and Dey, 1990). The inferior development of single embryos was improved by addition of epidermal growth factor (EGF), transforming growth factor-α (TGF-α) or transforming growth factor-β_1 (TGF-β_1, which may be produced by T cells and macrophages) to the culture medium. All three growth factors enhanced development between the 8-cell/morula and blastocyst stages.

EGF and TGF-α bind to the same receptor and mediate similar effects (Roberts et al, 1981). This may be important in view of the findings that EGF is localized to the luminal epithelium on day 4 of pregnancy and TGF-α is produced by the morula and blastocyst present in the uterus on days 3–4 of pregnancy (Rappolee et al, 1988; Paria and Dey, 1990). It has been suggested that TGF-α produced by the embryo acts in an autocrine manner and participates in morula blastocyst transformation, zona shedding and blastocyst activation. As EGF binds to the trophectoderm at the 8-cell/morula stage but not at earlier embryonic stages, it is likely that EGF receptors are expressed by the embryo from the 8-cell stage (Paria and Dey, 1990). It has not been possible to carry out analogous studies in the human.

These findings demonstrate that preimplantation embryos are capable of promoting their own development if they are allowed to develop close to each other. During normal pregnancy in rodents, embryos are not distributed in close proximity to each other and in monotocous species there is only a single embryo, and thus growth factors of reproductive tract origin are a necessary supplement to embryo produced factors to enable successful development in vivo.

The preimplantation uterus produces several growth factors, including EGF, TGF-α, TGF-β₁ and insulin like growth factor-1 (IGF-1) (Paria and Dey, 1990). Murine embryos produce TGF-β₁ from the 2-cell stage, and platelet derived growth factor-A chain (PDGF-A) and TGF-α are expressed at the morula and blastocyst stages (Rappolee et al, 1988). In the rat, in contrast to the mouse, TGF-α mRNA is expressed in the maternal decidua but not by the embryo. The data of Han et al (1987) suggest that the embryo induces TGF-α production in the decidua, as the mRNA levels are highest in the region adjacent to the embryo. It is possible therefore that the embryo not only responds to maternal factors but may signal the mother to produce them; however, advanced embryos transferred to uteri of lesser development could not accelerate development of an implantation window.

EGF produced by the luminal epithelium presumably induces the same effects as TGF-α but in a paracrine manner (Paria and Dey, 1990). Evidence has also been obtained to suggest that uterine EGF secretion is induced by oestrogen, which in turn induces an oestrogen dependent synthesis/release of uterine and/or embryonic prostaglandins which initiate implantation (Gupta and Dey, 1989). EGF receptors are also present on trophoblast outgrowths (Adamson and Meek, 1984) and are present on first trimester human trophoblast (Kawagoe et al, 1990). EGF is produced in large amounts by the mouse submandibular gland and concentrations increase during pregnancy. Removal of the gland prior to pregnancy attenuates the rise in plasma EGF levels and reduces the pregnancy rate by 50% as assessed by successful birth (Tsutsumi and Oka, 1987). EGF replacement therapy significantly improves the pregnancy rate, and the administration of anti-EGF antibody during the peri-/postimplantation period completely ablates the pregnancy. EGF is thus essential for pregnancy maintenance during the pre-, peri- and postimplantation periods. IGF-1 is also produced by maternal uterine cells but has no direct effect on preimplantation embryo development (Paria and Dey, 1990). IGF-1 does potentiate the action of EGF and may therefore indirectly influence embryo development (Corps and Brown, 1988; Paria and Dey, 1990).

PREIMPLANTATION EMBRYO DERIVED FACTORS THAT MAY ACT ON THE MOTHER

In order for embryo development to synchronize with the uterus, signals in the form of diffusible substances may be passed between embryo and maternal endometrium. The secretion of ovine trophoblast protein-1 (oTP-1) by the sheep conceptus appears to be initially dependent on a signal from the endometrium (Ashworth and Bazer, 1989). Secretory products of pig endometrium stimulate protein secretion by the conceptus and (in this species) inhibit secretion of antiviral proteins (Beers et al, 1990).

Although a majority of embryo derived proteins in luminal fluid have not been characterized, changes in their pattern of secretion appear to occur at implantation. In the mouse, proteins secreted by late stage peri-implantation blastocysts (day 5) differ from those secreted from preimplantation (day 4) blastocysts both qualitatively and quantitatively (Nieder et al, 1987). Changes in embryo secreted proteins also occur when delayed implantation embryos are reactivated after an injection of oestrogen and when ovariectomized rats and mice are injected with ovarian steroids (Surani, 1977; Nieder et al, 1987). This suggests that the sequence of signals and responses essential for implantation are dependent on the endocrine status of the mother. In the mouse, both peri-implantation blastocysts and uteri synthesize and release a complex array of proteins. Embryos can stimulate or inhibit the synthesis of individual secreted uterine proteins (Nieder et al, 1987). In the rat, uterine luminal proteins from day 5 pregnant uteri have a higher binding affinity to blastocysts than do proteins from pro-oestrus rats (Tzartos and Surani, 1979). Such proteins may enhance metabolic activity and/or enhance specific adhesion at the onset of the implantation window.

EFFECTS OF MATERNAL IMMUNE/PARAIMMUNE CELLS ON THE PREIMPLANTATION PHASE EMBRYO

The antigenic nature of the pre-embryo renders it a potential target for maternal immune recognition. In the mouse, there are three main types of class I molecules, designated as H-2, Q and TL antigens. H-2 antigens, important in self versus non-self recognition, have been detected on unfertilized eggs, 1-cell, 2-cell, 8-cell and blastocyst stage embryos (Goldbard et al, 1985). H-2K mRNA has been detected in 8-cell mouse embryos, and blastocysts stripped of their H-2 antigens are able to regenerate the antigens after further incubation, proving that the H-2 antigens are synthesized by the embryo (Goldbard et al, 1985; Nagata et al, 1988). Although it was not established in these studies whether the H-2 antigens were maternally or paternally encoded, it has been reported elsewhere that paternally derived β_2-microglobulin (a molecule which associates with H-2 antigens) is present on 2-cell mouse embryos (Sawicki et al, 1981). This suggests that a proportion of those H-2 antigens synthesized by the blastocyst are likely to be paternally encoded.

The functions of class I antigens encoded by the Q/TL region of the mouse MHC are less well defined. The Q/TL region encodes four distinct class I protein products, designated as Qa-1, Qa-2, Q10 and Tla (Soloski et al, 1986; Warner et al, 1987b). Recent studies on murine pre-embryos, using a monoclonal antibody specific for Qa-2 antigens in a sensitive ELISA assay, have revealed that Qa-2 antigens are present on oocytes, 2-cell, 8-cell and blastocyst stage embryos (Warner et al, 1987b). Qa-2 antigens appear to be involved in the regulation of growth and development of the early embryo (see earlier section on intrinsic cell properties of the embryo). In contrast to the mouse, human preimplantation embryos from the 8-cell stage to implantation do not appear to express MHC class I antigens (Desoye et al, 1988). No class II antigens have been detected on human or murine embryos.

Minor histocompatibility antigens have been detected on murine oocytes, zygotes and 8-cell stage embryos but not on 2-cell stage embryos (Heyner et al, 1980). Although previous studies showing antigen expression on 2-cell stage embryos lacked the specificity shown in Heyner's work, it is possible that minor histocompatibility antigens are present before the 8-cell stage, but at lower levels.

Despite its antigenicity, the preimplantation embryo is free floating and of small size and cell number and thus the chance of cell surface antigen interaction with the maternal immune system is limited. Maternal cytotoxic T lymphocytes directed against paternal class I MHC can kill blastocysts (but only if the zona pellucida is removed) (Ewoldsen et al, 1987). Pre-embryos are also resistant to the effects of antibody and complement (Croy et al, 1985; Head, 1989). In IVF patients receiving partially zona dissected embryos, the pregnancy success rate was enhanced with low dose immuno-suppression (Cohen et al, 1990). This suggests that the preimplantation embryo is most susceptible to maternal immune rejection if the zona is removed sooner than occurs physiologically. Cytokines such as IFN-γ, GM-CSF and IL-1 may also impair early embryo growth. IFN-γ and GM-CSF may be produced by maternal T cells, and GM-CSF and IL-1 may be produced by macrophages. Survival of the preimplantation embryo may require alteration of the maternal immune and paraimmune cells by the embryo via factors such as polyamines.

Glycogen induced leukocytosis in the pregnant rat uterus before and during the implantation stage (days 3 through 5, where day 5 = implantation) resulted in a complete prevention of implantation. However, leukocytosis induced after day 6 of pregnancy (postimplantation) had no effect on the maintenance of pregnancy (Anderson and Alexander, 1979). These results suggest that preimplantation and attachment stage embryos are susceptible to the toxic effects of intraluminal leukocytes, but postimplantation embryos are not. Similarly, the intrauterine administration of heat-desaggregated glycogen on day 2 of murine pregnancy resulted in leukocytosis and associated infertility (Waites and Bell, 1982). Blastocysts isolated from glycogen treated mice on day 4 of pregnancy developed normally in vitro but blastocysts from controls cultured in the presence of luminal cells (largely polymorphonuclear leukocytes, PMNLs) did not exhibit trophoblast out-growth. Blastocyst development was thus blocked at the hatching stage and the antifertility effect was attributed to a PMNL low molecular weight factor (Waites and Bell, 1982). The antifertility effects of intrauterine devices (IUDs) appear to be mediated by a similar influx of PMNLs. Analysis of the PMNL influx has shown that some mature T cells were recruited (both CD8[+] and CD8[-]). Mac-1 antigen bearing cells (monocytes/macrophages), mast cells and B cells were also recruited (Toder et al, 1988).

Human endometriosis involves the implantation and cyclic changes of endometrial tissue on ectopic sites in the peritoneum and this has been associated with infertility (Halme et al, 1987). Levels of total leukocytes, macrophages, T cells and NK cells are increased in the peritoneal fluid (Hill et al, 1988). Interestingly, women with unexplained infertility also exhibited increased numbers of total leukocytes, macrophages and T cells. This suggests that products of activated macrophages and lymphocytes could be responsible for some cases of unexplained infertility (Hill et al, 1988). Furthermore, in rabbits with induced endometriosis normal embryos were present in the uterus 4 days after mating but the number of fetuses was dramatically reduced after implantation (Hahn et al, 1986). The injection of peritoneal fluid from animals with endometriosis into control rabbits 1 day before artificial insemination was similarly found to reduce the number of postimplantation embryos. This suggests that endometriosis associated infertility occurs at the implantation stage and can be attributed to a soluble factor.

Peritoneal fluid in patients with endometriosis contains increased macrophage derived IL-1 levels (Fakih et al, 1987). IL-1 stimulates T-cell production of lymphokines such as IL-2, and thus the effects of IL-1 and IL-2 on pre-embryo development have been investigated.

Fakih et al (1987) found that human recombinant IL-1 was toxic to the development of 2-cell mouse embryos when administered at concentrations compatible to that found in the peritoneal fluid of women with endometriosis. At about the same time, Hill et al (1987) reported that human IL-1 and r-IL-1β was toxic only at very high concentrations and that even the highest dosage did not kill all the embryos in the test culture. IL-1α and β are structurally distinct lymphokines and may therefore exert different effects. A number of purified preparations of IL-1 (hr-IL-1α, mr-IL-1α, hr-IL-1β: from two different suppliers) were reported to exert no toxic effects on the in vitro development of the murine embryo, even at high concentrations (Schneider et al, 1989). However, one batch of hr-IL-1β was highly embryotoxic, whereas another batch of the same biological IL-1 activity was not. It is likely therefore that a contaminating activity accounts for the IL-1 mediated toxicity reported by Fakih et al (1987). To overcome possible problems of using recombinant products (see Anderson and Hill, 1987), mouse embryos were co-cultured with peritoneal macrophages actively secreting IL-1 as well as other cytokines. The highest concentrations of IL-1 measured in monolayer culture were similar to the highest concentrations of purified IL-1 added to embryo cultures and, as before, there was no toxic effect on embryo development (Schneider et al, 1989).

IL-2 had no direct effect on embryo development (Hill et al, 1987; Schneider et al, 1989). Hill and Anderson (1989) reported that six out of eight women (75%) with unexplained infertility had elevated IL-2 levels in their peritoneal fluid, as compared with three out of 23 women (13%) with endometriosis, but the elevated IL-2 was unlikely to be a direct cause of the unexplained infertility.

Another lymphokine produced by activated T cells is IFN-γ. In purified form, this factor has been shown to inhibit growth of a number of human tumour cell lines, virally infected cells and trophoblast proliferation (Baron et al, 1980; Trinchieri and Perussia, 1985; Berkowitz et al, 1988). Both recombinant and purified natural IFN-γ were found to inhibit development of the murine pre-embryo in vitro (Hill et al, 1987). In the same system, TNF-α, a product of activated macrophages was found *not* to inhibit murine pre-embryo development, except at very high concentrations. This contrasts with the cytotoxic effects of TNF-α on tumour cells and the ability to inhibit the proliferation of a malignant trophoblast cell line (Berkowitz et al, 1988; Hunt, 1989). IFN-γ and TNF-α are reported to produce toxicity synergistically but this was not tested in the pre-embryo culture system (Trinchieri and Perussia, 1985). TNF-α can also promote the production of IFN-γ and thus could enhance the toxic effects of IFN-γ on the development of the pre-embryo (Kohase et al, 1986). Carthew et al (1986) induced interferon production in vivo by injecting mice with polyinosinin-polycytidylic acid (poly I : C). Two hours later serum was collected, titrated for interferon and used to supplement in vitro cultures of murine pre-embryos. Preimplantation, growth, implantation and trophoblast outgrowth were completely unaffected.

IFN-γ may indirectly inhibit implantation by altering the expression of surface antigens on the embryo; however, the transfer of embryos treated with in vivo produced interferon to pseudopregnant foster mothers resulted in normal implantation (Carthew et al, 1986). Although IFN-γ does not affect development of the preimplantation embryo, it is possible that IFN inhibits development of the embryo after it has begun to develop following the initial attachment to the uterine epithelium. Indeed, poly I : C can cause very early abortion in mice (Chaouat et al, 1990).

Lymphocyte derived colony stimulating factor (human and mouse GM-CSF) and B-cell growth factor (BCGF: purified, IL-4?) both inhibited development of the pre-embryo over a wide concentration range (Hill et al, 1987). The cytocidal effects of BCGF are without precedent but are preliminary and await confirmation.

In summary, there appear to be maternal cell derived toxic molecules in tubal and peritoneal fluid of patients with infertility due to endometriosis. The nature and exact origin of these molecules is uncertain. Similar molecules may be present in uterine fluid in association with IUDs. There do not appear to be any direct cell–cell contact mechanisms whereby maternal cells kill preimplantation embryos.

THE 'IMPLANTATION WINDOW' AND CELL PHYSIOLOGY OF PERI-IMPLANTATION DEVELOPMENT

At implantation, rabbit uterine epithelial cells became junctionally coupled and cell to cell communication via gap junctions is initiated locally in the vicinity of the blastocyst (Winterhager et al, 1988). In contrast, the uterine epithelium of non-pregnant and pseudopregnant animals remains uncoupled in comparable phases of hormone conditioning and thus the presence of the blastocysts is necessary for the induction of epithelial gap junctions. This phenomenon is considered as being one of the earliest signs for blastocyst derived signals that may be involved in preparing the endometrium for implantation (Winterhager et al, 1988).

Uterine epithelial cells line the surface of the uterus and thus, in addition to forming close contacts with the neighbouring cells, they must present functionally distinct cell surfaces to differing environments. The apical plasma membrane of the uterine epithelial cells is exposed to the uterine lumen and thus, in response to progesterone and oestrogen, the composition of the membrane must change to allow attachment of the embryo (Anderson et al, 1986). In addition, prior to attachment, the apical secretions must support development of the preimplantation embryo (Salamonsen et al, 1985). The basal plasma membrane is integrated with the basal lamina, which compartmentalizes the uterine epithelial cells from the underlying stromal cells. Embryo attachment to the apical surface of the cell results in a stimulus being released from the basal surface of the cell, causing differentiation of the uterine stromal cells; a process known as the decidual cell response (Lejeune and Leroy, 1980). The decidual response is essential for subsequent success of the invading embryo. The uterine epithelial cell thus has a number of specialized functions and, what is more, exhibits clear differences between apical and basal function. The ability of the cells to carry out these specialized intercellular functions depends on the polarization of their plasma membranes to bring about the appropriate intracellular changes resulting in distinct apical and basal domains, which differ in both composition and function. Any factors interfering with the polarity of the cells would thus interfere with the ability of the cells to respond to external signals (direct and indirect) such as growth factors and lymphokines. Although the epithelial cells undergo asymmetric functional changes during the menstrual cycle, the differences between the opposite ends of the cell are most evident during early pregnancy. Changes in the apical plasma membrane must be synchronized with alterations in the embryo (as previously discussed), and these modifications are crucial for the development of a transient period or 'implantation window', during which the blastocyst can attach to the apical surface of the uterine epithelial cell.

Glasser et al (1988) developed an in vitro culture system whereby the implantation window can be studied in terms of changes in apical and basal secretions. Homogeneous populations of immature rat uterine epithelial cells were cultured on porous filter supports impregnated with Engelbreth–Holm–Swarm tumour matrix. Using the millicell apparatus, which allowed access to apical and basal secretions independently, Glasser established conditions which enhanced attachment, proliferation and growth but, most importantly, maintained the polarity of the cells.

The polarized epithelial cell monolayer was hormonally responsive and oestrogen treatment resulted in the polarized secretion of a number of proteins, including apical secretion of a 130 kDa molecule and the basal secretion of an 88 kDa molecule previously identified in oestrogen treated uterine strips (Glasser et al, 1988). In addition to proteins, the cells exhibited polarity dependent secretion of proteoglycans. Keratan sulphate proteoglycans (KSPG) and heparan sulphate containing molecules (HS(PG)) were both found in apical secretions (Carson et al, 1988). The in vitro attachment of blastocysts to the apical surface of the epithelial cells is clearly limited to a short period, dependent on hormonal conditioning. In contrast, blastocysts will attach to virtually any surface without discrimination, even to plastic. The expression of blastocyst attachment is likely a specialized function of polarized epithelial cells. Polarized uterine epithelial cells have been shown to exhibit basal secretion of the extracellular matrix components laminin and heparan sulphate glycoproteins, and apical secretion of KSPG and HS(PG) (Carson et al, 1988). Laminin is a heparan sulphate binding protein which is expressed at the apical surface of the murine embryonic trophectoderm (Leivo et al, 1980). This shows that trophectoderm laminin and epithelial HS(PG) act as important cell adhesion molecules during the initial stages of attachment. HS(PG) expressed by the trophectoderm can also participate in embryo adhesion, and high affinity heparin receptors appear to be present on epithelial cells (Farach et al, 1988; Carson et al, 1988). In humans, laminin appears to be a highly effective substate adhesion molecule, as first trimester trophoblast attaches to laminin in preference to collagen type IV or bovine serum albumin (Loke et al, 1989). Laminin is produced by uterine epithelial cells and its secretion is under hormonal control, with elevated stromal concentrations occurring during the midluteal phase and early pregnancy (Loke et al, 1989). Furthermore, extravillous trophoblast has been reported to express the laminin receptor (Wewer et al, 1987). Lactosaminoglycans are cell surface components of murine uterine epithelial cells which appear to mediate cell adhesion by binding to the cell surface enzyme galactosyl transferase (Gal Tase) on adjacent cell surfaces (Bayna et al, 1986; Dutt et al, 1987). Gal Tase is present on the surface of murine pre-embryos and is elevated just prior to implantation (Sato et al, 1984). Epithelial lactosaminoglycans and trophectoderm Gal Tase are therefore also important cell adhesion molecules during the initial stages of implantation. Interestingly, mice bearing certain T/t-complex mutations exhibit elevated levels of Gal Tase which would account for the characteristic defective cellular interactions (Bayna et al, 1986). The Glasser in vitro model will allow investigations of the role of luminal and stromal cell-derived products on attachment. Some of these factors may be products of lymphocytes and macrophages.

In 1989, Kliman et al proposed a four-step model to account for the process of human nidation:

1. Contact occurs between the trophoblast cell surface and appropriately receptive apical plasma membranes of the uterine epithelial cells. This is facilitated by cell adhesion molecules present on trophoblast and/or epithelial cells.
2. The trophoblast cells then interdigitate between the epithelial cells and make contact with extracellular matrix proteins, such as fibronectin, laminin, collagen and proteoglycans. This is facilitated by substrate adhesion molecules.
3. Trophoblast–extracellular matrix interaction induces trophoblast protease secretion, which degrades the pre-existing extracellular matrix. Trophoblast membrane associated and secreted protease inhibitors control the extent of degradation.
4. Once the trophoblast cells reach their final destination (in close proximity to a maternal spiral artery) they synthesize extracellular matrix proteins, which facilitate attachment to the surroundings.

Steps 2–4 represent postattachment events that constitute the peri-implantation phase of implantation (reviewed in Kliman et al, 1989).

EMBRYO DERIVED FACTORS AFFECTING INVASION AND OUTGROWTH AFTER ATTACHMENT

Certain factors dependent on the preimplantation embryo may affect later development. Murine and human preimplantation embryos have been reported to produce a platelet activating factor (PAF) which is homologous to 1-0-alkyl-2-acetyl-sn-glyceryl-3-phosphocholine (PAF acether) (reviewed in O'Neill et al, 1989a). Amiel et al (1989), however, detected a platelet activating factor, which was not identical to PAF acether, in human and mouse embryo culture media. Whatever the structure of embryo derived PAF (EDPAF), it appears to be responsible for an early pregnancy associated thrombocytopenia, evident from days 1 to 6 of pregnancy in mice and humans (reviewed in O'Neill et al, 1989a). PAF production by human pre-embryos has been reported to correlate with the pregnancy potential of embryos produced by in vitro fertilization, suggestive of an essential role in the establishment of pregnancy (O'Neill, 1987). Although PAF may be produced at the preimplantation stage of pregnancy, its effects may occur at later stages of the implantation process. For example, PAF increases vascular permeability, which is an important aspect of the decidual response. Inhibition of decidualization (using prostaglandin (PG) synthesis blocks such as indomethacin) inhibits implantation (Kennedy, 1983). Uterine ischaemia produced by injection of serotonin (Mitchell and Hammer, 1983) or by uncertain factors (Goswamy et al, 1988) has been related to infertility (implantation failure).

The importance of PAF during pre-embryo development and implantation has been extensively tested in the mouse. The administration of a PAF antagonist (SRI-63-441) inhibited implantation in the mouse and the inhibition was overcome by simultaneous administration of PAF (Spinks and O'Neill, 1988). The treatment of embryo donors before embryo transfers, but not recipients, with the PAF antagonist (SRI-63-441) reduced implantation rates, indicating that the antagonist was acting at the embryonic rather than the maternal level (Spinks et al, 1990). Further evidence that the factor acted at the embryonic level was obtained by supplementing in vitro cultures of murine embryos with PAF. Although the proportion of 2-cell mouse embryos reaching the blastocyst stage was unaffected (a polyamine-dependent process), the metabolic rate, cleavage rate and implantation potential of the embryos were increased (Ryan et al, 1990). PAF supplementation was only beneficial when the control embryos had a low pregnancy potential, suggesting that such embryos were deficient in PAF. Similarly, the supplementation of human IVF embryo culture media with PAF has been reported to increase the pregnancy success rate after embryo transfer, presumably due to supplementing PAF levels in that proportion of embryos normally PAF deficient (O'Neill et al, 1989b). Despite these findings, PAF does not appear to be essential for the survival of the preimplantation embryo, since murine pre-embryo cultures from the 2-cell to blastocyst stage cultured with PAF antagonists, which inhibit implantation in vivo, developed normally in vitro (O'Neill, 1987). The addition of PAF antagonists to in vitro cultures of murine blastocysts did, however, markedly inhibit trophoblast outgrowth (Spinks et al, 1990). It has been suggested that the exposure of the embryo to PAF at the blastocyst stage 'is essential for initiating the events that lead to the production of an invasive trophoblast' (Spinks et al, 1990). The authors also propose that, prior to the blastocyst stage, receptor mediated responses to PAF are not essential but PAF acts as an essential autocrine growth factor for the early embryo.

In contrast to O'Neill's work, Milligan and Finn (1990) found that the in vivo treatment of ovariectomized progesterone treated mice with PAF antagonists did not inhibit implantation. Even when the antagonist SRI-63-441 was administered using the highest dose but the same regimen as used by Spinks et al (1990), no effect was seen on pregnancy or implantation rate. The authors conclude that their results are not consistent with an indispensable role of PAF in the peri-implantation period (Milligan and Finn, 1990).

PAF has also been implicated in the conditioning of the uterus for implantation; indeed, PAF mediates the production and actions of prostaglandins and leukotrienes (arachidonic acid metabolites) which respectively induce vasodilatation and increase vascular permeability (Jouvin-Marche et al, 1982; Tawfik et al, 1987; Smith and Kelly, 1988). In the mouse, the deciduomal response to an intrauterine oil stimulus was not, however, inhibited by PAF antagonists, and uterine intraluminal instillation of PAF did not trigger a decidual response (Milligan and Finn, 1990; Spinks et al, 1990). The role of PAF in the decidual response is thus controversial.

The in vitro culture of human endometrial cells has revealed that PAF is also produced by the stromal cells and that progesterone enhances its secretion (Alecozay et al, 1989). In the rabbit, uterine PAF levels increase during the preimplantation period and then decline rapidly by day 7 in the pregnant, but not the pseudopregnant, uterus (Angle et al, 1988). It is possible that PAF is important for implantation and that levels of the factor must be high within close proximity to the embryo. In this regard, the source of PAF would be unimportant and uterine PAF secretion may make up for deficient embryos' PAF secretion. This may account for the apparently successful implantation of a proportion of PAF negative embryos (C. O'Neill, personal communication). Prostaglandin E_2 (PGE_2) was found to enhance PAF secretion by progesterone exposed cells, and PGE_2 was released by cultures of glandular cells on addition of PAF and oestrogen together (Smith and Kelly, 1988; Alecozay et al, 1989). The interaction between stromal cells, epithelial cells, PAF and PGE_2 suggests a possible paracrine control system. In conclusion, PAF appears to be important in early pregnancy in that it increases both the implantation potential of pre-embryos and the vascular permeability of the endometrium in preparation for the decidual reaction and implantation. PAF also has some immunosuppressive actions, that is, it reduces proliferation of lymphocytes, decreases IL-2 production and increases suppressor cell activity (Braquet et al, 1987). In contrast, however, it enhances responsiveness of lymphocytes to IL-2 and increases NK activity. Some of these actions may confer some protection to the early embryo; however, as embryos develop normally in antagonist treated mice, the significance is uncertain. This will be discussed later.

The administration of PAF to oestrous mice results in the appearance of EPF in the serum, which is reported to bring about an immunosuppressive effect (Orozco et al, 1986; Rolfe et al, 1988). EPF is induced by production of a factor by the fertilized oocyte within 24 h of fertilization. Antibodies to EPF may lead to abortion.

REJECTION/NON-REJECTION OF THE EARLY INVADING EMBRYO

Can active rejection of the embryo during the first 2–3 days after implantation occur and, if so, how? Only embryonic and minor antigens are expressed during this period. If such antigens were taken up by antigen presenting cells (APC) and presented to sensitized T_{DTH} cells, release of 'toxic' cytokines might be possible. A similar release of toxins such as TNF-α from macrophages (paracrine) or NK cells (IFN-γ) could be inhibitory. There is no experimental evidence that sensitization to minor antigens is normally dangerous. Indeed, it has been shown that blastocysts transferred to the kidney capsule of immunized mice were rejected (probably by ADCC but delayed type hypersensitivity is possible), whereas blastocysts placed in the uterus survived and developed normally after implantation (Searle et al, 1974). This normal survival may be explained by antirejection mechanisms operating in the uterus. There is now good evidence that peri-implantation failure in mice can be produced by asialo-GM1$^+$ killer cells (NK–LAK) activated by poly I:C or by lipopolysaccharide (LPS). IL-2 and indomethacin administration $\pm$ IL-2 has also been reported to cause failure in the peri-implant period in mice (Lala et al, 1990). Indeed, recombinant IL-2 injected into syngeneically or allogeneically mated mice during the preimplantation period caused 100% early resorption and an apparent lack of implants (Tezabwala et al, 1989). In this case, IL-2 may indirectly induce the secretion of other cytokines, such as IFN-γ, which may influence embryo implantation and development. Alternatively, IL-2 may directly activate cytotoxic cells, such as LAKs to kill trophoblast. Normal levels of resistance/protection against rejection can therefore be overcome.

How are deleterious maternal anti-embryo effects prevented? The potential role of embryo derived factors, such as derived polyamines, has already been discussed. As already mentioned, another activity stimulated by the embryo is EPF. The immunization of mice with polyclonal anti-EPF immunoglobulin G (IgG) has been shown to reduce embryonic viability significantly (Athanasas-Platsis et al, 1989). Suppressor factors released from EPF bound T lymphocytes (suppressor T cells) have been proposed to play a major role in inhibiting maternal antifetal interactions at the time of implantation (Rolfe et al, 1988). Passive immunization of mice on days 2–6 with a monoclonal antibody which binds a T suppressor cell inducing factor also results in embryonic loss (Beaman and Hoversland, 1988). It is possible that the suppressor factors are related to those induced by EPF.

Another set of potentially important embryo derived suppressor molecules are the interferons. oTP-1 and bovine trophoblast protein-1 (bTP-1) are products of the preimplantation ovine and bovine conceptus and are believed to mediate pregnancy recognition by inhibiting endometrial production or release of the luteolysin prostaglandin F_{2a} (reviewed in Roberts, 1989). The cloning and sequencing of cDNAs for oTP-1 and bTP-1 has shown that the proteins exhibit 85% identity and are structurally related to α-interferons (IFN-alphas) (Imakawa et al, 1989). Of particular interest is that both proteins have greater than 80% nucleotide sequence identity with a gene representing bovine IFN which belongs to a subfamily categorized as IFN-α-II or IFN-ω (Imakawa et al, 1989). At the primary level, both oTP-1 and bTP-1 have also been shown to have about 70% amino acid sequence identity with bovine IFN-α-II (Imakawa et al, 1989). The proteins are produced by the trophectoderm (the first epithelium of the conceptus) and synthesis is restricted to the period when the conceptus must signal its presence to the mother (Roberts, 1989). In the human, pregnancy syncytiotrophoblast has been shown to produce IFN-α and it has been suggested that it may have an antiluteolytic role similar to that observed in ruminants (Bulmer et al, 1990). The IFN-α-like proteins may, however, have two other functions. Firstly, the localization of oTP-1 to the trophectoderm of the ovine pre-embryo suggests that the proteins may provide a barrier to viral infection. Secondly, the interferons may have immuno-modulatory roles. Indeed, human syncytiotrophoblast produces a potent suppressive molecule that has been shown to be α-interferon (Bulmer et al, 1990). Interferons prolong allograft survival, inhibit lymphocyte activation and alter antigen expression (Baron et al, 1980). In support of this idea, oTP-1 has been found to inhibit both the growth of bovine kidney epithelial cells and the mitogen stimulation of ovine lymphocytes.

The ability of the blastocyst to attach to substrates in vitro and to exhibit outgrowth of trophectodermal and inner cell mass cells has enabled antigen expression to be examined during the implantation process. During the time between hatching from the zona pellucida and invasion after initial attachment, the expression of both MHC and non-MHC minor H antigens on the trophoblast cell membrane is shut off (Leclipteux and Remacle, 1983). Embryonic antigens such as EC-1 may be expressed, however (Hamilton et al, 1985). The inhibition of trophoblast histocompatibility antigen expression lasts about 3–4 days in the mouse, i.e. throughout the peri-implantation period. At day 7.5, the conceptus consists of an embryonic sac surrounded by trophoblast, with a proliferating cap of cells known as ectoplacental cone trophoblast (EPC). Only the smaller diploid trophoblast of the EPC core and the embryonic sac cells are MHC positive but they are surrounded by trophoblast giant cells which are devoid of MHC antigens (Billington, 1988). The allogeneic fetus can, in theory, develop safely within its cocoon of trophoblast shielding it from maternal specific and non-specific effector mechanisms. To what extent is the trophoblast susceptible to rejection and what mechanism prevents interaction with maternal effector cells in the decidua? It has already been mentioned that attachment of blastocyst trophoblast to uterine epithelium may be inhibited by toxins in tubal/uterine fluid. Once contact is made between uterine cells and the embryos, positive and negative effects of uterine stromal cells and intraepithelial lymphocytes become important (Table 3).

In the preimplantation rat uterus, cells bearing T lymphocyte and granulocyte–macrophage surface markers have been identified in endometrium and myometrium (Noun et al, 1989). One day before implantation, both types of cells migrated away from the uterine surface epithelia to the deep endometrium, and during the early implantation period there was a total lack of T cells, granulocytes and macrophages around the conceptus. Shortly after implantation in the rat, macrophages are numerous around the implantation site but none are found within the decidua (Tachi and Tachi, 1989). When macrophages are co-cultured with blastocysts, there is no evidence for their accumulation or repulsion from the blastocysts; however, the macrophages appear to adopt a different cellular morphology, that is, they look more rounded rather than their characteristic elongated or spread shape (Tachi and Tachi, 1989). Interestingly, the authors have obtained preliminary evidence to suggest that the two macrophage populations differ in terms of function as well as morphology. Tachi and Tachi (1989) found that the secretion of leukotriene C_4 by macrophages in response to calcium ionophore was associated with macrophage elongation. In contrast, the rounding of macrophages in response to cytochalasin B or colchicine was associated with inactivity. It is possible therefore that the more rounded macrophages in contact with blastocysts in vitro, and probably present in vivo, are inactive and thus unable to present antigen or recruit/activate other immunocompetent cells or phagocytose (see Hunt, 1989). Active paralysis of certain macrophage function is consistent with the intimate and benign association seen between macrophages and trophoblast cells (in the chorion laevae) later in pregnancy (Bulmer et al, 1987).

Early pregnancy also affects uterine lymphatics. Indeed, lymphatics do not appear near the uterine lumen after mating, or near the conceptus during or after implantation. This lack of lymphatics probably functions to restrict access of antigenic material to the uterine draining lymph nodes (Head and Billingham, 1986). In addition, early pregnancy in the rat is characterized by a reduction in the density of Ia^+ antigen presenting cells (dendritic morphology), particularly in the central decidua near the implanting blastocyst (Head and Billingham, 1986). Similar antigen presenting cells have been identified in murine and human decidua, although to date no preimplantation phase distribution data are available (reviewed in Lea and Clark, 1989). In total, these observations suggest that an important immunoregulatory mechanism operating to protect the pre-/peri-implantation conceptus is a block of alloantigen handling and processing which occurs locally at the fetomaternal interface.

A subset of unusual endometrial granular lymphocytes of T lineage is also present in luteal phase endometrium and early pregnancy decidua (Table 3; Clark and Daya, 1990). These cells lack the classical T-cell surface markers

CD3,4,5,8 and lack the NK cell surface markers Leu7 and OKM-1, but the cells do express Leu19 (CD56: marker of NK activated lymphocytes) and CD7 (T cell marker). The density of the cells increases during the luteal phase and early pregnancy and they possess NK activity that would include them among the intraepithelial T lineage NK-like cells described at other mucosal surfaces, such as the gut, and referred to as intraepithelial lymphocytes (IELs) (Tagliabue et al, 1982). IELs have been identified as common components of both luminal and glandular epithelium of the non-pregnant rat uterus (Sawicki et al, 1988). The number of IELs decreased from dioestrus to pro-oestrus and this was attributed to hormonal influences. In the pregnant rat uterus, the number of cells markedly decreased from as early as day 5, that is before implantation. This contrasts with the increase in number of endometrial granular lymphocytes in the human but is in agreement with a reduction in luminal epithelium IEL number reported to occur during early pregnancy in the cow (Vander Wielen and King, 1984). Of particular interest in the rat was that the reduction in lymphocyte number, as measured on days 7 and 9, occurred exclusively at the implantation sites, while interimplantation site cell numbers remained relatively constant. It appears therefore that this localized reduction in cell numbers is associated with an embryonic rather than a maternal factor. The authors suggest that the increase/decrease in the numbers of IELs probably results from an influx or efflux of cells from the lamina propria into the epithelium and back (Sawicki et al, 1988). The function of reproductive tract IELs is uncertain but the IELs of the gastrointestinal tract may have suppressor, cytotoxic or NK activities (Dobbins, 1986). The reduction in cell numbers in the local environment of the implanting embryo may represent a protective redistribution of immunocompetent and paraimmune effector cells.

In mice, uterine IgA secretion and the number of IgA plasma cells in the stroma increase in uteri containing normal or delayed embryos but decrease in pseudopregnant uteri (Rachman et al, 1986). IgG secretion was only increased during pregnancy. No plasma cells bearing IgA, IgG or IgE are, however, found closer to the embryo in the postimplantation murine decidua (Tachi and Tachi, 1989). Uterine IgA secretion during implantation may act to nourish or activate the blastocyst or may act to prevent passage of bacteria, virus or other antigens through the epithelium at the implantation site, along with the embryo. The lack of decidual immunocytes after implantation may represent an immunoprotective mechanism with respect to the peri-implantation embryo (reviewed in Lea and Clark, 1989).

While embryo produced factors may be primarily responsible for inhibiting its rejection, certain cell populations in the maternal decidua/endometrium may contribute. A population of $CD2^+3^+8^+$ cells is present in decidual tissue, and probably in luteal phase preimplantation endometrium (Clark and Daya, 1990; Clark et al, 1990). Despite expressing the CD3 marker, the cells appear to lack the antigen recognitive component of the T cell receptor complex, the α/β or γ/δ chains (Dietl et al, 1990). These cells are thus incapable of recognizing antigen and do not express the IL-2 receptor in early pregnancy.

Suppressor cells in endometrial/decidual tissue may also play a role in protecting the embryo against potential effector cell activation. In the mouse, whole preimplantation endometrial tissue and peri-implantation phase tissue contain suppressor cells (Brierley and Clark, 1987; Clark et al, 1989b). Further, human secretory phase endometrial explants release more suppressive activity into the culture supernatant than analogous proliferative phase explants (Wang et al, 1987). This has been largely attributed to the presence of a novel population of hormone induced suppressor cells identified in both the mouse and human preimplantation uterus (Brierley and Clark, 1987; Daya and Clark, 1985). The cells are large in size and, in the mouse, they have been shown to bear the Lyt 2^+ (CD8) antigen characteristic of suppressor T cells. These T lineage cells are unusual in that they are restricted to the uterine lining, hormone induced and fail to release any soluble suppressor factors for mice responses (Brierley and Clark, 1987). At the end of the peri-implantation phase in the mice, the $CD8^+$ suppressor cells are replaced by a population of non-specific, non-T suppressor bone marrow derived natural cells, which release a factor closely related to TGF-β_2 (Clark et al, 1990; R. G. Lea et al, unpublished data).

Alloantigen specific Lyt 2^+ cells have also been identified in the uterine draining lymph nodes of day 6.5 pregnant Balb/c mice (Thomas and Erickson, 1986). Recent data have also revealed that hormone dependent intrauterine suppressor cell activity may be manifest in the uterine draining lymph nodes of pregnant CBA/J mice (Clark et al, 1989b). It has been suggested that the uterine non-specific Lyt 2^+ suppressor cells may migrate downstream and become antigen specific suppressor cells on exposure to fetal antigens in the lymph node (Clark et al, 1989b). Antigen specific peptide factors secreted by T suppressor cells (TsF) may also be important. Beaman and Hoversland (1988) described an immunoreactive molecule in murine reproductive tissues which had physicochemical properties similar to TsF, was localized to the uterus, spleen and regional lymph nodes, and was elevated during early pregnancy. Levels of TsF in uterus and spleen are further elevated in response to implantation, whereas draining lymph node TsF levels were unaffected (Hoversland and Beaman, 1990). Monoclonal antibodies specific for a TsF from an L3T4 (CD4) cell line have been found to block implantation when administered to mice during the pre- and early peri-implantation period (Beaman and Hoversland, 1988). Monoclonal antibodies raised against a 'newly described 150 kD cytokine' present in uterine draining lymph nodes have recently been found to bind to the TsF described above, as well as to $L3T4^+$ splenic lymphocytes, and to completely ablate pregnancy when administered at or about the time of implantation (Beaman et al, 1990). The hormone-dependent Lyt 2^+ cells described by Clark et al (1989b) might bind.

It has been proposed that decidual/endometrial suppressor cells may be recruited and/or activated by signals from the embryo. Mayumi et al (1985) reported that factors released from 8-cell stage blastocysts can induce the generation of suppressor T cells from splenocytes. Whether these factors are involved in generating $CD8^+$ cells in the uterine nodes is unknown.

Lymphocytes of healthy pregnant women possess specific progesterone binding sites and demonstrate an unusually high progesterone sensitivity as compared with non-pregnancy lymphocytes (Szekeres-Bartho et al, 1990).

In the presence of progesterone, receptor bearing pregnancy lymphocytes release a 34 kDa protein which exhibits NK and NC blocking activity (Szekeres-Bartho et al, 1990). As progesterone increases the release of immunosuppressive activity from human endometrial cultures, it has been suggested that the Lyt 2^+ (CD8$^+$) cells described by Clark et al (1989b) may be stimulated by progesterone to release similar factor(s) (Chaouat et al, 1989). Given that it is the natural effector system that has the ability to kill the embryo, these CD8$^+$ cell derived factors may be of key importance in preventing pregnancy failure. However, the depletion of CD8$^+$ cells in rodents with normal pregnancy success rates does not alter the abortion rate (Sulila et al, 1988). It has been suggested that the effect of the dose of antibody administered may not be sufficient to affect pregnancy in animals with high pregnancy success rates (Athanassakis et al, 1987).

Various maternally derived cytokines may act as important growth factors for the growing embryo. A small binding protein for IGF (Mr 29–35 kDa) is localized to the extracellular matrix and is suggested to regulate trophoblast invasion (Bell, 1989). IGF-1 and -2 mRNA together with IGF receptors have been detected in a wide range of fetal tissues and it is interesting that IGF-2 mRNA expression is a postimplantation event (Bell, 1989; Ohlsson et al, 1989). Colony stimulating factor (CSF) can also act on trophoblast and activity is high in the pregnant mouse uterus. Most, if not all, of the activity can be attributed to CSF-1 (Pollard, 1990). Steroid hormones regulate CSF-1 synthesis through the induction of CSF-1 mRNA in epithelial cells, and in the preimplantation murine uterus CSF-1 mRNA levels were elevated before implantation on day 3 of pregnancy (Arceci et al, 1989; Pollard, 1990). The levels of CSF-1 then increased, reaching a peak at days 14–15, but its expression was not localized to implantation sites. CSF-1 receptor mRNA was first detected on maternal decidua at day 6 and on trophectodermal cells at day 7.5 (Arceci et al, 1989). It seems unlikely that CSF-1 is acting on the embryo before the receptor is expressed. CSF-1 is chemotactic for macrophages, and thus its lack of expression at implantation sites may help to reduce macrophage numbers in the close vicinity of the conceptus. CSF-1 also regulates survival and differentiation of macrophages and induces them to synthesize other cytokines, including IL-2, GM-CSF, IFNs and TNF-α (Pollard, 1990). Injection of semi-purified CSF-1 into pregnant mice during the preimplantation phase of pregnancy has been reported to induce a high rate of fetal resorption, although the number of implant sites was not significantly different to controls (Tartakovsky, 1989). Given that the CSF-1 was semi-purified, the effect may be due to endotoxin or production of excessive levels of IL-2 and TNF-α that may lead to damage to the implantating embryo, as discussed below. GM-CSF may, however, be important in embryo outgrowth on endometrial stromal cells; this was enhanced by GM-CSF in vitro, and superovulated mice (similar to IVF oocyte donors who have suboptimal implantation rates with ET) were unable to produce GM-CSF (Robertson et al, 1990).

Alloimmunization (or normal IgG) or injection of cytokines such as GM-CSF or IL-3 can prevent spontaneous abortion in DBA/2-mated CBA/J mice. CD8$^+$ cells appear to be required for protection, and the effect of the

IgG occurs in the peri-implantation period and suppresses infiltration by asialo-GM1$^+$ cells. Production of cytokine growth factors by maternal uterine lymphomyeloid cells may also, therefore, play a role in success in the peri- and postimplantation period. Couples with recurrent unexplained clinical abortion may also be treated by allogeneic stimulation by paternal or third-party leukocyte injection (Clark, 1989). Interestingly, the time to achieve clinical pregnancy seems to shorten with treatment and, on this basis, it has been suggested that occult abortions are being prevented. Since immunization can also protect against LPS and poly I:C mediated pregnancy failure in mice (Chaouat et al, 1990), it may be possible to treat peri-implant occult rejection after it is diagnosed.

SUMMARY AND CONCLUSIONS

The implantation of an appropriately developed embryo into a suitably conditioned uterine lining depends on the synchronous maturation of the preimplantation embryo and uterine lining. The pre- and postimplantation embryo also requires protection from immunocompetent maternal immune effectors. Preimplantation embryo development is affected by genotype, intercellular communication and autocrine growth factors (polyamines, TGF-α, TGF-β1, PAF). Factors of maternal origin may also enhance embryo development (EGF, TGF-α, TGF-β1, IGF, polyamines). The preimplantation embryo signals its presence to the mother by release of factor(s) such as IFN-α-II and a PAF-like factor. PAF may induce EPF in the mother and enhances vascular permeability at the implantation site. Uterine or peritoneal leukocytosis may inhibit development via toxic effects of lymphokines/monokines (IL-2, IL-1 ?, IFN-γ, TNF-α). Immuno-protection of the preimplantation embryo is conferred by embryo derived maternal factors (EPF, T-cell suppressor factors).

The uterus is receptive during a limited period of time (implantation window) and the substrate adhesion molecules produced by uterine and embryonic trophectoderm cells are crucial for the initial stages of implantation. At implantation, trophoblast expression of MHC and non-MHC antigens is shut off and both immunocompetent maternal cells (macrophages, dendritic cells, granulocytes, IELs, immunocytes) and lymphatics become sparse at implantation sites. Peri-implantation cytokines of maternal origin, such as CSF-1, GM-CSF and IGF-1 binding protein, are probably important for trophoblast growth and development. Immuno-protection of the embryo at this stage may be mediated by embryo derived factors that inactivate macrophages and by a population of large, hormone dependent Lyt 2$^+$ (CD8$^+$) suppressor cells. It is possible that these CD8$^+$ cells respond to progesterone and secrete molecules that inactivate natural effector (NK-type) cells against trophoblast. Prostaglandins (PGE$_2$) may play a brief role in immunosuppression at the time of implantation but its role is probably more important with respect to the decidual response. Defects in the pre- and peri-implantation stages of pregnancy may lead to delayed failure in the form of clinical miscarriage.

Acknowledgements

We thank Corinne Lea for her excellent secretarial assistance in the preparation of the manuscript.

REFERENCES

Adamson ED & Meek J (1984) The ontogeny of epidermal growth factor receptors during mouse development. *Developmental Biology* **103**: 62–70.

Alberman E (1988) The epidemiology of repeated abortion. In Beard RW & Sharp F (eds) *Early Pregnancy Loss: Mechanisms and Treatment*, pp 9–17. Ashton-under-Lyne: Peacock Press.

Alecozay AA, Casslen BG, Riehl RM et al (1989) Platelet-activating factor in human luteal phase endometrium. *Biology of Reproduction* **41**: 578–586.

Allen JC, Smith CJ & Curry MC (1977) Identification of a thymic inhibitor ('chalone') of lymphocyte transformation as a spermine complex. *Nature* **267**: 623–625.

Allen RD & Roberts TK (1987) Role of spermine in the cytotoxic effects of seminal plasma. *American Journal of Reproductive Immunology and Microbiology* **13**: 4–8.

Amiel ML, Duquenne C, Benveniste J & Testart J (1989) Platelet aggregating activity in human embryo culture media free of PAF-acether. *Human Reproduction* **4**: 327–330.

Anderson DJ & Alexander NJ (1979) Induction of uterine leukocytosis and its effect on pregnancy in rats. *Biology of Reproduction* **21**: 1143–1152.

Anderson DJ & Hill JA (1987) Interleukin-1 and endometrium. *Fertility and Sterility* **48**: 894–895.

Anderson TL, Olson GE & Hoffman LH (1986) Stage-specific alterations in the apical membrane glycoproteins of endometrial epithelial cells related to implantation in rabbits. *Biology of Reproduction* **34**: 701–720.

Angle MJ, Jones MA, McManus LM, Pinckard RN & Harper MJK (1988) Platelet-activating factor in the rabbit uterus during early pregnancy. *Journal of Reproduction and Fertility* **83**: 711–722.

Arceci RJ, Shanahan F, Stanley ER & Pollard JW (1989) Temporal expression and location of colony-stimulating factor 1 (CSF-1) and its receptor in the female reproductive tract are consistent with CSF-1-regulated placental development. *Proceedings of the National Academy of Sciences of the USA* **86**: 8818–8822.

Asch RH, Balmaceda JP, Cittadini E et al (1988) Gamete intrafallopian transfer: international cooperative study of the first 800 cases. *Annals of the New York Academy of Sciences* **541**: 722–727.

Ashworth CJ & Bazar FW (1989) Changes in ovine conceptus endometrial function following asynchronous embryo transfer or administration of progesterone. *Biology of Reproduction* **40**: 425–434.

Athanasas-Platsis S, Quinn KA, Wong T-Y et al (1989) Passive immunization of pregnant mice against early pregnancy factor causes loss of embryonic viability. *Journal of Reproduction and Fertility* **87**: 495–502.

Athanassakis I, Bleackley RC, Paetkau V et al (1987) The immunostimulatory effect of T cells and T cell lymphokines on murine fetally derived placental cells. *Journal of Immunology* **138**: 37–44.

Barkley MS & FitzGerald R (1990) Influence of embryonic and maternal genotype on gestational events in the mouse. *Journal of Reproduction and Fertility* **89**: 285–291.

Baron S, Blalock JE, Dianzani F et al (1980) Immune interferon: some properties and functions. *Annals of the New York Academy of Sciences* **350**: 130–144.

Bayna EM, Runyan RB, Scully NF, Reichner J, Lopez LC & Shur BD (1986) Cell surface galactosyltransferase as a recognition molecule during development. *Molecular and Cellular Biochemistry* **72**: 141–151.

Beaman K, Lee C-K, Ghoshal K & Gilman-Sachs A (1990) Expression of an allogeneic suppressor peptide by the decidual lymph nodes of the uterus. *FASEB Journal* **85** (abstract).

Beaman KD & Hoversland RC (1988) Induction of abortion in mice with a monoclonal antibody specific for suppressor T-lymphocyte molecules. *Journal of Reproduction and Fertility* **82:** 691–696.

Beers S, Mirando MA, Pontzer CH et al (1990) Influence of endometrium, protease inhibitors and freezing on antiviral activity of proteins secreted by pig conceptuses. *Journal of Reproduction and Fertility* (in press).

Bell SC (1989) Decidualization and insulin-like growth factor (IGF) binding protein: implications for its role in stromal cell differentiation and the decidual cell in haemochorial placentation. *Human Reproduction* **4:** 125–130.

Bellinge BS, Copeland CM, Thomas TD et al (1986) The influence of patient insemination on the implantation rate in an in vitro fertilization and embryo transfer program. *Fertility and Sterility* **46:** 252–256.

Ben-Nun I, Siegal A, Ghetler Y et al (1990) Effect of preovulatory progesterone administration on the endometrial maturation and implantation rate after in vitro fertilization and embryo transfer. *Fertility and Sterility* **53:** 276–281.

Berkowitz RS, Hill JA, Kurtz CB & Anderson DJ (1988) Effects of products of activated leukocytes (lymphokines and monokines) on the growth of malignant trophoblast cells in vitro. *American Journal of Obstetrics and Gynecology* **158:** 199–203.

Billington WD (1988) Antigen expression by cells of the conceptus before, during and after implantation. In Beard RW & Sharp F (eds) *Early Pregnancy Loss: Mechanisms and Treatment*, pp 205–212. Ashton-under-Lyne: Peacock Press.

Boue J, Boue A & Lazar P (1975) Retrospective and prospective epidemiological studies of 1500 karyotyped spontaneous human abortions. *Teratology* **12:** 11–26.

Braquet P, Touqui L, Shen TY & Vargaftig BB (1987) Perspectives in platelet-activating factor research. *Pharmacological Reviews* **39:** 97–145.

Brierley J & Clark DA (1987) Characterization of hormone-dependent suppressor cells in the uterus of pregnant and pseudopregnant mice. *Journal of Reproductive Immunology* **10:** 201–218.

Buehr M, Lee S, McLaren & Warner A (1987) Reduced gap junctional communication is associated with the lethal condition characteristic of DDK mouse eggs fertilized by foreign sperm. *Development* **101:** 449–459.

Bulmer JN, Smith JC & Wells M (1987) Maternal and fetal cellular relationships in the human placental basal plate. *Placenta* **9:** 237–246.

Bulmer JN, Morrison L, Johnson PM & Meager A (1990) Immunohistochemical localization of interferons in human placental tissues in normal, ectopic, and molar pregnancy. *American Journal of Reproductive Immunology* **22:** 109–116.

Bustillo M, Cohen SW, Thorneycroft IH & Buster JE (1986) Use of combination oral contraceptives to synchronize recipient–donor LH peaks for ovum transfer. *Abstract of the 42nd Annual Meeting of the Canadian Fertility and Andrology Society*, Toronto, p 54.

Butler JE & Biggers JD (1989) Assessing the viability of preimplantation embryos in vitro. *Theriogenology* **31:** 115–126.

Carson DD, Tang J-P, Julian J & Glasser SR (1988) Vectorial secretion of proteoglycans by polarized rat uterine epithelial cells. *Journal of Cell Biology* **107:** 2425–2435.

Carthew P, Wood M & Kirby C (1986) Mouse interferon produced in vivo does not inhibit the development of preimplantation mouse embryos. *Journal of Reproduction and Fertility* **77:** 75–79.

Chang MC (1950) Development and fate of transferred rabbit ova or blastocysts in relation to the ovulation time of recipients. *Journal of Experimental Zoology* **114:** 197–225.

Chaouat G, Menu E, Szekeres-Bartho J et al (1989) Lymphokines, steroids, placental factors and trophoblast intrinsic resistance to immune-cell-mediated lysis are involved in pregnancy success or immunologically mediated pregnancy failure. In Gill TJ & Wegmann TG (eds) *Molecular Immunology of the Feto-maternal Interface*. London: Oxford University Press (in press).

Chaouat G, Menu E, Clark DA et al (1990) Control of fetal survival in CBA × DBA/2 mice by lymphokine therapy. *Journal of Reproduction and Fertility* **89:** 447–458.

Chartier M, Roger M, Barrat J & Michelob B (1979) Measurement of plasma human chorionic gonadotrophin (hCG) and β-hCG activities in the late luteal phase: evidence of the occurrence of spontaneous menstrual abortions in infertile women. *Fertility and Sterility* **31:** 134–137.

Clark DA (1989) The immunology of recurrent abortion. In Bonnar J (ed.) *Recent Advances in Obstetrics and Gynaecology*, chap. 2, pp 25–42. Edinburgh: Churchill Livingstone.

Clark DA & Chaouat G (1989) Determinants of embryo survival in the peri- and post-implantation period. In Yoshinoga K (ed.) *Blastocyst Implantation*, pp 171–178. Boston: Adams Publishing.

Clark DA & Daya S (1990) Macrophages and their migratory cells in endometrium: relevance to endometrial bleeding. In WHO Symposium *Contraception and Mechanisms of Uterine Bleeding*, pp 363–382. Cambridge: Cambridge University Press.

Clark DA, Lee S, Fishell S et al (1989a) Immunosuppressive activity in human in vitro fertilization (IVF) culture supernatants and prediction of the outcome of embryo transfer: a multicenter trial. *Journal of In vitro Fertilization and Embryo Transfer* **6**: 51–58.

Clark DA, Brierley J, Banwatt D & Chaouat G (1989b) Hormone-induced preimplantation Lyt 2$^+$ murine uterine suppressor cells persist after implantation and may reduce the spontaneous abortion rate in CBA/J mice. *Cellular Immunology* **123**: 334–343.

Clark DA, Lea RG, Podor T et al (1990) Cytokines determining the success or failure of pregnancy. *Annals of the New York Academy of Sciences* (in press).

Cohen J, Kort H, Malter H et al (1990) Immunosuppression supports implantation of zona pellucida dissected human embryos. *Fertility and Sterility* **53**: 662–665.

Corps AN & Brown KD (1988) Ligand-receptor interactions involved in the stimulation of Swiss 3T3 fibroblasts by insulin-like growth factor. *Biochemical Journal* **252**: 119–125.

Croy BA, Gambel P, Rossant J & Wegmann TG (1985) Characterization of murine decidual natural killer (NK) cells and their relevance to the success of pregnancy. *Cell Immunology* **93**: 315–326.

Daya S & Clark DA (1985) Preliminary characterization of two types of suppressor cells in the human uterus. *Fertility and Sterility* **44**: 778–785.

Daya S & Clark DA (1986) Production of immunosuppressor factor(s) by pre-implantation embryos. *American Journal of Reproductive Immunology and Microbiology* **11**: 98–101.

Desoye G, Dohr GA, Motter W et al (1988) Lack of HLA class I and class II antigens on human preimplantation embryos. *Journal of Immunology* **140**: 4157–4159.

Dietl J, Horny H-P, Rcuk P et al (1990) Intradecidual T lymphocytes lack immunohistochemically detectable T-cell receptors. *American Journal of Reproductive Immunology* **24**: 33–36.

Dobbins WO (1986) Human intestinal intraepithelial lymphocytes. *Gut* **27**: 972–985.

Dutt A, Tang J-P & Carson DD (1987) Lactosaminoglycans are involved in uterine epithelial cell adhesion in vitro. *Developmental Biology* **119**: 27–37.

Eades DK, Cornelius P & Pekala PHJ (1988) Characterization of the tumor necrosis factor receptor in human placenta. *Placenta* **9**: 247–251.

Edmonds DK, Lindsay K, Miller JF, Williamson E & Wood PJ (1982) Early embryonic mortality in women. *Fertility and Sterility* **38**: 447–453.

Edwards RG (1985) In vitro fertilization and embryo replacement opening lecture. *Annals of the New York Academy of Sciences* **442**: 1–22.

Ewoldson MA, Ostlie NS & Warner CM (1987) Killing of mouse blastocyst stage embryos by cytotoxic T lymphocytes directed to major histocompatibility complex antigens. *Journal of Immunology* **138**: 2764–2770.

Fakih H, Baggett B, Holtz G et al (1987) Interleukin-1: a possible role in the infertility associated with endometriosis. *Fertility and Sterility* **47**: 213–217.

Farach MC, Tang J-P, Deecker GL & Carson DD (1988) Heparin-heparan sulfate is involved in attachment and spreading of mouse embryos in vitro. *Developmental Biology* **123**: 401–410.

Fischer B (1989) Effects of asynchrony on rabbit blastocyst development. *Journal of Reproduction and Fertility* **86**: 479–491.

Forman R, Fries N, Testart J et al (1988) Evidence for an adverse effect of elevated serum estradiol concentrations on embryo implantation. *Fertility and Sterility* **49**: 118–122.

Garcia JE, Acosta AA, Hsui J-G & Jones HW (1984) Advanced endometrial maturation after ovulation induction with human menopausal gonadotropin/human chorionic gonadotropin for in vitro fertilization. *Fertility and Sterility* **41**: 31–35.

Gidley-Baird A, O'Neill C, Sinosich M et al (1986) Failure of implantation in human in vitro fertilization and embryo transfer patients: the effect of altered progesterone estrogen ratios in humans and mice. *Fertility and Sterility* **45**: 69–74.

Glasser ST, Julian JA, Decker GL, Tang J-P & Carson DD (1988) Development of morphological and functional polarity in primary cultures of immature rat uterine epithelial cells. *Journal of Cell Biology* **107**: 2409–2423.

Goldbard SB, Gollnick SO & Warner CM (1985) Synthesis of H-2 antigens by preimplantation mouse embryos. *Biology of Reproduction* **33**: 30–36.

Goodall H & Johnson MH (1984) The nature of intercellular coupling within the preimplantation mouse embryo. *Journal of Embryology and Experimental Morphology* **79**: 53–76.

Goswamy RK, Williams G & Steptoe PC (1988) Decreased uterine perfusion—a cause of infertility. *Human Reproduction* **3**: 955–959.

Grey HM & Chesnut R (1985) Antigen processing and presentation to T cells. *Immunology Today* **6**: 101–106.

Hahn DW, Carraher RP, Foldesy RG & McGuire JL (1986) Experimental evidence for failure to implant as a mechanism of infertility associated with endometriosis. *American Journal of Obstetrics and Gynecology* **155**: 1109–1113.

Halme J, Becker S & Skill S (1987) Altered maturation and function of peritoneal macrophages: possible role in pathogenesis of endometriosis. *American Journal of Obstetrics and Gynecology* **156**: 783–788.

Hamilton MS, Vernon RB & Eddy EM (1985) A monoclonal antibody, EC-1, derived from a syngeneically multiparous mouse alters in vitro fertilization and development. *Journal of Reproductive Immunology* **8**: 45–60.

Han VKM, Hunter ES, Pratt RM, Zendegui JG & Lee DC (1987) Expression of rat transforming growth factor alpha mRNA during development occurs predominantly in the maternal decidua. *Molecular and Cellular Biology* **7**: 2335–2343.

Haney AF, Misukoni MA & Weinberg JB (1983) Macrophages and infertility: oviductal macrophages as potential mediators of infertility. *Fertility and Sterility* **39**: 310–315.

Head JR (1989) Can trophoblast be killed by cytotoxic cells?: in vitro evidence and in vivo possibilities. *American Journal of Reproductive Immunology* **20**: 100–105.

Head JR & Billingham RE (1986) Concerning the immunology of the uterus. *American Journal of Reproductive Immunology and Microbiology* **10**: 76–81.

Heyner S, Hunziker RD & Zink GL (1980) Differential expression of minor histocompatibility antigens on the surface of the mouse oocyte and preimplantation developmental stages. *Journal of Reproductive Immunology* **2**: 269–279.

Hill JA & Anderson DJ (1989) Lymphocyte activity in the presence of peritoneal fluid from fertile women and infertile women with and without endometriosis. *American Journal of Obstetrics and Gynecology* **161**: 861–864.

Hill JA, Haimovici F & Anderson DJ (1987) Products of activated lymphocytes and macrophages inhibit mouse embryo development in vitro. *Journal of Immunology* **139**: 2250–2254.

Hill JA, Faris HM, Schiff I & Anderson DJ (1988) Characterization of leukocyte subpopulations in the peritoneal fluid of women with endometriosis. *Fertility and Sterility* **50**: 216–222.

Hoversland RC & Beaman KD (1990) Embryo implantation associated with increase in T-cell suppressor factor in the uterus and spleen of mice. *Journal of Reproduction and Fertility* **88**: 135–139.

Huet-Hudson YM, Andrews GK & Dey SK (1990) Epidermal growth factor and pregnancy in the mouse. In Heyner S & Miley L (eds) *Early Embryo Development and Paracrine Relationships*, pp 125–136. New York: Alan R. Liss.

Hull MGR, Joyce DN, McLeod FN, Ray BD & McDermott A (1985) An economic and ethical way to introduce in vitro fertilization to infertility practice, and findings related to post-coital sperm/mucus penetration in isolated tubal, 'cervical', and unexplained infertility. *Annals of the New York Academy of Sciences* **442**: 318–323.

Hunt JS (1989) Cytokine networks in the uteroplacental unit: macrophages as pivotal regulatory cells. *Journal of Reproductive Immunology* **16**: 1–17.

Imakawa K, Hansen TR, Malathy P-V et al (1989) Molecular cloning and characterization of complementary deoxyribonucleic acids corresponding to bovine trophoblast protein-1: a comparison with ovine trophoblast protein-1 and bovine interferon-a. *Molecular Endocrinology* **3**: 127–139.

Joseph S, Krishnamurthi S & Kakkar VV (1987) Effect of the polyamine-spermine on agonist-induced human platelet activation-specific inhibition of 'aggregation independent' events induced by thrombin, but not by collagen, thromboxane mimetic, phorbol ester or calcium ionophore. *Thrombosis and Haemostasis* **57**: 191–195.

Jouvin-Marche E, Poitevin B & Benveniste J (1982) Platelet-activating factor (PAF-acether), an activator of neutrophil functions. *Agents and Actions* **12**: 716–720.

Kawagoe K, Akiyama J, Kawamoto T, Morishita Y & Mori S (1990) Immunohistochemical demonstration of epidermal growth factor (EGF) receptors in normal human placental villi. *Placenta* **11**: 7–15.

Kennedy TG (1983) Embryonic signals and the initiation of blastocyst implantation. *Australian Journal of Biological Sciences* **36**: 531–543.

Kliman HJ, Coutifaris C, Feinberg RF, Strauss JF & Haimowitz JE (1989) Implantation: in vitro models utilizing human tissues. In Yoshinaga K (ed.) *Blastocyst Implantation*, pp 83–91. Boston: Adams Publishing.

Kohase M, Henriksen-De Stefano D, May LT, Vilcek J & Sehgal PB (1986) Induction of beta 2-interferon by tumour necrosis factor: a homeostatic mechanism in the control of cell proliferation. *Cell* **45**: 659–666.

Kuo B-S, Korner G, Dryjski M & Bjornsson TD (1988) Role of polyamines in the stimulation of synthesis and secretion of plasminogen activator from bovine aortic endothelial cells. *Journal of Cellular Physiology* **137**: 192–198.

Lala PK, Scodras JM, Graham CH, Lysiak JJ & Parhar RS (1990) Activation of maternal killer cells in the pregnant uterus with chronic indomethacin therapy, IL-2 therapy, or a combination therapy is associated with embryonic demise. *Cellular Immunology* **127**: 368–381.

Lea RG & Clark DA (1989) The immune function of the endometrium. *Baillière's Clinical Obstetrics and Gynaecology* **3(2)**: 293–313.

Lea RG, Daya S & Clark DA (1990) Identification of low molecular weight immunosuppressor molecules in human in vitro fertilization supernatants predictive of implantation as a polyamine—possibly spermine. *Fertility and Sterility* **53**: 875–881.

Leclipteux T & Remacle J (1983) Disappearance of paternal histocompatibility antigens from hybrid mouse blastocyst at the time of implantation. *FEBS Letters* **157**: 277–281.

Lee S, Gilula NB & Warner AE (1987) Gap junctional communication and compaction during preimplantation stages of mouse development. *Cell* **51**: 851–860.

Leivo I, Vaheri A, Timpl R & Wartiovaara J (1980) Appearance and distribution of collagens and laminin in the early mouse embryo. *Developmental Biology* **76**: 100–114.

Lejeune B & Leroy F (1980) Role of the uterine epithelium in inducing the decidual reaction. *Progress in Reproductive Biology* **7**: 92–101.

Loke YW, Gardner L, Burland K & King A (1989) Laminin in human trophoblast–decidua interaction. *Human Reproduction* **4**: 457–463.

Marconi G, Auge L, Oses R et al (1989) Does sexual intercourse improve pregnancy rates in gamete intrafallopian transfer? *Fertility and Sterility* **51**: 357–359.

Mayumi T, Bitoh S, Anan S et al (1985) Suppressor T lymphocyte induction by a factor released from cultured blastocysts. *Journal of Immunology* **134**: 404–409.

Medawar PB (1953) Some immunological and endocrinological problems raised by the evolution of viviparity in vertebrates. *Symposium of the Society of Experimental Biology* **7**: 320–338.

Mendez JD (1989) Polyamines and human reproduction. In Bachrach UM & Heimer YM (eds) *The Physiology of Polyamines*, vol. 1, pp 23–38. Boca Raton, FL: CRC Press.

Miller JF, Williamson E, Glue J et al (1980) Fetal loss after implantation. A prospective study. *Lancet* **ii**: 554–556.

Milligan SR & Finn CA (1990) Failure of platelet-activating factor (PAF-acether) to induce decidualization in mice and failure of antagonists of PAF to inhibit implantation. *Journal of Reproduction and Fertility* **88**: 105–112.

Mitchell JA & Hammer RE (1983) Serotonin-induced disruption of implantation in the rat. I. Serum progesterone, implantation site blood flow, and intrauterine pO_2. *Biology of Reproduction* **28**: 830–835.

Morgan DML (1982) Commentary: amine oxidases and pregnancy. *British Journal of Obstetrics and Gynaecology* **89**: 177–178.

Nagata T, Nozaki M, Morita T & Matsushiro A (1988) Detection of H-2k mRNA in mouse 8-cell embryo by cDNA cloning. *Japanese Journal of Genetics* **63**: 465–469.

Nieder GL, Weitlauf HM & Suda-Hartman M (1987) Synthesis and secretion of stage-specific proteins by peri-implantation mouse embryos. *Biology of Reproduction* **36:** 687–699.

Noun A, Acker GM, Chaouat G, Antoine JC & Garabedian M (1989) Cells bearing granulocyte-macrophage and T lymphocyte antigens in the rat uterus before and during ovum implantation. *Clinical and Experimental Immunology* **78:** 494–498.

Ohlsson R, Larsson E, Nilsson O, Wahlstrom T & Sundstrom P (1989) Blastocyst implantation precedes induction of insulin-like growth factor II gene expression in human trophoblasts. *Development* **106:** 555–559.

O'Neill C (1987) Embryo-derived platelet activating factor: a preimplantation embryo mediator of maternal recognition of pregnancy. *Domestic Animal Endocrinology* **4:** 69–86.

O'Neill C, Collier M, Ryan JP & Spinks NR (1989a) Embryo-derived platelet-activating factor. *Journal of Reproduction and Fertility* **37:** 19–27.

O'Neill C, Ryan JP, Collier M et al (1989b) Supplementation of in vitro fertilisation culture medium with platelet activating factor. *Lancet* **ii:** 769–772.

Orozco C, Pekins T & Clarke FM (1986) Platelet-activating factor induces the expression of early pregnancy factor activity in female mice. *Journal of Reproduction and Fertility* **78:** 549–555.

Papadopoulos G, Randall J & Templeton AA (1989) The frequency of chromosome anomalies in human unfertilized oocytes and uncleaved zygotes after insemination in vitro. *Human Reproduction* **4:** 568–573.

Papaioannou VE & Ebert KM (1986) Development of fertilized embryos transferred to oviducts of immature mice. *Journal of Reproduction and Fertility* **76:** 603–608.

Paria BC & Dey SK (1990) Preimplantation embryo development in vitro: cooperative interactions among embryos and role of growth factors. *Proceedings of the National Academy of Sciences of the USA* **87:** 4756–4760.

Paulson RJ, Sauer MV & Lobo RA (1990) Embryo implantation after human in vitro fertilization: importance of endometrial receptivity. *Fertility and Sterility* **53:** 870–874.

Pollard JW (1990) Regulation of polypeptide growth factor synthesis and growth factor-related gene expression in the rat and mouse uterus before and after implantation. *Journal of Reproduction and Fertility* **88:** 721–731.

Porat O & Clark DA (1990) Analysis of immunosuppressive molecules associated with murine in vitro fertilization embryos. *Fertility and Sterility* **54:** 1154–1161.

Rachman F, Casimiri V, Psychoyos A & Bernard O (1986) Influence of the embryo on the distribution of maternal immunoglobulins in the mouse uterus. *Journal of Reproduction and Fertility* **77:** 257–264.

Ramsewak SS, Barratt CLR, Li T-C, Gooch H & Cooke ID (1990) Peritoneal sperm can be consistently demonstrated in women with unexplained infertility. *Fertility and Sterility* **53:** 1106–1108.

Rappolee DA, Brenner CA, Schultz R, Mark D & Werb Z (1988) Developmental expression of PDGF, TGF-a, and TGF-b genes in preimplantation mouse embryos. *Science* **241:** 1823–1825.

Roberts AB, Anazano MA, Lam LC, Smith JM & Sporn MB (1981) New class of transforming growth factors potentiated by epidermal growth factor: isolation from non-neoplastic tissues. *Proceedings of the National Academy of Sciences of the USA* **75:** 1864–1866.

Roberts CJ & Lowe CR (1975) Where have all the conceptions gone? *Lancet* **i:** 498–499.

Roberts RM (1989) Conceptus interferons and maternal recognition of pregnancy. *Biology of Reproduction* **40:** 449–452.

Robertson SA & Seamark RF (1990) Granulocyte macrophage colony stimulating factor (GM-CSF) in the murine reproductive tract: Stimulation by seminal factors. *Reproduction, Fertility and Development* **2:** 359–368.

Roblero LS & Caravagno AC (1979) Effect of oestradiol-17b and progesterone on oviductal transport and early development of mouse embryos. *Journal of Reproduction and Fertility* **57:** 91–95.

Rogers PAW & Murphy CR (1989) Uterine receptivity for implantation: human studies. In Yoshinoga K (ed.) *Blastocyst Implantation*, pp 231–238. Boston: Adams Publishing.

Rolfe BE (1982) Detection of fetal wastage. *Fertility and Sterility* **37:** 655–660.

Rolfe BE, Cavanagh AC, Quinn KA & Morton H (1988) Identification of two suppressor factors induced by early pregnancy factor. *Clinical and Experimental Immunology* **73:** 219–225.

Ryan JP, O'Neill C & Wales RG (1990) Oxidative metabolism of energy substrates by preimplantation mouse embryos in the presence of platelet-activating factor. *Journal of Reproduction and Fertility* **89**: 301–307.

Salamonsen LA, Sum W, Doughton B & Kindlay JK (1985) The effects of estrogen and progesterone in vivo on protein synthesis and secretion by cultured epithelial cells from sheep endometrium. *Endocrinology* **117**: 2148–2159.

Sato M, Muramatsu T & Berger EG (1984) Immunological detection of cell surface galactosyltransferase in preimplantation mouse embryos. *Developmental Biology* **102**: 514–518.

Sawicki JA, Magnuson T & Epstein CJ (1981) Evidence for expression of the paternal genome in the two-cell mouse embryo. *Nature* **294**: 450–451.

Sawicki W, Choroszewska A, Bem W & Strojny P (1988) Lymphocyte number and distribution in the rat uterine epithelium during estrous cycle and early pregnancy. *Cell and Tissue Research* **253**: 241–244.

Schneider EG, Armant DR, Kupper TS & Polan ML (1989) Absence of a direct effect of recombinant interleukins and cultured peritoneal macrophages on early embryonic development in the mouse. *Biology of Reproduction* **40**: 825–833.

Searle RF & Matthews CJ (1988) Differential expression of class II major histocompatibility complex and Thy 1.2 antigens on mouse decidua. *Placenta* **9**: 57–64.

Searle RF, Johnson MH, Billington WD, Elson J & Clutterbuck-Jackson S (1974) Investigation of H-2 and non-H-2 antigens on the mouse blastocyst. *Transplantation* **18**: 136–141.

Serhal PF & Craft IL (1989) Oocyte donation in 61 patients. *Lancet* **i**: 1185–1187.

Sharp NC, Anthony F, Miller JF & Masson GM (1986) Early conceptual loss in subfertile patients. *British Journal of Obstetrics and Gynaecology* **93**: 1072–1077.

Smart YC, Fraser IS, Roberts TK et al (1982) Fertilization and early pregnancy loss in healthy women attempting conception. *Clinical Reproduction and Fertility* **1**: 177–184.

Smith SK & Kelly RW (1988) Effect of platelet-activating factor on the release of PGF-2α and PGE-2 by separated cells of human endometrium. *Journal of Reproduction and Fertility* **82**: 271–276.

Soloski MJ, Vernachio J, Einhorn G & Lattimore A (1986) Qa gene expression biosynthesis and secretion of Qa-2 molecules in activated T cells. *Proceedings of the National Academy of Sciences of the USA* **83**: 2949–2953.

Spinks NR & O'Neill C (1988) Antagonists of embryo-derived platelet-activating factor prevent implantation of mouse embryos. *Journal of Reproduction and Fertility* **84**: 89–98.

Spinks NR, Ryan JP & O'Neill C (1990) Antagonists of embryo-derived platelet-activating factor act by inhibiting the ability of the mouse embryo to implant. *Journal of Reproduction and Fertility* **88**: 241–248.

Sulila P, Holmdane R, Hansson I et al (1988) An investigation of allogeneic pregnancy in multiparous mice subjected to in vivo depletion of CD8 (ly2)-positive lymphocytes by monoclonal antibody treatment. *Journal of Reproductive Immunology* **14**: 235–246.

Surani MAH (1977) Radiolabeled rat uterine luminal proteins and their regulation by estradiol and progesterone. *Journal of Reproduction and Fertility* **50**: 289–296.

Szekeres-Bartho J, Varga P, Kinsky R & Chaouat G (1990) Progesterone-mediated immunosuppression and the maintenance of pregnancy. FORUM 1990. *Research in Immunology* (Institut Pasteur) **141**: 175–181.

Tachi C & Tachi S (1989) Role of macrophages in the maternal recognition of pregnancy. *Journal of Reproduction and Fertility* **37**: 63–68.

Tagliabue A, Befus AD, Clark DA & Bienenstock J (1982) Characteristics of natural killer cells in the murine intestinal epithelium and lamina propria. *Journal of Experimental Medicine* **155**: 1785–1796.

Tartakovsky B (1989) CSF-1 induces resorption of embryos in mice. *Immunology Letters* **23**: 65–70

Tawfik OW, Huet YM, Malathy PV, Johnson DC & Dey SK (1987) Release of prostaglandin and leukotrienes from rat uterus is an early oestrogenic response. *Prostaglandins* **34**: 805–815.

Testart J, Lasalle B, Belaish-Allart J et al (1986) Cryopreservation does not affect the future of human fertilized eggs. *Lancet* **ii**: 569.

Tezabwala BU, Johnson PM & Rees RC (1989) Inhibition of pregnancy viability in mice following IL-2 administration. *Immunology* **67**: 115–119.

Thomas IK & Erickson KL (1986) Gestational immunosuppression is mediated by specific Lyt 2⁺ T cells. *Immunology* **57**: 201–206.

Toder V, Madanes A & Gleicher N (1988) Immunologic aspects of IUD action. *Contraception* **37**: 391–403.

Trinchieri G & Perussia B (1985) Immune interferon: a pleiotopic lymphokine with multiple effects. *Immunology Today* **6**: 131–136.

Tsutsumi O & Oka T (1987) Epidermal growth factor deficiency during pregnancy causes abortion in mice. *American Journal of Obstetrics and Gynecology* **156**: 241–244.

Tzartos SJ & Surani MAH (1979) Affinity of uterine luminal proteins for rat blastocysts. *Journal of Reproduction and Fertility* **56**: 579–586.

Vanderhyden BC & Armstrong DT (1988) Decreased embryonic survival of in vitro fertilized oocytes in rats is due to retardation of preimplantation development. *Journal of Reproduction and Fertility* **83**: 851–857.

Vander Wielen AL & King GJ (1984) Intraepithelial lymphocytes in the bovine uterus during the oestrous cycle and early gestation. *Journal of Reproduction and Fertility* **70**: 457–462.

Waites GT & Bell SC (1982) Glycogen-induced intrauterine leucocytosis and its effect on mouse blastocyst implantation in vivo and in vitro. *Journal of Reproduction and Fertility* **66**: 563–569.

Wakasugi N (1973) Studies on fertility of DDK mice: reciprocal crosses between DDK and C57BL/6J strains and experimental transplantation of the ovary. *Reproduction and Fertility* **14**: 7–21.

Walters DE, Edwards RG & Meistrich ML (1985) A statistical evaluation of implantation after replacing one or more human embryos. *Journal of Reproduction and Fertility* **74**: 557–563.

Wang H-S, Kanzaki H, Yoshida M et al (1987) Suppression of lymphocyte reactivity in vitro by supernatants of explants of human endometrium. *American Journal of Obstetrics and Gynecology* **157**: 956–963.

Warner CM, Gollnick SO & Goldbard SB (1987a) Linkage of the preimplantation-embryo-development (Ped) gene to the mouse major histocompatibility complex (MHC). *Biology of Reproduction* **36**: 606–610.

Warner CM, Gollnick SA, Flaherty L & Goldbard SB (1987b) Analysis of Qa-2 antigen expression by preimplantation mouse embryos: possible relationship to the preimplantation-embryo-development (Ped) gene product. *Biology of Reproduction* **36**: 611–616.

Wewer UM, Taraboleti G, Sobel ME, Albrechtsen R & Liotta LA (1987) Role of laminin receptor in tumor cell migration. *Cancer Research* **47**: 5691–5698.

Whittaker PG, Taylor A & Lind T (1983) Unsuspected pregnancy loss in healthy women. *Lancet* **i**: 1126–1127.

Wilcox AJ, Weinberg CR, Wehmann RE et al (1985) Measuring early pregnancy loss: laboratory and field methods. *Fertility and Sterility* **44**: 366–374.

Williams-Ashman HG, Bell RE, Wilson J et al (1980) Transglutaminases in mammalian reproductive tissues and fluids: relation to polyamine metabolism and semen coagulation. *Advances in Enzyme Regulation* **18**: 239–258.

Wilmut I & Sales DI (1981) Effect of an asynchronous environment on embryonic development in sheep. *Journal of Reproduction and Fertility* **61**: 179–184.

Wilmut I, Sales DI & Ashworth CJ (1985) Physiological criteria for embryo mortality—is asynchrony between embryo and ewe a significant factor. In Lard RB & Robinson D (eds) *The Genetics of Reproduction in Sheep*, pp 275–289. London: Butterworths.

Winterhager E, Brummer F, Dermietzel R, Husler DF & Denker H-W (1988) Gap junction formation in rabbit uterine epithelium in response to embryo recognition. *Developmental Biology* **126**: 203–211.

Wolpert L (1978) Gap junctions: channels for communication in development. In Feldman J, Gilula NB & Pitts JD (eds) *Intercellular Junctions and Synapses*, pp 83–94. London: Chapman & Hall.

Yovich JL (1985) Embryo quality and pregnancy rates in in vitro fertilization. *Lancet* **i**: 283–284.

Zwierzchowski L, Czlonkowska M & Guszkiewicz A (1986) Effect of polyamine limitation on DNA synthesis and development of mouse preimplantation embryos in vitro. *Journal of Reproduction and Fertility* **76**: 115–121.

4

Human endometrial protein secretion relative to implantation

MARKKU SEPPÄLÄ
MAARIT ANGERVO
RIITTA KOISTINEN
LEENA RIITTINEN
MERVI JULKUNEN

Human endometrium undergoes cyclical changes during the menstrual cycle. Proliferation ends after ovulation and secretory changes appear. The two major cell types of the endometrium are epithelial cells and stromal cells. Morphological changes appear in endometrial glands (epithelial cells) after ovulation, and the stromal cells differentiate into predecidual cells during the second week of the luteal phase. These changes are accompanied by changing patterns in protein secretion. This chapter will review studies on two major endometrial protein products, one of which represents stromal cells and the other glandular cells. The synthesis of either protein is markedly increased during the peri-implantation period.

INSULIN-LIKE GROWTH FACTORS AND THEIR BINDING PROTEINS

Insulin-like growth factors IGF-1 and IGF-2 are mitogenic peptides expressed in various tissues (D'Ercole et al, 1984). IGFs regulate cell growth and differentiation, and have insulin-like effects. IGFs show remarkable structural homology with proinsulin and insulin (Rinderknecht and Humbel, 1978). The IGF-1 gene and the circulating IGF-1 level are regulated by growth hormone (GH) (Baxter, 1986; Mathews et al, 1986), whereas IGF-2 is less GH dependent and appears to play its major role during fetal life.

The human endometrium contains IGF-1 and type 1 IGF receptor (Nissley and Rechler, 1984). On the basis of its mitogenic effects on a number of tissues (Froesch et al, 1985), IGF is believed to have similar effects on the endometrium, although its action(s) in this respect are yet to be studied. IGF-1 increases prolactin secretion by human decidual cells (Thrailkill et al, 1988). In serum, IGFs are bound to specific binding proteins (IGFBPs) (Hintz and Liu, 1977). According to the current classification the three major groups of

Baillière's Clinical Obstetrics and Gynaecology—
Vol. 5, No. 1, March 1991
ISBN 0–7020–1533–4

binding proteins are IGFBP-1, IGFBP-2 and IGFBP-3. IGFBP-3 is the major carrier in serum, regulated by GH (Baxter, 1986). IGFBP-1 appears to have a minor role as a carrier, and it rather serves as a modulator of IGF actions in tissue. IGFBP-2 is abundant in cerebrospinal fluid (Rosenfeld et al, 1989). The cDNAs encoding all three binding proteins have been cloned and sequenced (Brinkman et al, 1988; Julkunen et al, 1988a; Lee et al, 1988; Wood et al, 1988; Binkert et al, 1989). While there is a certain degree of homology between the deduced amino acid sequences of all three IGFBPs, they have non-homologous parts distinct from each other and they are different from type 1 and type 2 IGF receptors (Lee et al, 1988; Ullrich et al, 1986).

Before the above nomenclature was established, IGFBP-1 appeared under several names in the literature. Based on immunological comparisons (Bell and Bohn, 1986), N-terminal sequence analyses (Povoa et al, 1984; Koistinen et al, 1986; Bell and Keyte, 1988) and cloning (Julkunen et al, 1988a; Lee et al, 1988), IGFBP-1 appears to be the same as placental protein 12 (PP12), $\alpha 1$ pregnancy associated endometrial globulin ($\alpha 1$-PEG), BP25, low molecular weight 34 kDa IGF–binding protein, and amniotic fluid IGF–binding protein. There is DNA polymorphism in the IGFBP-1 gene which resides in chromosome 7p12–p13 (Alitalo et al, 1989). IGFBP-1 binds IGF-1 with high affinity similar to that of type 1 IGF receptor (Marshall et al, 1974; Koistinen et al, 1987; Rutanen et al, 1988).

Previous studies indicate that IGFBP-1 isolated from amniotic fluid inhibits the insulin-like and mitogenic effects of IGFs (Drop et al, 1979), and it also inhibits binding of IGF-1 to its endometrial membrane receptor (Rutanen et al, 1988). Amniotic fluid IGFBP enhances the DNA synthesis in fibroblast and smooth muscle cells (Elgin et al, 1987). Busby and his co-workers (1988) have isolated two low molecular weight IGFBPs from human amniotic fluid. One enhances and the other inhibits the IGF-1 stimulated DNA synthesis. These authors maintain that the difference depends on attachment of the binding protein to the cell membrane. The IGFBP that attaches to cell membrane is stimulatory, whereas the IGFBP that does not attach is inhibitory. While the observation of two forms of low molecular weight IGFBPs in amniotic fluid with opposite biological activities remains to be confirmed, it is noteworthy that the sequence of IGFBP-1/PP12, the major amniotic fluid IGF–binding protein, contains the RGD adhesion sequence (Ruoslahti and Pierschbacher, 1987; Julkunen et al, 1988), and yet this protein inhibits the binding of IGF-1 to its cell membrane receptors (Rutanen et al, 1988). IGFBP-1 also inhibits DNA amplification in ovarian granulosa cells (Koistinen et al, 1990a), but it may enhance DNA amplification in some other cell types (R. Koistinen et al, unpublished data). Thus it seems that the stimulatory or inhibitory actions of IGFBP-1 depend on the target tissues rather than on the protein itself. It will be important to understand the role the other IGF–binding proteins may play locally, as all three binding proteins may appear in the same tissue (see below). It is of interest to note that, depending on the incubation procedure, IGFBP-3 has also been reported to have either stimulatory or inhibitory effects on thymidine incorporation into neonatal human skin fibroblasts (De Mellow and Baxter, 1988).

Human endometrium contains mRNAs of all three types of IGFBPs (Giudice et al, 1990). IGFBP-1 mRNA can be detected in secretory and decidualized endometrium, but not in proliferative endometrium (Julkunen et al, 1988a; Giudice et al, 1990). This corresponds to the content of IGFBP-1 in tissue: there is no detectable IGFBP-1 in the endometrium during the proliferative phase when the endometrium is growing rapidly, and the IGFBP-1 content in tissue increases only after ovulation towards the end of the cycle (Rutanen et al, 1984a; Wahlström and Seppälä, 1984). While occasional staining by the immunoperoxidase method has been detected in glandular luminal epithelial cells (Wahlström and Seppälä, 1984), the staining is mainly localized into the stromal cells (Waites et al, 1988a). It is noteworthy that both glandular and stromal cells can release IGFBP-1 in culture (Ren and Braunstein, 1990). Julkunen and her co-workers (1990) have demonstrated IGFBP-1 mRNA in endometrial secretory stromal cells but not in endometrial glands, thereby substantiating that the stromal cells are the site of IGFBP-1 synthesis. The reason why the glandular cells are also stained remains to be clarified. It may be a reflection of antibody specificity. The fact that glandular staining can only be found with high antibody concentrations indicates that the IGFBP-1 concentration in the glands is clearly smaller than in the stroma. It is not impossible that the stroma and the glands interact in vivo, whereby IGFBP-1 comes into contact with the glands.

Studies by Rutanen and her co-workers (1986) indicate that progesterone stimulates IGFBP-1 secretion by cultured proliferative and secretory endometrium explants. This has not been found in all studies. Ren and Braunstein (1990) found no increasing effect of progesterone on IGFBP-1 release from decidual explants, or from enriched cultures of stromal or glandular cells. Furthermore, Giudice and her co-workers (1990) found no increased IGFBP-1 synthesis by progesterone in cultured endometrial stromal cells. It is possible that the effect of progesterone on IGFBP-1 synthesis is not direct and involves the whole sequence of events required for endometrial differentiation. In view of its inhibitory effect on binding of IGF-1 to its receptor, it is possible that, after ovulation, induction of IGFBP-1 synthesis plays a role in the proliferative/secretory transition of the endometrium.

As judged by immunoperoxidase staining, the first appearance of IGFBP-1 in the endometrium is seen on day 4 after ovulation (Wahlström and Seppälä, 1984). This is well before implantation of the blastocyst is expected to take place in a fertile cycle. The roles IGF-1 and IGFBPs may play in the implantation process are yet to be studied. It has been suggested that IGFBP-1 plays a part in human placentation by inhibiting the cellular binding and biological activity of trophoblastic IGF-1 (Ritvos et al, 1988).

The circulating levels of IGFBP-1 show a marked circadian rhythm, with a nocturnal peak. This has been seen during pregnancy as well as in the non-pregnant state (Rutanen et al, 1984b; Baxter and Cowell, 1987; Holly et al, 1988). The diurnal variation is unrelated to GH levels and is inversely related to insulin levels (Brismar et al, 1988; Holly et al, 1988; Suikkari et al, 1988). Insulin, not glucose, regulates the circulating IGFBP-1 concentration

(Suikkari et al, 1989). The IGFBP-1 levels fall with age, showing a pattern opposite to that of IGF-1 and IGFBP-3 during childhood and adolescence (Hall et al, 1988; Cianfarani and Holly, 1989).

No clue to the possible physiological role of IGFBP-1 in the implantation process has been obtained from studies on its circulating levels during the peri-implantation period. The levels show no regular variation in ovulatory cycles (Suikkari et al, 1987). During ovarian stimulation the levels rise as the multiple follicles develop at the time when the endometrium is still assumed to be in the proliferative phase (Seppälä et al, 1988a). After in vitro fertilization and embryo transfer the serum IGFBP-1 levels in the luteal phase do not distinguish between implantation and non-implantation cycles. This is not surprising in view of the multiple sites of IGFBP-1 synthesis. In addition to secretory and decidualized endometrium IGFBP-1 is produced in the liver and in the granulosa cells (Julkunen et al, 1988a; Koistinen et al, 1990b).

IGFBP-3 serves as a major carrier of IGFs in serum, thereby preventing IGFs freely crossing the capillary endothelium, extending the half-life of IGFs and stabilizing their plasma levels (Binoux and Hossenlopp, 1988). Heparin liberates IGFs from the binding proteins (Clemmons et al, 1983) and it also interacts with IGFBP-1 (Rutanen et al, 1984b). It is believed that IGF–IGFBP-3 complex serves as a reservoir from which IGFs are released by heparin-like substances and a fall in pH (Clemmons et al, 1983).

The physiological roles of IGFBP-2 and IGFBP-3 in the endometrium are yet to be determined. In their studies utilizing oligomeric cDNA probes encoding the non-homologous coding regions of the IGFBPs, Giudice and her co-workers (1990) found that, unlike IGFBP-1 mRNA, IGFBP-2 and IGFBP-3 mRNAs are also detectable in the proliferative endometrium, where these proteins are localized to endometrial glands. In their studies progesterone stimulated endometrial IGFBP-2 synthesis, and the expression of IGFBP-2 and IGFBP-3 was found to be higher in secretory than in proliferative endometrium. Thus, in addition to IGF-1 and type 1 IGF receptor, there are at least three different IGFBP species synthesized by secretory endometrium during the peri-implantation period. This study indicates that regulation of the actions of IGFs on the endometrium is under a complex control by a number of factors. Whether the implanting human embryo has IGF receptors or the capacity to produce IGFs or any of their binding proteins remains to be investigated.

ENDOMETRIAL PROTEIN PP14

This protein was originally isolated from the human placenta and its membranes and hence called placental protein 14 (PP14) (Bohn et al, 1982). The name appeared to be a misnomer on the basis of three lines of evidence: (1) incorporation of labelled methionine into immunoreactive PP14 was found to take place in secretory endometrium, not in placenta (Julkunen et al, 1986b); (2) after molecular cloning of the cDNA, Northern blot analysis showed PP14 mRNA in secretory and decidualized endometrium, not in placenta (Julkunen et al, 1988b); and (3) in situ hybridization using single stranded RNA probes demonstrated PP14 mRNA in endometrial secretory glands, not in the stroma (Julkunen et al, 1990). Thus, as far as the uterus is concerned, PP14 appears to be synthesized by endometrial secretory glands as exclusively as IGFBP-1 by the stroma. The uterus apart, the only tissue in which PP14 and its mRNA have been detected so far is the fallopian tubal mucosa (Julkunen et al, 1986d, 1990). This is not unexpected in the light of the common embryonic origin of the uterus and the fallopian tubes from the müllerian duct.

There are several names for this protein in the literature. Immunological comparisons and N-terminal sequence analyses indicate that pregnancy-associated endometrial $\alpha 2$-globulin ($\alpha 2$-PEG) (Bell and Bohn, 1986), progestagen associated endometrial protein (PEP) (Joshi et al, 1980; Julkunen et al, 1986c), α-uterine protein (AUP) (Sutcliffe et al, 1982) and chorionic $\alpha 2$-microglobulin (Petrunin et al, 1980) are the same protein as PP14. However, only the cDNA encoding PP14 has been cloned so far (Julkunen et al, 1988b), so the common identity of PP14 with these other proteins awaits confirmation from cloning studies. On the basis of sequence analysis PP14 contains 180 amino acids, 18 of which correspond to a putative signal peptide. The predicted molecular weight of the mature protein is 18 787. PP14 is encoded by a 1 kb mRNA expressed in human secretory and decidualized endometrium, but not in postmenopausal endometrium, placenta, liver, kidney and adrenals (Julkunen et al, 1988b). There is amino acid sequence homology between PP14 and β-lactoglobulins from various species (up to 53%), bilin binding protein (27%), human retinol binding protein (23%) and human protein HC (18%) (Julkunen et al, 1988b; Seppälä et al, 1988b). PP14 is a glycoprotein containing 17% carbohydrate (Bohn et al, 1982). On the basis of the above, PP14 appears to be an endometrium specific protein. However, not all tissues have been thoroughly investigated for their PP14 mRNA content at various phases of the menstrual cycle. This will be important before PP14 can be deemed exclusively an endometrial protein, particularly in view of the fact that even the endometrium can be devoid of PP14 mRNA in certain phases of the cycle.

Studies by immunoperoxidase staining have shown PP14/$\alpha 2$-PEG in deep basal glands during the first 5 days of the menstrual cycle, after which the protein is undetectable and reappears in some glands on day 5 after ovulation (Seppälä et al, 1988c; Waites, 1988b). All endometrial glands are strongly PP14 positive 10 days after ovulation. This is the time when significant amounts of PP14 are released by endometrial explants in tissue culture (Julkunen et al, 1986b) and the serum level also rises (Julkunen et al, 1986a).

In cycles stimulated by human menopausal gonadotrophins for IVF, endometrial maturation is often advanced (Garcia et al, 1984). This is also indicated by early appearance of both IGFBP-1 and PP14 in the endometrium after ovarian hyperstimulation and oocyte retrieval. Using immunoperoxidase staining, we have looked at the endometrium in normal (Seppälä et al, 1988c) and IVF cycles when no embryo was available for replacement (Wahlström et al, 1985). While in normal cycles only parts of some glands were PP14-positive on day 5, positive staining of glands was found as early as 28–96 h after aspiration of hyperstimulated follicles in six out of 18 women. If an implantation window exists in the human, then the early endometrial maturation should be favourable for implantation because in an IVF cycle embryo replacement is usually performed earlier (48–52 h after oocyte retrieval) than the time when a fertilized ovum arrives in the uterine cavity after spontaneous conception.

Biological role

Little is known about the biological action of PP14. In spite of its structural homologies with certain carrier proteins, notably retinol binding protein, we found no retinol binding property in PP14. Bolton and his co-workers have suggested that PP14 is immunosuppressive (Bolton et al, 1987; Pockley et al, 1988). Indeed, subsequent detailed studies by Okamoto and his co-workers (unpublished data), utilizing cultures of cells isolated from the human endometrium, have shown that purified PP14 suppresses natural killer cell activity and phytohaemagglutinin-stimulated T-cell proliferation in vitro. In view of the high concentration of PP14 in the endometrium during mid- and late secretory phases (Julkunen et al, 1986b), the immunosuppressive properties of PP14 could be important for the implantation process.

Serum PP14 levels

The PP14 levels are high in menstrual blood and serum during the menstrual period. In ovulatory cycles the serum PP14 levels show cyclical variation (Julkunen et al, 1986a). The levels are lowest at the time of ovulation, then rise during the last week of the luteal phase and peak at the onset of menstruation when the progesterone level has declined. High levels are maintained for the first days of the next cycle. No similar elevation is seen in anovulatory cycles. Therefore it is possible, on the basis of a single serum PP14 measurement done at the time of menstrual bleeding, to estimate whether the previous cycle was ovulatory or not and whether the endometrium had responded to the ovulatory progesterone levels or not. In cycles with inadequate luteal phase the serum PEP/PP14 levels are subnormal (Joshi et al, 1986), and the levels can be elevated by administration of micronized progesterone in the luteal phase (Seppälä et al, 1987b).

Elevated serum PP14 levels have been observed in patients with endometriosis (Telimaa et al, 1989), also at midcycle when the levels are usually low. Sustained treatment with danazol or medroxyprogesterone acetate brings the levels down. In endometriosis lesions, cyclical morphological changes are more irregular than in the normal endometrium. Whereas PP14 cannot be detected by immunoperoxidase staining in proliferative endometrium, endometriosis lesions from the proliferative phase may contain PP14 (Cornillie et al, 1990). High PP14 levels have been found in the peritoneal fluid of patients with endometriosis, and occasionally also in infertile patients with no apparent lesions. The source of peritoneal fluid PP14 remains to be identified.

A positive correlation has been observed between the serum oestradiol levels on day 9 of the cycle and the PP14 levels on day 22–23 during suppression of serum prolactin secretion by bromocriptine. This indicates that either the prolactin suppression or a more efficient oestrogen priming is important for subsequent endometrial protein secretion to take place (Seppälä et al, 1989). In postmenopausal women, oestrogen–progestogen replacement therapy brings about a 48% elevation in serum PP14 levels at the end of the last week of progestogen administration, whereas this elevation is much smaller (7%) in postmenopausal women who have undergone hysterectomy (Seppälä et al, 1987a; 1988b). These clinical studies indicate the importance of progesterone and of the uterus for PP14 secretion to take place. However, they also indicate that the uterus may not be the only site in the body contributing to serum PP14 because a small elevation was seen in some hysterectomized women taking oestrogen and progestogen. Remnants of the fallopian tubes, the peritoneum or the pleura may be the sources, as peritoneal and pleural fluids occasionally contain high concentrations of PP14. Homology between PP14 and β-lactoglobulins indicates the breast as being yet another source of PP14. Although no PP14 mRNA has been detected in the breast cancer cell lines examined so far (Julkunen et al, 1988b), normal breast tissues have not been studied in sufficient numbers; these should include specimens from women of reproductive age at various phases of the menstrual cycle.

The above considerations are necessary for the understanding of the clinical situations in which the serum PP14 levels may change. Normally, the serum PP14 level rises during the last week of the luteal phase (Julkunen et al, 1986a), and the rise continues and is even steeper if pregnancy ensues (Julkunen et al, 1985). The pattern of circulating levels of PP14 and chorionic gonadotrophin are strikingly similar throughout pregnancy, peaking at 10 weeks.

Could the circulating PP14 level allow one to predict whether the endometrium is prepared for implantation or not? In a joint study between groups working at Bourn Hall and Helsinki (R. G. Edwards and M. Seppälä, personal communication), in which blood samples were taken every second day over the peri-implantation period from women participating in an IVF programme, no difference was found in serum PP14 levels between conception and non-conception cycles. Two other studies indicate the same. Than and his colleagues (1988) found no difference in serum PP14 levels between women who did or did not conceive after artificial insemination, and similar conclusions were derived for α2-PEG in a recent study by Wood and his co-workers (1990). The latter authors maintain that serum α2-PEG levels do not necessarily reflect events at the implantation site in which increased decidual reaction may take place, and the results do not reflect a lack of function for this protein.

A recent study on a woman with Turner's syndrome who became pregnant after frozen embryo transfer reported subnormal elevation of serum PP14 level during early gestation, and yet her early pregnancy was uneventful at the time of reporting (Critchley et al, 1990). This study indicates that there may be interaction between the ovary and the endometrial PP14 secretion other than through progesterone, and it also indicates that PP14 may not be obligatory for maintenance of early pregnancy. As the authors point out, the subnormal PP14 levels may represent one extreme of a wide normal range, and thus this case awaits confirmation from other pregnancies of similar type.

CONCLUSIONS

The two major proteins of secretory endometrium are IGFBP-1 and endometrial protein PP14/α2-PEG/PEP. Both proteins have been purified from human midtrimester amniotic fluid, and their cDNAs have been cloned and sequenced. IGFBP-1 is a product of endometrial stromal cells, whereas PP14 is synthesized by the secretory glands. PP14 is more endometrium specific than IGFBP-1, whose synthesis has also been demonstrated in the liver and ovarian granulosa cells. Both proteins appear in the endometrium a few days before implantation is assumed to take place in a fertile cycle. Evidence is accumulating to indicate that IGFBP-1 modulates the biological action of IGFs at the cellular site by inhibiting, or sometimes enhancing, the action of IGF-1. Both proteins appear in menstrual fluid at high concentrations and they can also be detected in serum. There is no cyclical variation in serum IGFBP-1 levels, whereas PP14 levels rise during the last week of ovulatory cycles and remain high over the first days of the next period. No such pattern is seen in anovulatory cycles, indicating that a luteal phase is required before the circulating PP14 level becomes elevated. Lower levels have been found when the luteal phase is inadequate, and administration of oral progesterone can increase the luteal phase serum PP14 concentration. Disappointingly, serum PP14 measurement cannot be used for prediction of implantation after embryo replacement. After implantation, both PP14 and human chorionic gonadotrophin (hCG) levels rise steeply, peak around 10 weeks gestation, and decline thereafter. While the importance of PP14 for pregnancy maintenance has been questioned on the basis of subnormal serum PP14 levels in an overtly normal early gestation, a local immunoregulatory role at the implantation site is anticipated.

Acknowledgements

This work was supported by grants from the Sigrid Jusélius Foundation, the Academy of Finland and the Finnish Social Insurance Institution.

REFERENCES

Alitalo T, Kontula K, Koistinen R et al (1989) The gene encoding human low-molecular weight insulin-like growth factor binding protein (IGF-BP25): regional localization to 7p12–p13 and description of a DNA polymorphism. *Human Genetics* **83:** 335–338.
Baxter RC (1986) The somatomedins: insulin-like growth factors. *Advances in Clinical Chemistry* **25:** 49–115.
Baxter RC & Cowell CT (1987) Diurnal rhythm of growth hormone-independent binding

protein for insulin-like growth factors in human plasma. *Journal of Clinical Endocrinology and Metabolism* **65**: 432–440.

Bell SC & Bohn H (1986) Immunochemical and biochemical relationship between human pregnancy-associated secreted endometrial alpha-1- and alpha-2-globulins (alpha-1- and alpha-2-PEG) and the soluble placental proteins 12 and 14 (PP12 and PP14). *Placenta* **7**: 283–294.

Bell SC & Keyte JW (1988) N-terminal amino acid sequence of human pregnancy-associated endometrial alpha-1 globulin, an endometrial insulin-like growth factor (IGF) binding protein—evidence for two small molecular weight IGF binding proteins. *Endocrinology* **123**: 1202–1204.

Binkert C, Landmehr J, Mary J-L et al (1989) Cloning, sequence analysis and expression of a cDNA encoding a novel insulin-like growth factor binding protein IGFBP-2. *EMBO Journal* **8**: 2497–2502.

Binoux M & Hossenlopp P (1988) Insulin-like growth factor (IGF) and IGF-binding proteins: comparison of human serum and lymph. *Journal of Clinical Endocrinology and Metabolism* **67**: 509–514.

Bohn H, Kraus W & Winckler W (1982) New soluble placental tissue proteins: their isolation, characterization, localization and quantification. *Placenta* **4 (supplement)**: 67–81.

Bolton AE, Pockley AG, Clough KJ et al (1987) Identification of placental protein 14 as an immunosuppressive factor in human reproduction. *Lancet* **i**: 593–595.

Brinkman A, Groffen C, Kortleve DJ, Van Kessel AG & Drop SLS (1988) Isolation and characterization of a cDNA encoding the low molecular weight insulin-like growth factor binding protein (IBP-1). *EMBO Journal* **7**: 2417–2423.

Brismar K, Gutniak M, Povoa G, Werner S & Hall K (1988) Insulin regulates the 35 Kda IGF-binding protein in patients with diabetes mellitus. *Journal of Endocrinological Investigation* **11**: 599–602.

Busby WH Jr, Klapper DG & Clemmons DR (1988) Purification of a 31 000 dalton insulin-like growth factor binding protein from human amniotic fluid. Isolation of two forms with different biologic actions. *Journal of Biological Chemistry* **263**: 14203–14210.

Cianfarani S & Holly JMP (1989) Somatomedin-binding proteins: what role do they play in the growth process? *Pediatrics* **149**: 76–79.

Clemmons DR, Underwood LE, Chatelain PG & Van Wyk JJ (1983) Liberation of immuno-reactive somatomedin-C from its binding proteins by proteolytic enzymes and heparin. *Journal of Clinical Endocrinology and Metabolism* **56**: 384–389.

Cornillie FJ, Seppälä M, Riittinen L & Koninckx PR (1990) Deep infiltrating pelvic endo-metriotic implants express endometrial protein PP14. *Proceedings of the VIIth World Congress on Human Reproduction*, abstract 614.

Critchley HOD, Chard T, Lieberman BA, Buckley CH & Anderson DC (1990) Serum PP14 levels in a patient with Turner's syndrome pregnant after frozen embryo transfer. *Human Reproduction* **5**: 250–254.

D'Ercole AJ, Stiles AD & Underwood LE (1984) Tissue concentrations of somatomedin C: further evidence for multiple sites of synthesis and paracrine or autocrine mechanisms of action. *Proceedings of the National Academy of Sciences of the USA* **81**: 935–939.

De Mellow JSM & Baxter RC (1988) Growth hormone-dependent insulin-like growth factor (IGF) binding protein both inhibits and potentiates IGF-I-stimulated DNA synthesis in human skin fibroblasts. *Biochemical and Biophysical Research Communications* **156**: 199–204.

Drop SLS, Valiquette G, Guyda HJ, Corvol MT & Posner BI (1979) Partial purification and characterization of a binding protein for insulin-like activity (ILAs) in human amniotic fluid: a possible inhibitor of insulin-like activity. *Acta Endocrinologica* **90**: 505–518.

Elgin RG, Busby WH Jr & Clemmons DR (1987) An insulin-like growth factor (IGF) binding protein enhances the biologic response to IGF-1. *Proceedings of the National Academy of Sciences of the USA* **84**: 3254–3258.

Froesch ER, Schmid C, Scwander J & Zapf J (1985) Actions of insulin-like growth factors. *Annual Review of Physiology* **47**: 443–467.

Garcia JE, Acosta AA, Hsui J-G & Jones HW (1984) Advanced endometrial maturation after ovulation induction with human menopausal gonadotropin/human chorionic gonado-tropin for in-vitro fertilization. *Fertility and Sterility* **41**: 31–35.

Giudice LC, Lamson G, Rosenfeld RG et al (1990) Insulin-like growth factor binding proteins

(IGF-BP-1, BP-2, BP-3) in human endometrium: mRNA expression, protein synthesis, and cellular localization. *Proceedings of the VIIth World Congress on Human Reproduction*, abstract 457.

Hall K, Lundin G & Povoa G (1988) Serum levels of the low molecular weight form of insulin-like growth factor binding protein in healthy subjects and patients with growth hormone deficiency, acromegaly, and anorexia nervosa. *Acta Endocrinologica* **118:** 321–326.

Hintz RL & Liu F (1977) Demonstration of specific plasma protein binding sites for somatomedin. *Journal of Clinical Endocrinology and Metabolism* **45:** 988–995.

Holly JMP, Biddlecombe RA, Dunger DB et al (1988) Circadian variation of GH independent IGF-binding protein in diabetes mellitus and its relationship with insulin. A new role for insulin? *Clinical Endocrinology* **29:** 667–675.

Joshi SG, Ebert KM & Swartz DP (1980) Detection and synthesis of a progestagen-dependent protein in human endometrium. *Journal of Reproduction and Fertility* **59:** 273–285.

Joshi SG, Rao R, Henriques EE, Raikar RS & Gordon M (1986) Luteal phase concentration of a progestagen-associated endometrial protein (PEP) in the serum of cycling women with adequate or inadequate endometrium. *Journal of Clinical Endocrinology and Metabolism* **63:** 1247–1249.

Julkunen M, Rutanen E-M, Koskimies A et al (1985) Distribution of placental protein 14 in tissues and body fluids during pregnancy. *British Journal of Obstetrics and Gynaecology* **92:** 1145–1151.

Julkunen M, Apter D, Seppälä M, Stenman U-H & Bohn H (1986a) Serum levels of placental protein 14 reflect ovulation in nonconceptional menstrual cycles. *Fertility and Sterility* **45:** 47–50.

Julkunen M, Koistinen R, Sjöberg J et al (1986b) Secretory endometrium synthesizes placental protein 14. *Endocrinology* **118:** 1782–1786.

Julkunen M, Raikar RS, Joshi SG, Bohn H & Seppälä M (1986c) Placental protein 14 and progestagen-dependent endometrial protein are immunologically indistinguishable. *Human Reproduction* **1:** 7–8.

Julkunen M, Wahlström T & Seppälä M (1986d) Human fallopian tube contains placental protein 14. *American Journal of Obstetrics and Gynecology* **154:** 1076–1079.

Julkunen M, Koistinen R, Aalto-Setälä K et al (1988a) Primary structure of human insulin-like growth factor-binding protein/placental protein 12 and tissue specific expression of its mRNA. *FEBS Letters* **236:** 295–301.

Julkunen M, Seppälä M & Jänne OA (1988b) Complete amino acid sequence of human placental protein 14: a progesterone-regulated uterine protein homologous to beta-lactoglobulins. *Proceedings of the National Academy of Sciences of the USA* **85:** 8845–8849.

Julkunen M, Koistinen R, Suikkari A-M, Seppälä M & Jänne OA (1990) Identification by hybridization histochemistry of human endometrial cells expressing mRNAs encoding a uterine beta-lactoglobulin homologue and an insulin-like growth factor-binding protein-1. *Molecular Endocrinology* **4:** 700–707.

Koistinen R, Kalkkinen N, Huhtala M-L et al (1986) Placental protein 12 is a decidual protein that has an identical N-terminal amino acid sequence with somatomedin-binding protein from human amniotic fluid. *Endocrinology* **118:** 1375–1378.

Koistinen R, Huhtala M-L, Stenman U-H & Seppälä M (1987) Purification of placental protein PP12 from human amniotic fluid and its comparison with PP12 from placenta by immunological, physicochemical and somatomedin-binding properties. *Clinica Chimica Acta* **164:** 293–303.

Koistinen R, Angervo M & Seppälä M (1990a) Expression and effects of IGFBP-1 on human granulosa-luteal cells. *Proceedings of the VIIth World Congress on Human Reproduction*, abstract 453.

Koistinen R, Suikkari A-M, Tiitinen A, Kontula K & Seppälä M (1990b) Human granulosa cells contain insulin-like growth factor binding protein (IGFBP-1) mRNA. *Clinical Endocrinology* **32:** 635–640.

Lee Y-L, Hintz RL, James PM et al (1988) Insulin-like growth factor (IGF) binding protein complementary desoxyribonucleic acid from human HP G2 hepatoma cells: predicted protein sequence suggests an IGF binding domain different from those of the IGF and IGF II receptors. *Molecular Endocrinology* **2:** 404–411.

Marshall RN, Underwood LE, Voina SJ, Foushee DB & Van Wyk JJ (1974) Characterization of the insulin and somatomedin-C receptors in human placental cell membranes. *Journal of Clinical Endocrinology and Metabolism* **39**: 283–292.

Mathews LS, Norstedt G & Palmiter R (1986) Regulation of insulin-like growth factor I gene expression by growth hormone. *Proceedings of the National Academy of Sciences of the USA* **83**: 9343–9347.

Nissley SP & Rechler MM (1984) Insulin-like growth factors: biosynthesis, receptors and carrier proteins. In Li CH (ed.) *Hormones, Proteins and Peptides*, vol. XII, pp 127–203. New York: Academic Press.

Petrunin DD, Kozlyaeva GA, Mesnyankina NV & Shevchenko OP (1980) Detection of chorionic alpha.2 microglobulin in the endometrium in the secretory phase of the menstrual cycle and in the male sperm. *Akusherstvo i Ginekologiia* **3**: 22–23 (in Russian).

Pockley AG, Mowles EA, Stocker RJ et al (1988) Suppression of in vitro lymphocyte reactivity to phytohaemagglutinin by placental protein 14. *Journal of Reproductive Immunology* **13**: 31–39.

Povoa G, Enberg G, Jörnvall H & Hall K (1984) Isolation and characterization of a somatomedin-binding protein from mid-term human amniotic fluid. *European Journal of Biochemistry* **144**: 199–204.

Ren SG & Braunstein GD (1990) Progesterone and human chorionic gonadotropin do not stimulate placental proteins 12 and 14 or prolactin production by human decidual cells in vitro. *Journal of Clinical Endocrinology and Metabolism* **70**: 983–989.

Rinderknecht E & Humbel RE (1978) The amino acid sequence of human insulin-like growth factor I and its structural homology with proinsulin. *Journal of Biological Chemistry* **253**: 2769–2776.

Ritvos O, Ranta T, Jalkanen J et al (1988) Insulin-like growth factor (IGF) binding protein from human decidua inhibits the binding and biological action of IGF-I in cultured choriocarcinoma cells. *Endocrinology* **122**: 2150–2157.

Rosenfeld RG, Pham H, Conover CA, Hintz L & Baxter R (1989) Structural and immunological comparison of insulin-like growth factor binding proteins of cerebrospinal and amniotic fluids. *Journal of Clinical Endocrinology and Metabolism* **68**: 638–646.

Ruoslahti E & Pierschbacher MD (1987) New perspectives in cell adhesion: RGD and integrins. *Science* **238**: 491–497.

Rutanen E-M, Koistinen R, Wahlström T et al (1984a) Placental protein 12 (PP12) in the human endometrium: tissue concentration in relation to histology and serum levels of PP12, progesterone and oestradiol. *British Journal of Obstetrics Gynaecology* **91**: 277–381.

Rutanen E-M, Seppälä M, Pietilä R & Bohn H (1984b) Placental protein 12 (PP12): factors affecting levels in late pregnancy. *Placenta* **5**: 243–248.

Rutanen E-M, Koistinen R, Sjöberg J et al (1986) Synthesis of placental protein 12 by human endometrium. *Endocrinology* **118**: 1067–1071.

Rutanen E-M, Pekonen F & Mäkinen T (1988) Soluble 34K binding protein inhibits the binding of insulin-like growth factor I to its cell receptors in human secretory phase endometrium: evidence for autocrine/paracrine regulation of growth factor action. *Journal of Clinical Endocrinology and Metabolism* **66**: 173–180.

Seppälä M, Alfthan H, Vartiainen E & Stenman U-H (1987a) The post-menopausal uterus: the effect of hormone replacement therapy on the serum levels of secretory endometrial protein PP14/beta-lactoglobulin homologue. *Human Reproduction* **2**: 741–743.

Seppälä M, Rönnberg L, Karonen S-L & Kauppila A (1987b) Micronized oral progesterone increases the circulating level of endometrial secretory PP14/beta-lactoglobulin homologue. *Human Reproduction* **2**: 453–455.

Seppälä M, Julkunen M, Koskimies A et al (1988a) Proteins of the human endometrium: basic and clinical studies toward a blood test for endometrial function. *Annals of the New York Academy of Sciences* **541**: 432–444.

Seppälä M, Riittinen L, Julkunen M et al (1988b) Structural studies, localization in tissue and clinical aspects of human endometrial proteins. *Journal of Reproduction and Fertility* **36 (supplement)**: 127–141.

Seppälä M, Wahlström T, Julkunen M, Vartiainen E & Huhtala M-L (1988c) Endometrial proteins as indicators of endometrial function. In Tomoda Y, Mizutani S, Narita O & Klopper A (eds) *Placental and Endometrial Proteins: Basic and Clinical Aspects*, pp 35–42. Utrecht: VNU Science Press.

Seppälä M, Martikainen H, Rönnberg L, Riittinen L & Kauppila A (1989) Suppression of prolactin secretion during ovarian hyperstimulation is followed by elevated serum levels of endometrial protein PP14 in the late luteal phase. *Human Reproduction* **4**: 389–391.

Suikkari A-M, Rutanen E-M & Seppälä M (1987) Circulating levels of immunoreactive insulin-like growth factor-binding protein in non-pregnant women. *Human Reproduction* **2**: 297–300.

Suikkari A-M, Koivisto VA, Rutanen E-M et al (1988) Insulin regulates the serum levels of low molecular weight insulin-like growth factor-binding protein. *Journal of Clinical Endocrinology and Metabolism* **66**: 266–272.

Suikkari A-M, Koivisto VA, Koistinen R et al (1989) Dose–response characteristics for suppression of low molecular weight plasma insulin-like growth factor-binding protein by insulin. *Journal of Clinical Endocrinology and Metabolism* **68**: 135–140.

Sutcliffe RG, Joshi SG, Paterson WF & Bank JF (1982) Serological identity between human uterine protein and human progestagen-dependent endometrial protein. *Journal of Reproduction and Fertility* **65**: 207–209.

Telimaa S, Kauppila A, Rönnberg L et al (1989) Elevated serum levels of endometrial secretory protein PP14 in patients with advanced endometriosis. Suppression by treatment with danazol and high dose medroxyprogesterone acetate. *American Journal of Obstetrics and Gynecology* **161**: 866–871.

Than GN, Tatra G, Arnold L et al (1988) Serum PP12, PP14, SP1 and hCG values in the 28 days after the LH-surge in patients who do and do not conceive after artificial insemination. *Archives of Gynecology and Obstetrics* **243**: 139–144.

Thrailkill KM, Golander A, Underwood LE & Handwerger S (1988) Insulin-like growth factor I stimulates the synthesis and release of prolactin from human decidual cells. *Endocrinology* **123**: 2930–2934.

Ullrich A, Gray A, Tam AW et al (1986) Insulin-like growth factor I receptor primary structure: comparison with insulin receptor suggests structural determinants that define functional specificity. *EMBO Journal* **5**: 2503–2512.

Wahlström T & Seppälä M (1984) Placental protein 12 (PP12) is induced in the endometrium by progesterone. *Fertility and Sterility* **41**: 781–784.

Wahlström T, Koskimies AI, Tenhunen A et al (1985) Pregnancy proteins in the endometrium after follicle aspiration for in vitro fertilization. *Annals of the New York Academy of Sciences* **442**: 402–407.

Waites GT, James RFL & Bell SC (1988a) Immunohistochemical localization of the human endometrial secretory protein pregnancy-associated endometrial alpha-1-globulin, an insulin-like growth factor-binding protein, during the menstrual cycle. *Journal of Clinical Endocrinology and Metabolism* **67**: 1100–1104.

Waites GT, Wood PL, Walker RA & Bell SC (1988b) Immunohistological localization of human secretory 'pregnancy-associated endometrial alpha-2 globulin' (alpha-2 PEG) during the menstrual cycle. *Journal of Reproduction and Fertility* **82**: 665–672.

Wood PK, Iffland CA, Allen E et al (1990) Serum levels of pregnancy-associated endometrial alpha-2 globulin (alpha-2 PEG), a glycosylated beta-lactoglobulin homologue, in successful and unsuccessful assisted conception. *Human Reproduction* **5**: 421–426.

Wood WI, Cachianes G, Henzel WJ et al (1988) Cloning and expression of the growth hormone-dependent insulin-like growth factor-binding protein. *Molecular Endocrinology* **2**: 1176–1185.

5

The role of prostaglandins in implantation

S. K. SMITH

The mechanism of implantation is perhaps the least well understood aspect of reproduction in our species. Successful implantation in women is a complex event requiring the correct development of the early embryo, the preparation of a receptive endometrium, the attachment of the embryo to the epithelial surface, the recognition by the mother of the presence of the embryo, decidualization of the endometrium and the maintenance of the corpus luteum (Csapo et al, 1973). Our knowledge of these events is inevitably hampered by ethical and practical constraints on experimentation at this stage of the reproductive cycle. Nevertheless disorders of implantation have serious consequences for human fertility and may even be the cause of life-threatening complications in later pregnancy (Reginald et al, 1987).

The exact figures for early pregnancy loss are difficult to determine but probably constitute about 30% of pregnancies (Wilcox et al, 1988). Assisted fertilization has helped many thousands of women who are infertile, but in most centres, sufficient oocytes are obtained in about 80% of patients and fertilization rates of around 70% of oocytes are achieved. Despite the transfer of multiple embryos, 90% of these embryos do not thrive. Although poor quality of oocytes and developing embryos are partly responsible, there is increasing evidence that the high rate of failure of these procedures arises because of impaired implantation (Wilcox et al, 1988; Yovich and Matson, 1988).

Several mammalian strategies have evolved that permit the necessary developmental changes to occur in the endometrium under the influence of ovarian steroids. The precise relationship between the embryo and the endometrium may be broadly divided into those with epitheliochorial placentation, in which the trophoblast does not invade into the endometrium, and haemochorial placentation in which trophoblastic penetration occurs to a greater or lesser degree depending on the species studied. In primates it is this latter type of placentation that occurs and is thus most relevant to the human (Hearn, 1986).

EICOSANOIDS AND EARLY PREGNANCY

Eicosanoids appear to be involved in at least two of these important aspects of early pregnancy. Firstly, increased synthesis of prostaglandins (PGs)

Baillière's Clinical Obstetrics and Gynaecology—
Vol. 5, No. 1, March 1991
ISBN 0–7020–1533–4

appears to be necessary at the site of implantation to facilitate the very early embryo–maternal interactions. Conversely, once attachment and early invasion have occurred, the release of PGs from the endometrial surface as a whole needs to be suppressed to prevent corpus luteal regression and in women to prevent the onset of menstruation. In this chapter these two aspects of the establishment of pregnancy will be considered separately. Before addressing these questions it is important to consider in brief detail the pathways of eicosanoid synthesis.

Eicosanoid synthesis and metabolism

Prostaglandin and leukotriene synthesis

Prostaglandins are the products of cyclo-oxygenase and endoperoxidase breakdown of free intracellular arachidonic acid (AA). Less than 5% of cellular AA is present in the free form, most being bound to the membrane phospholipids. The rate limiting step in the synthesis of PGs is the release of

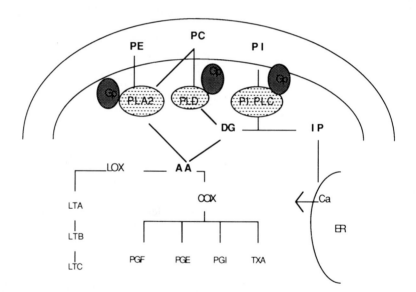

Figure 1. Schematic representation of the synthesis and metabolism of arachidonic acid. Arachidonic acid (AA) is released by the action of phospholipase A_2 (PLA$_2$), phospholipase D (PLD), and PLC (PLC) from a group of phospholipid precursors which include phosphatidyl-ethanolamine (PE), phosphatidylcholine (PC) and phosphatidylinositol (PI). Arachidonic acid is further converted by cyclo-oxygenase (COX) to the various prostaglandins (PGF, PGE, PGI and thromboxane). Alternatively, arachidonic acid is converted by lipoxygenase enzymes (LOX) to the leukotrienes (LTA, LTB, LTC). Arachidonic acid is part of a wider mechanism of second messenger induction. Hydrolysis of PI by phosphatidylinositol specific phospholipases (PI-PLC) results in the formation of diacylglycerol (DG) and inositol phosphates (IP). These affect intracellular events as IP induces the release of calcium from intracellular stores and endoplasmic reticulum (ER). DG alternatively activates protein kinase C, resulting in wide-spread phosphorylation.

AA from the membranes (Lapetina, 1982). At least two groups of phospho-diesterases are responsible for this effect and are therefore central to the understanding of PG release (see Figure 1).

Endometrial phospholipases

Phospholipase A_2 (PLA_2) cleaves AA from the C-2 position of 3-sn-phosphoglycerides like phosphatidylethenolamine and phosphatidylcholine. PLA_2s are a diverse family of enzymes which hydrolyse the sn-2 fatty acyl ester bond of phosphatidylethanolamine and phosphatidylcholine to release AA. Two broad groups of enzymes have been identified. Type I PLA_2s are found in *Elapid* snake venom and type II enzymes in *Viperid* and *Crotalid* snake venoms. These enzymes are characterized by the alignment of their cysteine residues and the subsequent formation of disulphide bridges. In the human, pancreatic PLA_2 is a type I enzyme, but transcripts for this enzyme have also been found in human lung (Seilhamer et al, 1986), suggesting a wider distribution than just pancreas. In addition, a 124 amino acid peptide is present in human rheumatoid arthritic synovial fluid (Seilhamer et al, 1989a), platelets (Kramer et al, 1989) and placental membranes (Lai and Wada, 1988); it is a type II enzyme, similar to other mammalian non-pancreatic PLA_2s. However, the structure of this enzyme is slightly different from the other sequenced human non-pancreatic PLA_2 (Seilhamer et al, 1989b) and, in addition, the same author has found multiple forms of PLA_2 in synovial fluid (Seilhamer et al, 1989a). Several mechanisms regulate PLA_2 activity but the levels of intracellular Ca^{2+} appear to be of particular importance (Van den Bosch, 1980).

Arachidonic acid is also released from membrane phospholipids by the action of another phosphodiesterase, phospholipase C (PLC). PLC is also a diverse enzyme family and large numbers of bacterial and mammalian phospholipases have been purified and characterized (Little, 1989). Particular interest has centred on the inositol phospholipid PLC (PI-PLC) whose substrate is phosphatidylinositol (PI). Several PI-PLC isozymes have been purified to homogeneity and their nucleotide sequence determined. Three isozymes, PI-PLC β, γ and δ (Rhee et al, 1989) derived from rat and bovine brain, are similar in that they contain two conserved regions with significant sequence homology. The first region (X) being 150 amino acids in length and the second 120 amino acids long. The fourth PI-PLC ($PLC\alpha$) does not contain these homologous regions but interestingly has been identified in guinea-pig uterus (Bennett and Crooke, 1987).

PLC cleaves diacylglycerol (DG) from phosphatidylinositol 4,5-bisphosphate (PIP_2), which serves as a substrate for diacyl and monoacyl glycerol lipases, which eventually release AA (Lapetina, 1982). The other products released from the hydrolysis of PIP_2 are the inositol phosphates (Berridge and Irvine, 1984). Inositol 1,4,5-trisphosphate ($InsP_3$) promotes the release of intracellular Ca^{2+} from endoplasmic reticulum (Streb et al, 1983), an action possibly enhanced by kinase mediated conversion of $InsP_3$ to inositol 1,3,4,5-tetrakisphosphate ($InsP_4$), which promotes the transfer of extracellular Ca^{2+} into the cell (Morris et al, 1987). Both DG

and the inositol phosphates are important receptor stimulated signal transduction messengers which alter endometrial PG synthesis. Elevation of
intracellular Ca^{2+} levels activates both PLA_2 and PLC, whereas DG
influences PG release not only by its own degradation to AA, but because in
combination with Ca^{2+} and phosphatidylserine it activates protein kinase C
(Nishizuka, 1988), which could stimulate PLA_2 activity by phosphorylating
and inactivating lipocortin (Khanna et al, 1986), an inhibitor of AA release.
Human endometrium contains both PLA_2 and PLC activity (Bonney, 1985;
Bonney and Franks, 1987) but it is not known which pathway is predominant. Studies are underway to resolve this issue, which is inevitably complicated by the possible heterogeneity of phospholipases in endometrium.

Metabolism of arachidonic acid

Free AA is converted to the various PGs by the action of cyclo-oxygenase,
which has been demonstrated immunohistochemically in the glandular cells
of human endometrium (Rees et al, 1982) and at the site of implantation in
the rat (Parr et al, 1988). Prostaglandin endoperoxide is further converted to
a series of PGs including PGE_2, $PGF_{2\alpha}$, PGI_2, PGD_2 and thromboxanes.
Prostaglandin E_2 and $PGF_{2\alpha}$ are inactivated by PG dehydrogenase to their
metabolites 15-keto,13-14 dihydro PGs.

Prostaglandin synthesis by human endometrium

The ability of endometrium to synthesize PGs has been studied extensively
in many animal species over the past 15 years. Initially most studies
measured the endogenous content of tissue PGs by radioimmunoassay. This
was thought to reflect rapid de novo synthesis caused by the trauma of tissue
collection. Levels of $PGF_{2\alpha}$ but not PGE_2 rose in secretory endometrium
(Downie et al, 1974; Singh et al, 1975), an effect presumed to reflect the
action of the ovarian steroids on PG release, particularly because the effects
could be mimicked by giving oestrogen and progesterone to postmenopausal women (Smith et al, 1984). However, decidua removed in early
pregnancy synthesizes very low levels of PGs (Maathuis and Kelly, 1978),
irrespective of whether the embryo is in the uterine cavity or in the fallopian
tube (Abel et al, 1980).

Studies of PG synthesis by endometrium in vitro have served to increase
our understanding of the complexity of PG synthesis. Abel and Baird (1980)
found that secretory endometrium released more $PGF_{2\alpha}$ and PGE_2 than
proliferative endometrium but Tsang and Ooi (1982) and Schatz et al (1985)
found the converse to be true. The technique of partial digestion of endometrium and separation of the tubular gland structures on a fine membrane
prepared the way for the study of different capacities of epithelial and
stromal cells to synthesize PGs (Satyaswaroop et al, 1979) (Figure 2). Schatz
et al (1985) and Smith and Kelly (1988a) found that epithelial cells synthesized more PGs than stromal cells, although it must be remembered that
these preparations are not pure. However, Gal et al (1982) found that
stromal cells maintained in culture for 7 days released more PGs than did

epithelial cells maintained for the same amount of time. As with all in vitro studies, caution must be used when ascribing physiological events to these findings. Cyclo-oxygenase enzyme has been demonstrated immunohisto-chemically to be present predominantly in the epithelial cells, suggesting the principal source of PGs is the epithelium (Rees et al, 1982). This is important because Lejeune et al (1981) has shown in rodents that the epithelial cells are required for the decidual response, which suggests that it is the PGs released from the endometrium which are the ones which promote decidualization, at least in rodents. Further support for this hypothesis is the observation (Glasser et al, 1988; Cherny and Findlay, 1990) that PG secretion arises principally from the basal aspect of the endometrium.

The ability of separated cells of human endometrium to release PGs changes throughout the cycle, with lower amounts being released in the

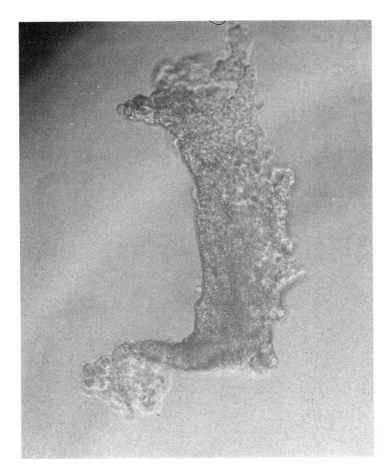

Figure 2. Uterine gland isolated by partial digestion of endometrium as described by Satyaswaroop et al (1979).

secretory phase of the cycle compared with the proliferative phase (Smith and Kelly, 1988). These observations in the human appear at first sight to contradict those in rodents, where increased PG synthesis is required to induce decidualization and implantation. This is compounded by the finding that decidua removed in early human pregnancy has a still further reduction in its capacity to metabolize AA (Ishihara et al, 1986), which is reflected in a grossly reduced release of PGs by epithelial cells taken from decidua (Smith and Kelly, 1988a) (Figure 3).

This paradox could be explained by the ability of the embryo to locally increase PG synthesis whilst not altering the synthesis of PGs from the non-implantation site. This putative effect of the embryo will be discussed first, followed by the actual need and mechanisms for inhibition of PG release from endometrium.

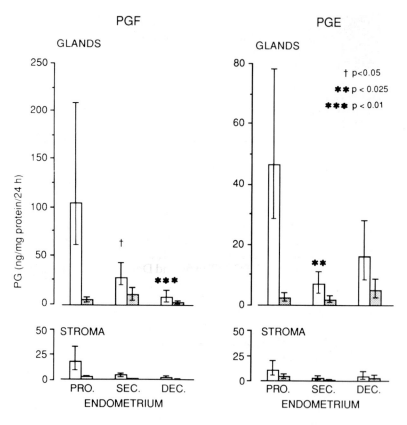

Figure 3. Release of $PGF_{2\alpha}$ and PGE (ng/mg protein for 24 h) from separated enriched fractions of glandular and stromal cells obtained from human endometrium in the proliferative (PRO) and secretory (SEC) stages of the cycle and in early pregnancy (DEC). Clear histograms demonstrate primary PG; the hatched histogram the principal metabolite, 13,14-dihydro-15-keto-PG. From Smith and Kelly (1988a) with permission.

Eicosanoids and implantation

Animal studies

In rodents, the site of implantation may be characterized before the embryo implants and appears as an area of increased vascular permeability, demonstrated by the extravasation of macromolecular dyes (Psychoyos and Martel, 1985). Further changes involving stromal differentiation require the presence of an embryo acting on a steroid primed endometrium (Finn, 1983; Bell, 1985). These changes appear to require the presence of the epithelial cells (Lejeune et al, 1981). It is not known in women whether preferential implantation sites develop in the same way, yet the principal site of implantation appears to be the fundus, suggesting some mechanism of preferment.

Animal studies clearly demonstrate a role for PGs in the increased vascular permeability and decidual changes that arise at the site of implantation (Kennedy, 1983, 1985). The increased vascular permeability described above is abolished in the mouse (Lundqvist and Nilsson, 1980), hamster (Evans and Kennedy, 1978), rat (Phillips and Poyser, 1981) and rabbit (El-Banna, 1980) by inhibitors of PG synthesis. Furthermore, these agents prevent implantation in the mouse (Saksena et al, 1976), rabbit (El-Banna, 1980) and pig (Kraeling et al, 1985). Increased levels of PGE_2, $PGF_{2\alpha}$ and PGI_2 are found at the site of implantation when compared with levels at non-implantation sites (Kennedy, 1985). Decidual cells contain receptors for PGE_2 in the rat (Kennedy, 1983), pig (Kennedy et al, 1986) and human (Hofman et al, 1985). PGE_2 also induces decidual change in rodents (Rankin et al, 1979; Kennedy and Lukich, 1982) and stimulates expression of alkaline phosphatase, a marker of decidualization (Daniel and Kennedy, 1987).

However, PGs do not appear to exert this action alone. Products of the lipoxygenase pathway of AA metabolism are involved at least in the uterus of the rat. FPL, a specific leukotriene receptor antagonist (Levinson, 1984), prevents the decidual cell reaction in the rat, an action antagonized by the infusion of leukotriene C_4 (LTC_4) (Tawfik and Dey, 1988). PGE_2 appears to act with LTC_4 to enhance this decidual cell reaction (Tawfik et al, 1987).

Such studies are not available in women because of obvious ethical constraints and may only be inferred as part of the mechanism of implantation in the human. However, many of the aspects of implantation are similar to that of inflammation in both rodents and humans and it is likely that at least similar mechanisms are involved.

Eicosanoid synthesis by the embryo

Blastocysts of mice (Marshburn et al, 1990), rabbits (Kasamo et al, 1986), rats (Parr et al, 1988), sheep (Hyland et al, 1982), cows (Lewis et al, 1982) and human preimplantation embryos (Shutt and Lopata, 1981; Holmes et al, 1989) release PGE_2 and/or $PGF_{2\alpha}$. In the preimplantation embryos there is some difficulty in establishing the site of PG synthesis as both seminal fluid and corona cells contain or synthesize considerable amounts of PGs.

However, viewed overall it appears that the embryo and trophoblast can synthesize PGs.

Role of eicosanoids at implantation

The evidence above clearly indicates that PGs play an important role in the mechanism of implantation. The principal role suggested by these studies is that of promoting a mild inflammatory reaction at the site of implantation, which presumably acts by providing a receptive milieu for the very early embryo. The oedema associated with this reaction probably provides the nutrition for the embryo, which at this stage has not undergone the profound differentiation and development of the trophoblast with the formation of lacunae that occurs later in the pregnancy. However, PGs most certainly play other roles. They have been implicated in the proliferation of rabbit endometrium, where inhibitors of PG synthesis attenuate DNA synthesis, an effect reversed by the addition of $PGF_{2\alpha}$ (Orlicky et al, 1987). This action of PGs is complicated, as PGE_2 inhibits the action of $PGF_{2\alpha}$ on endometrial proliferation (Orlicky et al, 1986). Furthermore, PGE_2 has been implicated in the immune response that occurs in the endometrium at implantation (Clarke, 1989) and the synthesis of PGs may be involved in the recruitment of the natural killer-like cells which invade the endometrium at implantation. This aspect of PG synthesis and implantation will not be dealt with in this chapter.

Eicosanoids synthesized by the embryo could have wide-ranging effects but this must only be speculation at this stage. They could be involved in the proliferative changes of the embryo and trophoblast, whilst alternatively they may be involved in the embryonic signalling to the local endometrium.

In rodents, implantation and decidualization require the action of an independent agent, which can be the presence of the embryo, the injection of oil or trauma on a steroid primed endometrium (Finn, 1983). It is possible that in women a similar type of mechanism may be involved. Epithelial cells are the principal source of PG synthesis in women but, contrary to there being a general increase in PG release at the time of implantation, there is a reduced capacity of endometrial epithelial cells to synthesize PGs (Smith and Kelly, 1988a). If successful implantation is dependent on the local release of PGs, as occurs in rodents, then the preimplantation human embryo must signal its presence to the mother by a local mechanism. Such a mechanism is suggested in the sheep, where the asynchronous transfer of an advanced staged blastocyst (day 10) to day 6 postoestrous ewes results in the stimulation of PGE_2 synthesis from the uterus (Vincent et al, 1986). Several agents could be responsible, including embryo derived PGs, histamine, bradykinin or oestrogen. However, most attention has focused on the putative role of 1-alkyl-2(R)-acetyl-glycero-3-phosphocholine (platelet activating factor, PAF).

PLATELET ACTIVATING FACTOR AND IMPLANTATION

Platelet activating factor is an unsymmetrically substituted derivative of

D-glycerol. The biosynthesis of PAF involves the action of phospholipase A_2 on alky-acyl-glycero-3-phosphocholine to release lyso-PAF which is metabolized to PAF by acetyl transferase (Braquet et al, 1987). PAF is an important mediator in the inflammatory response and stimulates release of PGs from platelets, neutrophils, mesangial cells and human amnion (reviewed in Braquet et al, 1987). PAF binds to high affinity cell surface receptors which have been identified in platelets, neutrophils and lung membranes and have recently been demonstrated in the endometrium of the rabbit (Harper, 1989). The primary biological signal induced by PAF is the breakdown of phosphatidylinositol from the cell membrane, with the consequent release of DG, inositol 1,4,5-trisphosphate ($InsP_3$) and PGs.

There is reasonable evidence to suggest that PAF may be the first physiological signal produced by the embryo for the maternal recognition of pregnancy. Mice and human preimplantation embryos synthesize PAF (O'Neill, 1985; O'Neill et al, 1987). The culture fluid from mice embryos induces platelet activation and thrombocytopenia, the active agent being PAF, and in both species transient thrombocytopenia occurs in the mother in early pregnancy. Murine and rat implantation is abolished by PAF antagonists (Spinks and O'Neill, 1987; Acker et al, 1988) and successful implantation of human embryos broadly correlates with their ability to synthesize PAF in culture (O'Neill et al, 1987). These findings suggest that PAF acts as an early embryonic signal in the maternal recognition of pregnancy. In the light of the requirement for local elevation of endometrial PG synthesis and the presence of PAF receptors in endometrium, it is likely that embryo derived PAF facilitates implantation by stimulating PG synthesis from endometrium in close proximity to the embryo.

PAF has been shown to stimulate PGE_2 release from separated glandular cells from human endometrium (Smith and Kelly, 1988b). This effect was only found when cells were obtained from secretory endometrium, the action being absent in cells taken from proliferative endometrium. However, stromal cells taken from endometrium removed at either stage of the cycle failed to respond to PAF (Figure 4). $PGF_{2\alpha}$ release was not altered by PAF, indicating preferential stimulation of PGE_2 release. As already described, in rodents it is PGE_2 which seems to be most necessary for implantation. Recent studies have begun to determine the mechanism of action. PAF stimulates accumulation of inositol phospholipids with an initial rise in $InsP_3$ levels, followed by a rise in total inositol phosphate levels. Of particular interest is the observation that this action does not occur in proliferative endometrium, only arising in secretory endometrium, as does the rise of PGE_2 synthesis (Ahmed et al, 1990). These findings indicate that PAF does stimulate the activity of a uterine PLC, though it does not exclude the possibility that PLA_2 activity is also elevated. In addition to the embryo, human luteal phase endometrium synthesizes PAF, suggesting a further source of PAF in the endometrium at implantation (Angle et al, 1988). This raises the interesting prospect as to the differential effects of PAF when administered to the alternate poles of the endometrial epithelial cell. Endometrial polarity has particularly important effects on epithelial cell function (Glasser et al, 1988; Cherny and Findlay, 1990). It is of particular

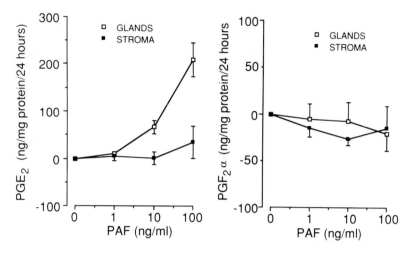

Figure 4. Release of PGE_2 and PGF from separated enriched fractions of glandular and stromal cells obtained from human endometrium in the secretory phase of the menstrual cycle. PAF induced a significant rise in PGE release from glandular cells but not stromal cells, whilst $PGF_{2\alpha}$ levels were unaltered. From Smith and Kelly (1988b) with permission.

interest that, in endometrial cells maintained on a permeable membrane, PG secretion is primarily from the basal region, increasing the possibility that epithelial derived PGs pass into the stroma.

More recently, doubt has been cast as to the site of action of PAF. PAF does have a direct effect on the embryo, enhancing the oxidative metabolism of glucose and lactate by mouse embryos (O'Neill et al, 1989; Ryan et al, 1990). Supplementation of culture medium with PAF enhances the ability of embryos to implant in both murine and human pregnancies (O'Neill et al, 1989; Ryan et al, 1990). Treatment of embryo donors before transfer results in impaired implantation when the recipients do not receive PAF antagonists (Spinks et al, 1990), suggesting an effect of the PAF antagonist on the embryo, not on the endometrium.

Regrettably, it is not possible for ethical reasons to give patients PAF antagonists to prevent implantation, and at this stage most of the putative effects of PAF on human implantation remain speculative.

MAINTENANCE OF PREGNANCY

Animal studies

The continuation of pregnancy in laboratory and farm animals is dependent on the maintenance of the corpus luteum. $PGF_{2\alpha}$ seems to be the uterine luteolysin. Concentrations of $PGF_{2\alpha}$ are elevated in uterine vein blood at the time of luteolysis in the guinea-pig (Horton and Poyser, 1976), $PGF_{2\alpha}$, PGE_2 and 6-keto-PGF output is greater from the superfused guinea-pig uterus in vitro, and the release of these PGs is reduced from endometrium removed on day 15 of the oestrous cycle compared with that removed on day 7, in the case of $PGF_{2\alpha}$ the reduction being less by a factor of 48.7 (Leckie and Poyser, 1990).

In the sheep, levels of $PGF_{2\alpha}$ are elevated in the uterine vein at luteolysis (McCracken et al, 1984). In this species, $PGF_{2\alpha}$ is released in a pulsatile fashion under the influence of oxytocin (Hooper et al, 1986) and there is a reduction in this pulsatile release in early pregnancy (Zarco et al, 1984). In the bovine oestrous cycle there is an increase in the episodic release of PGFM from the uterus associated with falling levels of progesterone (Thatcher et al, 1984); this is prevented by the presence of a viable pregnancy (Betteridge et al, 1984). Similarly, the release of $PGF_{2\alpha}$ is reduced from cultured (Thatcher et al, 1984; Gross et al, 1988a) or perifused endometrium (Gross et al, 1988a) removed from day 17 of pregnancy compared with tissue obtained on day 17 of oestrous. Finally, in the pig the prevention of uterine PGs reaching the ovary is achieved by a redirection of its release from the endometrium, PGs being released into the uterine cavity away from the uterine vein (Bazer et al, 1986).

Conceptus secretory proteins

Conceptus secretory proteins from both the sheep and cow prolong the oestrous cycle when instilled into the uterine cavity (Ellinwood et al, 1979; Martal et al, 1979). The active molecules appear to be a group of interferon-like, N-linked glycoproteins of molecular weights between 18 and 26 kDa (Helmer et al, 1987) derived from at least three mRNA transcripts (Imakawa et al, 1987; Anthony et al, 1988; Helmer et al, 1989). Ovine and bovine trophoblastic proteins (TPs) demonstrate immunological cross-reactivity (Helmer et al, 1987; Godkin et al, 1988) and 70% cDNA sequence homology (Imakawa et al, 1987). In addition, there is significant sequence homology in the 40 N-terminal amino acids between the ovine and bovine TPs and human α-interferon (Stewart et al, 1987) and 40% homology of the cDNA sequences, all molecules containing the highly conserved Cys-Ala-Trp-Glu sequence motif (Imakawa et al, 1987).

Conceptus secretory proteins and endometrial PG synthesis

Sheep

Ovine trophoblastic protein is secreted between days 12 to 22 of pregnancy (Godkin et al, 1982) and inhibits luteolysis (Vallet et al, 1988). Intrauterine infusion of conceptus secretory proteins (CSPs) or purified oTP-1 inhibits oestradiol or oxytocin stimulated release of $PGF_{2\alpha}$ (Fincher et al, 1986; Vallet et al, 1988). In this species, oxytocin appears to stimulate PG synthesis via the increased turnover of PI (Flint et al, 1986) but the mechanism of oTP-1 action on PG synthesis remains unclear and differs between cycling ewes and those ovariectomized ewes given exogenous steroids (Vallet and Bazer, 1989). Ovine TP does not inhibit basal PI turnover from endometrium removed on day 15 of the oestrous cycle but when administered in combination with oxytocin it attenuates oxytocin induced PI turnover. This effect is not seen when oTP-1 is given with oxytocin to ovariectomized ewes treated with progesterone followed by oestradiol. However PI turnover is reduced by oTP-1 in animals treated with ovarian steroids and receiving pretreatment with oxytocin. Contrary to these findings, pretreatment with oTP-1 stimulated PI turnover in endometrium taken from sheep treated with progesterone or progesterone and oestradiol. In concluding, the authors could not confirm that oTP-1 prevented luteolysis by attenuating oxytocin induced $PGF_{2\alpha}$ release from the ovine uterus; but it

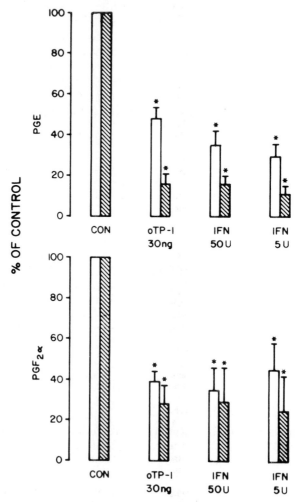

Figure 5. Change in release of PGE and PGF from sheep endometrium maintained in culture. Ovine trophoblastic protein (OTP-1) and interferon-α2 (IFN) significantly suppress prostaglandin E and $F_{2\alpha}$ release from sheep endometrium. From Salamonsen et al, 1988 with permission.

should be remembered that oTP-1 does prevent luteolysis and reduce $PGF_{2\alpha}$ synthesis from the uterus.

Additional evidence for a role of oTP-1 in the maintenance of pregnancy is provided by the observation that oTP-1 binds membrane receptors in the sheep and the finding that human α-interferon binds to similar receptors and that the binding is displaced by purified oTP-1 (Stewart et al, 1987). The release of $PGF_{2\alpha}$ and PGE_2 into culture medium from endometrium obtained from ovariectomized sheep treated with oestrogen and progesterone is significantly attenuated by oTP-1 and human α-interferon (Salamonsen et al, 1988) (Figure 5).

Cow

Bovine CSP extends the interoestrous interval in the cow (Knickerbocker et al, 1986a) and intrauterine instillation of bTP-1 delays luteolysis (Helmer et al, 1989). This action is probably mediated by the effects of the proteins on PG release, as bCSP attenuates $PGF_{2\alpha}$ release from the uterus (Knicker-bocker et al, 1986b) and endometrial explants (Gross et al, 1988b). Whilst both bCSP and bTP-1 inhibit $PGF_{2\alpha}$ release from endometrial explants, they do not alter PGE_2 release (Helmer et al, 1989). This could reflect different actions of the proteins, as Fortier et al (1988) showed that $PGF_{2\alpha}$ synthesis arises in epithelial cells in cow endometrium whilst PGE_2 arises predominantly from the stromal cells.

Pig

The situation in the pig seems to be completely different to that in the sheep and cow. Porcine CSPs do not alter the interoestrous interval and indeed stimulate both $PGF_{2\alpha}$ and PGE_2 synthesis by the uterus (Harney and Bazer, 1989). They do not act as the luteolytic agent, as in the other species.

HUMAN STUDIES OF THE MAINTENANCE OF EARLY PREGNANCY

Introduction

Unlike laboratory and farm animals, uterine PGs are not luteolytic in women. However, it is still the case that the maintenance of the corpus luteum is required for the successful establishment of pregnancy. Surgical removal of the corpus luteum in primates performed before about the seventh week of pregnancy results in abortion (Csapo et al, 1973). Evidence that PGs are involved in this mechanism is suggested by the finding that intrauterine instillation of PGs results in menstrual bleeding (Wiqvist et al, 1971; Toppozada et al, 1980), and administration of analogues of PGs results in abortion when given in early pregnancy.

Clearly the need to attenuate PG release from the uterus to prevent luteolysis does not arise in women but PGs are involved in the induction of menstrual bleeding which usually occurs with the withdrawal of progesterone from an oestrogen primed endometrium. Inhibition of luteolysis is required but, in addition, inhibition of menstruation is also needed to prevent dislodgement of the embryo, though this is not an absolute requirement as some women bleed in early pregnancy and retain the embryo. In the light of these observations progesterone appears to be the most likely agent for suppression of PG synthesis but it may not be the only agent. α_2-Interferon, which suppresses PG release from sheep endometrium, is present in amniotic fluid of human pregnancy (Lebon et al, 1982; Chard et al, 1986) and has been demonstrated by immunohistochemistry in human, chorionic villous syncytiotrophoblast from the eighth week of pregnancy (Bocci et al, 1985). In addition, provisional studies by Loke and King (1990) has shown staining for α_2-interferon in glandular cells of human endometrium. The putative roles for progesterone and α_2-interferon in the maintenance of early human pregnancy will be considered in the next section.

Progesterone and PG release from human endometrium and decidua

The effects of progesterone on endometrial synthesis of PGs in vivo and in vitro appears to be paradoxical. Endogenous levels of PGs are higher in secretory phase endometrium compared with proliferative endometrium (Downie et al, 1974), and endometrium exposed to oestradiol and progesterone in vivo has higher levels of $PGF_{2\alpha}$ than endometrium exposed to oestradiol alone (Smith et al, 1982, 1984). However, release of PGs from separated cells of human endometrium is greatest from proliferative endometrium compared with secretory endometrium (Smith and Kelly, 1987). The synthesis of PGs from decidua obtained in early pregnancy is different again. Endogenous levels are very low compared with non-pregnant endometrium (Maathuis and Kelly, 1978) and release of PGs from decidua is greatly suppressed compared to endometrium (Smith and Kelly, 1988).

One explanation for these observations is that progesterone enhances the capacity of the tissue to release PGs, which is reflected in the measurement of endogenous levels as the response to trauma. In vitro, progesterone suppresses basal release of PGs but the tissue retains the capacity to synthesize large amounts of PGs in response to other stimuli. Decidua is different in that it cannot release large amounts of PGs. One way of investigating the effect of progesterone on PG synthesis from decidua is to use antiprogestins. Antiprogestins combine with the nuclear progesterone receptor and compete with native progesterone. They probably act by stabilizing the complex formed between the receptor and heat shock protein, thus preventing the complex from adhering to the DNA binding site (Baulieu, 1987).

Antiprogestins stimulate $PGF_{2\alpha}$ and PGE_2 release from enriched fractions of glandular cells obtained from decidua of early pregnancy (Smith and Kelly, 1987). This action is abolished by the addition of the protein synthesis antagonist, actinomycin, and the Ca^{2+} channel blocker, verapamil (Smith and Kelly, 1990). This suggests that progesterone inhibits protein synthesis of the enzymes required for PG synthesis and that PG synthesis from human endometrium requires the passage of extracellular Ca^{2+} into the cell.

More recently, Mitchell and Smith (1990) demonstrated that progesterone suppressed both $PGF_{2\alpha}$ and PGE_2 synthesis from enriched glandular cells of proliferative endometrium in vitro, but did not alter PG synthesis from cells taken from proliferative endometrium. This action was attenuated by exogenous AA, suggesting that progesterone was preventing the release of AA from the cell membrane. In addition to its action on AA release, progesterone may alter cyclo-oxygenase (COX) activity. The increased release of PGs from glandular cells of decidua was enhanced by the addition of exogenous AA (Smith and Kelly, 1987), a conclusion reached by Jeremy and Dandona (1986) for PG release from rat myometrium. Thus progesterone may act on at least two parts of the PG synthetic pathway.

α_2-Interferon and PG release from endometrium

α_2-Interferon, at doses which did suppress $PGF_{2\alpha}$ and PGE_2 release from sheep endometrium, did not have the same action when incubated with separated cells of human endometrium (Mitchell and Smith, 1990). In the latter study, α_2-interferon not only failed to suppress PG synthesis from enriched glandular cells taken from proliferative endometrium, but abolished the inhibition of PG synthesis induced by progesterone (Figure 6). In this respect, human endometrium responds to α_2-interferon in the same way as does pig endometrium, i.e. there is an increased PG release.

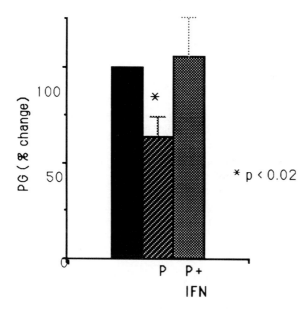

Figure 6. The effect of progesterone and interferon (IFN) on prostaglandin $F_{2\alpha}$ release from enriched fractions of human glandular cells obtained from peripheral endometrium. Progesterone (P) caused a significant reduction of PG release over 4 days and this effect was attenuated by the combined incubation with IFN.

88 S. K. SMITH

CONCLUSION

The role that PGs play at implantation and in the maintenance of early human pregnancy appear to be discrete. Considerable animal information points to a significant role for PGs at the very earliest days of the pregnancy, i.e. at implantation. In women, implantation occurs around day 5 to 8 after the midcycle luteinizing hormone surge. At this time, progesterone is suppressing basal PG release from the endometrium but the tissue retains its capacity to respond to other PG agonists. As in rodents, this could simply be due to the presence of the embryo itself, to molecules released by the embryo, such as PAF or interferons, or to agonists released from the endometrium itself. It is presumed that PGs induce oedema, increase vascular permeability and generally assist in increasing the provision of essential nutrients to the embryo before the establishment of the true placenta. However, the maintenance of the corpus luteum is required to prevent a decline in systemic levels of progesterone which would result in the onset of menstruation and the loss of the embryo. The suppression of PG synthesis is retained until it is reversed at the time of the onset of labour.

Our knowledge of the mechanism of human implantation is pitifully small and the hypothesis outlined above is certainly too simplistic. However, implantation remains one of the most intriguing enigmas in our understanding of human reproduction. The ability to improve implantation rates after in vitro fertilization and embryo transfer would significantly improve the success rates of this procedure and provide a reliable means of achieving pregnancy for the large number of couples yearning for the opportunity to have their own child.

Abel MH & Baird DT (1980) The effect of 17β-estradiol and progesterone on prostaglandin production by human endometrium maintained in organ culture. *Endocrinology* **106:** 1599–1606.
Abel MH, Smith SK & Baird DT (1980) Suppression of concentration of endometrial prostaglandin in early intra-uterine and ectopic pregnancy in women. *Journal of Endocrinology* **85:** 379–386.
Acker G, Hecquet F, Etienne A, Braquet P & Mercia-Huerata JM (1988) Role of platelet-activating factor (PAF) in ovoimplantation in the rat: effect of the specific PAF-acether antagonist, BN 52021. *Prostaglandins* **35:** 233–241.
Ahmed A, Littlewood CJ & Smith SK (1990) Stimulation of phosphoinositide (PI) hydrolysis by platelet activating factor (PAF) in human endometrium. *Journal of Reproduction and Fertility*, Abstract Series No. 5, Abstract 41, p 26, Society for the Study of Fertility Annual Conference, Sheffield, 1990.
Angle MJ, Jones MA, McManus LM, Pinckard RN & Harper MJK (1988) Platelet-activating factor in the rabbit uterus during early pregnancy. *Journal of Reproduction and Fertility* **83:** 711–722.
Anthony RV, Helmer SD, Sharif SF et al (1988) Synthesis and processing of ovine trophoblast protein-1 and bovine trophoblast protein-1, conceptus secretory proteins involved in the maternal recognition of pregnancy. *Endocrinology* **123:** 1224–1280.
Baulieu EE (1987) Contragestion by the progesterone antagonist RU 486 a novel approach to human fertility control. *Research Reviews* **19:** 3–4.

Bazer FW, Vallett JL, Roberts RM, Sharp DC & Thatcher WW (1986) Role of conceptus secretory products in establishment of pregnancy. *Journal of Reproduction and Fertility* **76:** 841–850.

Bell SC (1985) Comparative aspects of decidualization in rodents and humans: cell types, secreted products and associated function. In Edwards RG, Purdy JM & Steptoe PC (eds) *Implantation of the Human Embryo*, pp 71–122. London: Academic Press.

Bennett CF & Crooke ST (1987) Purification and characterisation of a phosphoinositide-specific phospholipase C from guinea pig uterus. *Journal of Biological Chemistry* **262:** 13789–13797.

Berridge MJ & Irvine RF (1984) Inositol trisphosphate, a novel second messenger in cellular signal transduction. *Nature* **312:** 315–321.

Betteridge KJ, Randall GCB, Eaglesome MD & Sugden EA (1984) The influence of pregnancy on $PGF_{2\alpha}$ secretion in cattle. I. Concentrations of 15-keto-13,14-dihydro-prostaglandin $F_{2\alpha}$ and progesterone in peripheral blood of recipients of transferred embryos. *Animal Reproductive Science* **7:** 195–216.

Bocci V, Paulesu L & Ricci MG (1985) The physiological interferon response: IV. Production of interferon by the perfused human placenta at term. *Proceedings of the Society of Experimental Biology and Medicine* **180:** 137–143.

Bonney RC (1985) Measurement of phospholipase A_2 activity in human endometrium during the menstrual cycle. *Journal of Endocrinology* **107:** 183–189.

Bonney RC & Franks S (1987) Phospholipase C activity in human endometrium: its significance in endometrial pathology. *Clinical Endocrinology* **27:** 307–320.

Braquet P, Touqui L, Shen TY & Vargaftig BB (1987) Perspectives in platelet-activating factor research. *Pharmacological Reviews* **39:** 97–145.

Chard T, Craig PH, Menabawey M & Lee C (1986) Alpha interferon in human pregnancy. *British Journal of Obstetrics and Gynaecology* **93:** 1145–1149.

Cherny RA & Findlay JK (1990) Separation and culture of ovine endometrial epithelial and stromal cells: evidence of morphological and functional polarity. *Biology of Reproduction* **43:** 241–250.

Clarke DA (1989) Macrophages and other migratory cells in endometrium: relevance to endometrial bleeding. In Newton JR & d'Arcangues C (eds) *Contraception and Mechanisms in Endometrial Bleeding.* Cambridge: Cambridge University Press (in press).

Csapo AI, Pulkinnen MO & Wiest WG (1973) Effects of luteectomy and progesterone therapy in early pregnant patients. *American Journal of Obstetrics and Gynecology* **115:** 759–765.

Daniel SAJ & Kennedy TG (1987) Prostaglandin E_2 enhances uterine stromal cell alkaline phosphatase activity in vitro. *Prostaglandins* **33:** 241–252.

Downie J, Poyser N & Wunderlich M (1974) Levels of prostaglandins in human endometrium during the normal menstrual cycle. *Journal of Physiology* **236:** 465–472.

El-Banna AA (1980) The degenerative effect on rabbit implantation sites by indomethacin. I. Timing of indomethacin action, possible effect of uterine proteins and the effect of replacement doses of $PGF_{2\alpha}$. *Prostaglandins* **20:** 587–599.

Ellinwood WE, Nett TM & Niswender GD (1979) Maintenance of the corpus luteum of early pregnancy in the ewe. II. Prostaglandin secretion by the endometrium in vitro and in vivo. *Biology of Reproduction* **21:** 845–856.

Evans CA & Kennedy TG (1978) The importance of prostaglandin synthesis for the initiation of blastocyst implantation in the hamster. *Journal of Reproduction and Fertility* **54:** 255–261.

Fincher KB, Bazer FW, Hansen PJ, Thatcher WW & Roberts RM (1986) Proteins secreted by the sheep conceptus suppress induction of uterine prostaglandin F-2α release by oestradiol and oxytocin. *Journal of Reproduction and Fertility* **76:** 425–433.

Finn CA (1983) Implantation of ova—assessment of the value of laboratory animals for the study of implantation in women. *Oxford Reviews of Reproductive Biology* **5:** 272–289.

Flint APF, Leat WMF, Sheldrick EL & Stewart HJ (1986) Stimulation of phosphoinositide hydrolysis by oxytocin and the mechanism by which oxytocin controls prostaglandin synthesis in the ovine endometria. *Biochemical Journal* **237:** 797–805.

Fortier MA, Guilbault LA & Grasso F (1988) Specific properties of epithelial and stromal cells from the endometrium of cows. *Journal of Reproduction and Fertility* **83:** 239–248.

Gal D, Casey ML, Johnston JM & Macdonald PC (1982) Mesenchyme–epithelial interactions in human endometrium. Prostaglandin synthesis in separated cell types. *Journal of Clinical Investigation* **70:** 798–805.

90   S. K. SMITH

Glasser SR, Julian J, Decker GL, Tang JP & Carson DD (1988) Development of morphological and functional polarity in primary cultures of immature rat uterine epithelial cells. *Journal of Cellular Biology* **107**: 2409–2423.

Godkin JD, Bazer FW, Moffat RJ, Sessions F & Roberts RM (1982) Purification and properties of a major, low molecular weight protein released by the trophoblast of sheep blastocysts at Day 13–21. *Journal of Reproduction and Fertility* **65**: 141–150.

Godkin JD, Lifsey BJ & Gillespie BE (1988) Characterization of bovine conceptus proteins produced during the peri- and postattachment periods of early pregnancy. *Biology of Reproduction* **38**: 703–711.

Gross TS, Thatcher WW, Hensen PJ & Lacroix MC (1988a) Prostaglandin secretion by perifused bovine endometrium: secretion towards the myometrial and luminal sides at day 17 post-estrus as altered by pregnancy. *Prostaglandins* **35**: 343–357.

Gross TS, Thatcher WW, Hansen PJ, Johnson JW & Helmer SD (1988b) Presence of an intracellular endometrial inhibitor of prostaglandin synthesis during early pregnancy in the cow. *Prostaglandins* **35**: 359–377.

Harney JP & Bazer FW (1989) Effect of porcine conceptus secretory proteins on interestrous interval and uterine secretion of prostaglandins. *Biology of Reproduction* **41**: 277–285.

Harper MJK (1989) Platelet activating factor: a paracrine factor in preimplantation stages of reproduction. *Biology of Reproduction* **40**: 907–913.

Hearn JP (1986) The embryo–maternal dialogue during early pregnancy in primates. *Journal of Reproduction and Fertility* **76**: 809–819.

Helmer SD, Hansen PJ, Anthony RV, Thatcher WW, Bazer FW & Roberts RM (1987) Identification of bovine trophoblasts protein 1, a secretory protein immunologically related to ovine trophoblast protein 1. *Journal of Reproduction and Fertility* **79**: 83–91.

Helmer SD, Gross TS, Newton GR, Hansen PJ & Thatcher WW (1989) Bovine trophoblast protein-1 complex alters endometrial protein and prostaglandin secretion and induces an intracellular inhibitor of prostaglandin synthesis in vitro. *Journal of Reproduction and Fertility* **87**: 421–430.

Hofman GE, Rao CV, De Leon FD, Toledo AA & Sanfilippo JS (1985) Human endometrial prostaglandin E_2 binding sites and their profiles during the menstrual cycle and in pathological states. *American Journal of Obstetrics and Gynecology* **151**: 369–375.

Holmes PV, Sjogren A & Hamberger L (1989) Prostaglandin-E_2 released by pre-implantation human conceptuses. *Journal of Reproductive Immunology* **17**: 79–86.

Hooper SB, Watkins WV & Thorburn GD (1986) Oxytocin, oxytocin-associated neurophysin, and prostaglandin F-2α concentrations in the utero-ovarian vein of pregnant and non-pregnant sheep. *Endocrinology* **119**: 2590–2597.

Horton EW & Poyser NL (1976) Uterine luteolytic hormone: a physiological role for prostaglandin $F_{2\alpha}$. *Physiology Reviews* **56**: 559–561.

Hyland JH, Manns JG & Humphrey WD (1982) Prostaglandin production by ovine embryos and endometrium in vitro. *Journal of Reproduction and Fertility* **65**: 299–304.

Imakawa K, Anthony RV, Kezemi M, Marotti KR, Polites HG & Roberts RM (1987) Interferon like sequence of ovine trophoblast protein secreted by embryonic trophectoderm. *Nature* **330**: 337–339.

Ishihara O, Tsutsumi O, Mizuno M, Kinoshita K & Satoh K (1986) Metabolism of arachidonic acid and synthesis of prostanoids in human endometrium and decidua. *Prostaglandins, Leukotrienes and Medicine* **24**: 93–102.

Jeremy JY & Dandona P (1986) RU 486 antagonises the inhibitory action of progesterone on prostacyclin and thromboxane A_2 synthesis in cultured rat myometrial explant. *Endocrinology* **119**: 65–69.

Kasamo M, Ishikawa M, Yamashita K, Senogoku K & Shimizu T (1986) Possible role of prostaglandin F in blastocyst implantation. *Prostaglandins* **31**: 321–336.

Kennedy TG (1983) Embryonic signals and the initiation of blastocyst implantation. *Australian Journal of Biological Sciences* **36**: 531–543.

Kennedy TG (1985) Prostaglandins and blastocyst implantation. *Prostaglandin Perspectives* **1**: 1:3.

Kennedy TG & Lukich LA (1982) Induction of decidualization in rats by the intrauterine infusions of prostaglandins. *Biology of Reproduction* **27**: 253–260.

Kennedy TG, Keys JL & King GJ (1986) Endometrial prostaglandin E_2-binding sites in the pig: characterization and changes during the estrous cycle and early pregnancy. *Biology of Reproduction* **35**: 624–632.

Khanna NC, Tokuda M & Waisman DM (1986) Phosphorylation of lipocortins in vitro by protein kinase C. *Biochemical and Biophysical Research Communications* **141**: 547–554.

Knickerbocker JJ, Thatcher WW, Bazer FW, Barron DH & Roberts RM (1986a) Inhibition of uterine prostaglandin $F_{2\alpha}$ production by bovine conceptus secretory proteins. *Prostaglandins* **31**: 777–793.

Knickerbocker JJ, Thatcher WW, Bazer FW et al (1986b) Proteins secreted by day 16 to 18 conceptuses extend corpus luteum function in cows. *Journal of Reproduction and Fertility* **77**: 381–391.

Kraeling RR, Rampacek GB & Fiorello NA (1985) Inhibition of pregnancy with indomethacin in mature gilts and prepubertal gilts induced to ovulate. *Biology of Reproduction* **32**: 105–110.

Kramer RM, Hession C, Johansen B et al (1989) Structure and properties of a human non-pancreatic phospholipase A_2. *Journal of Biological Chemistry* **264**: 5738–5775.

Lai CY & Wada K (1988) Phospholipase A_2 from human synovial fluid: Purification and structural homology of the placental enzyme. *Biochemical and Biophysical Research Communications* **157**: 488–493.

Lapetina EG (1982) Regulation of arachidonic acid production: role of phospholipase C and A_2. *Trends in Pharmacological Science* **3**: 115–118.

Lebon P, Girard S, Thepot F & Chany C (1982) The presence of γ-interferon in human amniotic fluid. *Journal of General Virology* **59**: 393–396.

Leckie CM & Poyser NL (1990) The effects of cholera toxin, pertussis toxin, sodium fluoride and α-interferon on prostaglandin production by the guinea-pig endometrium. *Journal of Reproduction and Fertility* **89**: 325–333.

Lejeune B, Van Hoeck J & Leroy F (1981) Transmitter role of the luminal uterine epithelium in the induction of decidualization in rats. *Journal of Reproduction and Fertility* **61**: 235–240.

Levinson SL (1984) Peptidoleukotriene binding in guinea pig uterine membrane preparations. *Prostaglandins* **28**: 229–235.

Lewis GS, Thatcher WW, Bazer FW & Curl JS (1982) Metabolism of arachidonic acid in vitro by bovine blastocysts and endometrium. *Biology of Reproduction* **27**: 431–439.

Little C (1989) Phospholipase C. *Biochemical Society Transactions* **17**: 271–273.

Loke YW & King A (1990) Current Topic: Interferon and human placental development. *Placenta* **11**: 291–299.

Lundqvist O & Nilsson BO (1980) Ultrastructural changes of the trophoblast–epithelial complex in mice subject to implantation blocking treatment with indomethacin. *Biology of Reproduction* **22**: 719–726.

Maathuis JB & Kelly RW (1978) Concentration of prostaglandins $F_{2\alpha}$ and E_2 in endometrium throughout the menstrual cycle after the administration of clomiphene or an oestrogen–progesterone pill and in early pregnancy. *Journal of Endocrinology* **77**: 361–371.

McCracken JA, Schramm W & Okulicz WC (1984) Hormone receptor control of pulsatile secretion of $PGF_{2\alpha}$ from the ovine uterus during luteolysis and its abrogation in early pregnancy. *Animal Reproduction Science* **7**: 31–55.

Marshburn PB, Shabanowitz RB & Clark MR (1990) Immunohistochemical localization of prostaglandin H synthase in the embryo and uterus of the mouse from ovulation through implantation. *Molecular Reproduction Developments* **25**: 309–316.

Martal J, Lacroix MC, Loudes C, Saunier M & Winterberger-Torres S (1979) Trophoblastin, an antiluteolytic protein present in early pregnancy in sheep. *Journal of Reproduction and Fertility* **56**: 63–73.

Mitchell SN & Smith SK (1990) Progesterone and human interferon α-2 have a different effect on the release of prostaglandins $F_{2\alpha}$ from human endometrium. *Advances in Prostaglandin, Thromboxane and Leukotriene Research* (in press).

Morris AP, Gallacher DV, Irvine RF & Peterson OH (1987) Synergism of inositol trisphosphate and tetrakisphosphate in activating Ca^{2+}-dependent K^+ channels. *Nature* **330**: 653–655.

Nishizuka Y (1988) The molecular heterogeneity of protein kinase C and its implications for cellular regulation. *Nature* **334**: 661–665.

O'Neill C (1985) Partial characterisation of the embryo-derived platelet-activating factor in mice. *Journal of Reproduction and Fertility* **75**: 375–380.

O'Neill C, Gidley-Baird AA, Pike IL & Saunders DM (1987) Use of a bioassay for embryo-derived platelet-activating factor as a means of assessing quality and pregnancy potential of human embryos. *Fertility and Sterility* **47**: 969–975.

O'Neill C, Collier M, Ammit AJ, Ryan JP, Saunders DM & Pike IL (1989) Supplementation of in-vitro fertilisation culture medium with platelet activating factor. *Lancet* **ii:** 769–772.

Orlicky DJ, Lieberman R & Gerschenson LE (1986) Prostaglandin $F_{2\alpha}$ and E_1 regulation of proliferation in primary cultures of rabbit endometrial cells. *Journal of Cellular Physiology* **127:** 55–60.

Orlicky DJ, Lieberman R, Williams C & Gerschenson LE (1987) Requirement for prostaglandin $F_{2\alpha}$ in 17β estradiol stimulation of DNA synthesis in rabbit endometrial cultures. *Journal of Cellular Physiology* **130:** 292–300.

Parr MB, Parr EL, Munaretto K, Clark MR & Dey SK (1988) Immunohistochemical localisation of prostaglandin synthase in the rat uterus and embryo during the peri-implantation period. *Biology of Reproduction* **38:** 333–343.

Phillips CA & Poyser NL (1981) Studies on the involvement of prostaglandins in implantation in the rat. *Journal of Reproduction and Fertility* **62:** 73–81.

Psychoyos A & Martel D (1985) Embryo–endometrial interactions at implantation. In Edwards RG, Purdy JM & Steptoe PC (eds) *Implantation of the Human Embryo*, pp 197–219. London: Academic Press.

Rankin JC, Ledford BE, Jonsson HT & Baggett B (1979) Prostaglandins, indomethacin and the decidual cell reaction in the mouse uterus. *Biology of Reproduction* **249:** 399–404.

Rees MCP, Parry DM, Anderson ABM & Turnbull AC (1982) Immunohistochemical localisation of cyclooxygenase in the human uterus. *Prostaglandins* **23:** 207–214.

Reginald PW, Beard RW, Chapple J et al (1987) Outcome of pregnancies progressing beyond 28 weeks gestation in women with a history of recurrent miscarriages. *British Journal of Obstetrics and Gynaecology* **94:** 643–648.

Rhee SG, Suh PG, Ryu SH & Lee SY (1989) Studies of inositol phospholipid-specific phospholipase C. *Science* **244:** 546–550.

Ryan JP, Spinks NR, O'Neill C & Wales RG (1990) Implantation potential and fetal viability of mouse embryos cultured in media supplemented with platelet-activating factor. *Journal of Reproduction and Fertility* **89:** 309–315.

Saksena SK, Lau IF & Chang MC (1976) Relationship between oestrogen, prostaglandin $F_{2\alpha}$ and histamine in delayed implantation in the mouse. *Acta Endocrinologica* **42:** 225–232.

Salamonsen SA, Stuchbery SJ, O'Grady CM, Godkin JD & Findlay JK (1988) Interferon-α mimics effects of ovine trophoblast protein 1 on prostaglandin and protein secretion by ovine endometrial cells in vitro. *Journal of Endocrinology* **117:** R1–R4.

Satyaswaroop PG, Bressler RS, Delapina MM & Gurpide E (1979) Isolation and culture of human endometrial glands. *Journal of Clinical Endocrinology and Metabolism* **48:** 639–641.

Schatz F, Markiewicz L, Barg P & Gurpide E (1985) In vitro effects of ovarian steroids on prostaglandin $F_{2\alpha}$ output by human endometrium and endometrial epithelial cells. *Journal of Clinical Endocrinology and Metabolism* **61:** 361–367.

Seilhamer JJ, Randall TL, Yamanaka M & Johnson LK (1986) Pancreatic phospholipase A_2: isolation of the human gene and cDNAs from porcine pancreas and human lung. *DNA* **5:** 519–527.

Seilhamer JJ, Pruzanski W, Vadas P et al (1989a) Cloning and recombinant expression of phospholipase A_2 present in rheumatoid arthritic synovial fluid. *Journal of Biological Chemistry* **264:** 5335–5338.

Seilhamer JJ, Randall TL, Johnson LK et al (1989b) Novel gene exon homologous to pancreatic phospholipase A_2: sequence and chromosomal mapping of both human genes. *Journal of Cellular Biochemistry* **39:** 327–337.

Shutt DA & Lopata A (1981) The secretion of hormones during the culture of human preimplantation embryos with corona cells. *Fertility and Sterility* **35:** 413–416.

Singh EJ, Baccarini IM & Zuspan FP (1975) Levels of prostaglandins $F_{2\alpha}$ and E_2 in human endometrium during the menstrual cycle. *American Journal of Obstetrics and Gynecology* **121:** 1003–1006.

Smith SK & Kelly RW (1987) The effect of the antiprogestins RU486 and ZK98734 on the synthesis and metabolism of $PGF_{2\alpha}$ and PGE_2 in separated cells from early human decidua. *Journal of Clinical Endocrinology and Metabolism* **63:** 527–537.

Smith SK & Kelly RW (1988a) The release of $PGF_{2\alpha}$ and PGE_2 from separated cells of human endometrium and decidua. *Prostaglandins, Leukotrienes and Essential Fatty Acids* **33:** 91–96.

Smith SK & Kelly RW (1988b) Effect of platelet activating factor on the release of $PGF_{2\alpha}$ and PGE_2 by separated cells of human endometrium. *Journal of Reproduction and Fertility* **82:** 271–276.

Smith SK & Kelly RW (1990) The mechanisms of action of progesterone and the anti-progestin ZK 98734 on $PGF\alpha$ synthesis by early human decidua. *Prostaglandins* (in press).

Smith SK, Abel MK, Kelly RW & Baird DT (1982) The synthesis of prostaglandins from persistent proliferative endometrium. *Journal of Clinical Endocrinology and Metabolism* **55:** 284–289.

Smith SK, Abel MH & Baird DT (1984) Effects of 17 beta-estradiol and progesterone on the levels of prostaglandins F_2 alpha and E in human endometrium. *Prostaglandins* **27:** 591–597.

Spinks NR & O'Neill CO (1987) Embryo-derived PAF activity is essential for the establishment of pregnancy in the mouse. *Lancet* **i:** 106–107.

Spinks NR, Ryan JP & O'Neill CO (1990) Antagonists of embryo-derived platelet-activating factor act by inhibiting the ability of the mouse embryo to implant. *Journal of Reproduction and Fertility* **88:** 241–248.

Stewart HJ, McCann SHE, Barker PJ, Lee KE, Lamming GE & Flint APF (1987) Interferon sequence homology and receptor binding of ovine trophoblast antiluteolytic protein. *Journal of Endocrinology* **115:** R13–R15.

Streb H, Irvine RF, Berridge MJ & Schulz I (1983) Release of Ca^{2+} from a nonmitochondrial intracellular store in pancreatic acinar cells by inositol-1,4,5-trisphosphate. *Nature* **306:** 67–69.

Tawfik OW & Dey SK (1988) Further evidence for role of leukotrienes as mediators of decidualization in the rat. *Prostaglandins* **35:** 379–402.

Tawfik OW, Sagrillo C, Johnson DC & Dey SK (1987) Decidualization in the rat: role of leukotrienes and prostaglandins. *Prostaglandins, Leukotrienes and Medicine* **29:** 221–227.

Thatcher WW, Bartol FF, Knickerbocker JJ et al (1984) Maternal recognition of pregnancy in cattle. *Journal of Dairy Science* **67:** 2797–2811.

Toppozada M, El-Attar A, El-Ayatt MA & Khamis Y (1980) Management of uterine bleeding by PGs or their synthesis inhibition. *Advances in Prostaglandin and Thromboxane Research* **8:** 459–463.

Tsang BK & Ooi TC (1982) Prostaglandin secretion by human endometrium. *American Journal of Obstetrics and Gynecology* **142:** 626–633.

Vallet JL & Bazer FW (1989) Effect of ovine trophoblast protein-1, oestrogen and progesterone on oxytocin-induced phosphatidylinositol turnover in endometrium of sheep. *Journal of Reproduction and Fertility* **87:** 755–761.

Vallet JL, Bazer FW, Fliss MFV & Thatcher WW (1988) Effect of ovine conceptus secretory proteins and purified ovine trophoblast protein-1 on interoestrous interval and plasma concentrations of prostaglandins F-2α and E and 13,14-dihydro-15-keto prostaglandin F-2α in cyclic ewes. *Journal of Reproduction and Fertility* **84:** 493–504.

Van den Bosch H (1980) Intracellular phospholipase A_2. *Biochimica et Biophysica Acta* **604:** 191–195.

Vincent DL, Meredith S & Inskeep EK (1986) Advancement of uterine secretion of prostaglandin E_2 by treatment with progesterone and transfer of asynchronous embryos. *Endocrinology* **119:** 527–529.

Wilcox AJ, Weinberg CR, O'Connor JF et al (1988) Incidence of early pregnancy loss. *New England Journal of Medicine* **319:** 189–194.

Wiqvist N, Bygdeman M & Kirton K (1971) Non-steroidal infertility agents in the female. In Diczfalusy E & Borell B (eds) *Control of Human Fertility* **1:** 137, Nobel Symposium 15.

Yovich JL & Matson PL (1988) Early pregnancy wastage after gamete manipulation. *British Journal of Obstetrics and Gynaecology* **95:** 1120–1127.

Zarco L, Stabenfeldt GH, Kindahl H, Quirke JF & Granstrom E (1984) Persistence of luteal activity in the non-pregnant ewe. *Animal Reproduction Science* **7:** 245–267.

6

Endometrial prolactin and implantation

DAVID L. HEALY

The aim of this chapter is to review current knowledge regarding human endometrial prolactin, uterine receptivity and implantation. The study of human implantation is obviously restricted by many ethical considerations as well as many practical clinical restrictions. In spontaneous human implantation, the endometrial stroma undergoes terminal differentiation and this process is called decidualization. Decidualization is observed only in women and a few non-human primates, so limiting the opportunity of research in appropriate animal models. Furthermore, the study of human implantation following in vitro fertilization and embryo transfer have led to the concept of an 'implantation window' as the period of time when the uterine endometrium is receptive to an implanting blastocyst (Rogers et al, 1986). Uterine receptivity can now be defined morphologically following scanning electron micrograph studies (Rogers and Murphy, 1989) (Figures 1 and 2).

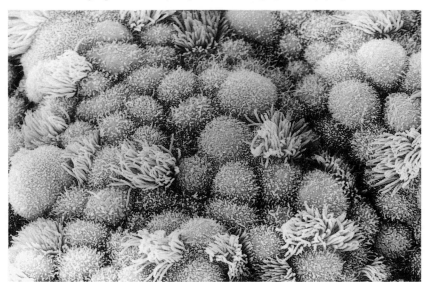

Figure 1. Scanning electron micrograph of a receptive human endometrium indicating bulging endometrial epithelial cell apices and short, sparse microvilli. (×3000, reduced to 68% on reproduction.) Courtesy of Dr Chris Murphy.

Baillière's Clinical Obstetrics and Gynaecology—
Vol. 5, No. 1, March 1991
ISBN 0–7020–1533–4

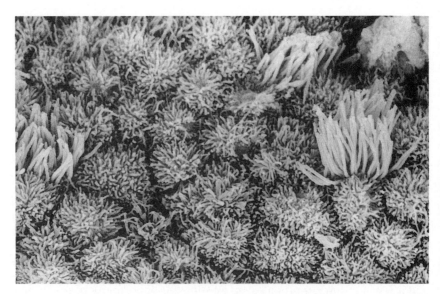

Figure 2. Scanning electron micrograph of a non-receptive human endometrial epithelial surface. Note that the epithelial surface is covered in microvilli. Note also that the microvilli are long, thin and regular, in contrast to those seen in a receptive endometrium shown in Figure 1. (×7200, reduced to 68% on reproduction.) Courtesy of Dr Chris Murphy.

PROLACTIN AND THE HUMAN UTERUS

Valid and sensitive radioimmunoassays for human prolactin (PRL) were initially reported in 1971 (Hwang et al, 1971). Application of this assay found PRL concentrations in human amniotic fluid up to 100-fold higher than in maternal blood. The major source of amniotic fluid PRL was initially thought to be either the maternal or the fetal pituitary, but no other maternal hormone with a molecular weight of approximately 20 kDa was known to cross the placenta to amniotic fluid in such concentrations. Furthermore, bromocriptine administration to pregnant women lowered maternal serum PRL values, but left amniotic fluid PRL values undisturbed. Whereas these data suggested the maternal pituitary was not the major source of amniotic fluid PRL, a major fetal source for amniotic fluid PRL was inconsistent with data that radiolabelled PRL injected into rhesus monkeys did not reach amniotic fluid. Moreover, fetal death in utero failed in lower amniotic fluid PRL values. It was therefore possible that amniotic fluid PRL was locally produced (Healy et al, 1977).

HUMAN ENDOMETRIAL AND DECIDUAL PROLACTIN SYNTHESIS

The placenta was the most obvious local source for high amniotic fluid PRL concentrations. However, placenta did not release PRL in organ culture and did not stain with anti-PRL antiserum when examined by immuno-fluorescence. Several groups then reported the identification of immuno-reactive material identical to pituitary PRL in chorion laeve freed from the amnion, but containing cells from the subjacent decidua parietalis (Golander et al, 1978; Healy et al, 1979). Active peptide synthesis of PRL was indicated, in that cyclohexamide and puromycin suppressed PRL secretion from this tissue. Moreover, labelled amino acid incorporation into a protein which behaved identically to human pituitary PRL in bioassay was demonstrated. Nevertheless, the precise tissue origin of this decidual chorionic PRL remained uncertain until Riddick and co-workers identified PRL, not only in the endometrium of women carrying an ectopic pregnancy, but also in normal secretory endometrium from day 22 of the menstrual cycle (Maslar and Riddick, 1979; Maslar et al, 1980).

The conclusion that endometrial decidua, a mesodermal tissue, normally synthesized and released PRL was heretical when first presented in 1977. Although PRL secretion had been reported from non-pituitary neoplasms, identification and release of classic pituitary hormones within a normal non-pituitary tissue were novel. More recently, other data along similar lines have considerably broadened our concepts of hormonal secretion and function and generated many new hypotheses of the evolutionary origins of chemical messengers. Corroboratory evidence for endometrial secretion of a functional PRL molecule came from interaction of milligram amounts of this protein from amniotic fluid and purification by affinity chromatography, which revealed that the 25 N-terminal amino acid sequence was identical to pituitary PRL (Shome and Parlow, 1977). Moreover, decidual amniotic fluid PRL molecules had potent bioactivities in vitro. In addition, expression of the PRL gene by identification of PRL messenger RNA (Clements et al, 1983) in decidua reinforced the view that decidual PRL was a functional molecule of endometrial origin. More recently, PRL synthesis and secretion have also been identified in myometrium (Walters et al, 1983; Rein et al, 1990).

GLYCOSYLATED PROLACTIN

Glycosylated PRL (G-PRL) is identical in aminoacid sequence to the major form of PRL but has a carbohydrate unit of 2 kDa molecular weight on an asparagine residue and accounts for 1–15% of pituitary PRL (Lewis et al, 1984). G-PRL has been identified in amniotic fluid, as a secretory product of luteal phase endometrium and in term decidual tissue. It appears that G-PRL is the predominant form of PRL secreted in the late luteal phase of the menstrual cycle (Markoff and Lee, 1987). It can be identified in the peripheral circulation at this time. The biological significance of G-PRL at this time is uncertain, although ovine G-PRL has been reported to have reduced lactogenic bioactivity compared with ovine PRL, while porcine G-PRL has been claimed to have enhanced activity compared with the non-glycosylated form of porcine PRL. These differences may relate to the differences in carbohydrate composition.

In pregnancy, decidual explants secrete less G-PRL than non-glycosylated PRL. As pregnancy advances, less and less G-PRL is secreted, as determined by sodium dodecyl sulphate polyacrylamide gel electrophoresis. Before pregnancy, serum G-PRL was the predominant PRL form in the peripheral circulation, and as pregnancy progressed, increasing amounts of PRL, compared with G-PRL, appeared in serum, reaching a maximum by the third trimester (Markoff et al, 1988).

REGULATION OF ENDOMETRIAL AND DECIDUAL PROLACTIN SECRETION

Although dopamine inhibits and thyrotrophin releasing hormone (TRH) stimulates the synthesis and release of pituitary PRL, neither dopamine nor TRH affects the synthesis or release of decidual PRL. Furthermore, the intracellular localization of PRL in decidual tissue is different from that in the pituitary. Pituitary PRL is localized in typical cytoplasmic secretory granules, while decidual PRL is localized in the postmicrosomal supernatant and not in granules at all. Anterior pituitary cells, which are of ectodermal origin, share common cell surface antigens such as chromogranin, a major soluble protein in secretory vesicles. Decidual cells do not contain chromogranin, consistent with their mesodermal origin, suggesting there are major differences in the cell surface antigens of these two PRL producing tissues (Markoff et al, 1982).

Despite these differences between pituitary and uterine PRL, calcium and progesterone appear capable of stimulating PRL secretion from both tissues (Table 1). While progesterone stimulation of decidual PRL secretion presumably acts via the decidual progesterone receptor, which is itself oestrogen dependent, the addition of oestradiol to the progesterone diminishes decidual PRL synthesis. Surprisingly, the reverse appears to be true for myometrial PRL secretion. Such an oestrogen–progesterone interdependence is similar to the oestrogen–progesterone synergy previously demonstrated to stimulate pituitary PRL secretion, and this stimulatory

Table 1. Regulation of human endometrial/decidual PRL secretion.

Effect	Agent	Concentration
Stimulation	Progesterone	$1–100$ ng/ml
	IGF-1	100 ng/ml
	Calcium	10^{-3} mol/litre
Inhibition	Arachidonic acid	$10^{-4}–10^{-5}$ mol/litre
No effect	TRH	$10^{-3}–10^{-9}$ mol/litre
	Dopamine	$10^{-5}–10^{-9}$ mol/litre
	Bromocriptine	$10^{-7}–10^{-10}$ mol/litre
	Oestradiol	10^{-6} mol/litre
	$PGF_{2\alpha}$ PGE_2	$10^{-5}–10^{-12}$ mol/litre
	Dibutyryl cyclic AMP	10^{-3} mol/litre
	Indomethacin	10^{-4} mol/litre

mechanism appears common at both sites of PRL secretion in women (Williams et al, 1981).

Calcium also appears to stimulate both pituitary and decidual PRL secretion, whereas arachidonic acid has been reported to inhibit decidual PRL release. More recently, insulin-like growth factor-1 (IGF-1), a polypeptide growth factor implicated in the oestrogen-promoted growth of reproductive tissues, has been found in high concentration in the pig uterus, and IGF-1 has been shown to stimulate the release and secretion of PRL from human decidua (Thrailkill et al, 1988).

PROLACTIN RECEPTORS IN PREGNANCY TISSUES

A mandatory prerequisite for any biological action of endometrial or decidual PRL upon human endometrium would be the demonstration of PRL receptors, since interaction with receptors is assumed to be the first step in the mechanism of action of protein hormones. No PRL receptors have been identified in human endometrium.

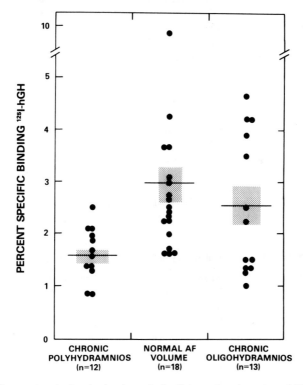

Figure 3. PRL receptors in the chorion laeve indicating a reduced number of PRL receptors from the chorion of patients with chronic polyhydramnios. Note the reduced percentage of specific binding from cases of chronic polyhydramnios when compared with pregnancies showing normal amniotic fluid volume or from patients with chronic oligohydramnios. From Healy et al (1985), with permission.

We have identified a PRL binding site in human chorion laeve. The binding affinity $(0.47 \times 10^9$ litres/pmol and capacity (175 fmol/ml) in this tissue are similar to those described for PRL receptors in liver and mammary gland. Small amounts of this receptor also appeared within placental preparations, in keeping with the identical origin of the chorion laeve and chorion frondosum. No PRL-binding sites were identified in decidua, amnion or umbilical cord. However, others have suggested the presence of PRL receptors in human amnion after studying water transport before and after in vitro exposure of amnion to an antibody directed towards a partially purified rabbit PRL receptor (Tyson et al, 1985). A reduced number of PRL receptors have been reported in patients with chronic polyhydramnios and may be responsible for the excess amniotic fluid in these women (Healy et al, 1985) (Figure 3).

PROLACTIN AND PROSTAGLANDINS

Prolactin stimulates prostaglandins E and $F_{2\alpha}$ (PGE and $PGF_{2\alpha}$) secretion from rat granulosa cells at low concentrations, while inhibiting their secretion at high concentrations (Knazek et al, 1981). Similar results have been obtained by infusing PRL into the isolated superior mesenteric artery vascular bed of the rat. We have previously hypothesized that a function of the chorionic PRL receptor may be to modulate prostaglandin synthesis from these fetal membranes. Indeed, ovine PRL has been reported to reduce PGE output from human amniochorion by 39–59% (Tyson et al, 1985), suggesting that endogenous PRL released by human decidual tissue might also inhibit the elaboration of PGE within the fetal membranes.

More recently, we examined the hypothesis that endometrial PRL may inhibit endometrial prostaglandin production. Human endometrial explants from the late luteal phase, incubated on stainless steel grids in 35-mm culture dishes in medium M199 with added progesterone or prolactin (460, 46, 4.6 units/litre) and maintained in culture for 3 days, with a medium change every 24 h, were assayed for PGE and $PGF_{2\alpha}$. Progesterone decreased PGE and $PGF_{2\alpha}$ production to within 64% of control cultures with no added treatments, as expected from earlier data. The response to PRL was variable. PRL (460 units/litre) increased PGE released in three of nine subjects (mean 144% of control). At a PRL concentration of 46 units/litre, PGE release was increased in tissue from only one of four subjects, decreased in one of four and not changed in the tissue from two remaining subjects tested at this concentration. By contrast, PGE was released by histamine in tissues from all subjects. It appears that PRL gives no clear dose–response changes in PGE or $PGF_{2\alpha}$ release and is not central in the control of human endometrial prostaglandin secretion.

PROLACTIN AND MENSTRUATION

It will now be clear to readers of this book that human endometrium is an active endocrine organ capable of secreting many substances (Healy and Hodgen, 1983). It is surprising how little information is available about the composition of menstrual blood, although PRL and prostaglandins are known to be two hormones or hormonal groups released from secretory endometrium into the menstrual fluid. Fraser and colleagues (Zhou et al, 1989) have demonstrated that PRL concentrations in menstrual fluid on day 1 of menses were fivefold higher than the median peripheral prolactin levels. Menstrual PRL concentrations decline quickly from the first to the third day of menstrual flow, showing an exponential fall with time from the onset of menstruation. Since it has been demonstrated that defective luteal phase endometrium produces significantly less PRL than normal endometrium, it is possible that endometrial PRL may have a role in the mechanism of normal or abnormal menstruation. However, menstrual PRL concentrations from patients with abnormal menstrual cycles are not yet determined and no clinical value of this measurement is yet clear (Daly et al, 1981; Ying et al, 1985).

Administration of PRL has been reported to increase blood pressure in rabbits and rats, suggesting that PRL is involved in blood pressure regulation or is vasoactive in mammals. Support for this view comes from studies in which administration of antiserum to PRL lowers blood pressure in neonatal rats (Mills et al, 1982). Nevertheless, the role of PRL in the pathophysiology of hypertension is controversial. While suppression of circulating PRL by bromocriptine can be associated with a decrease in blood pressure in hypertensive individuals, it remains to be established whether this is a central effect or a peripheral action of PRL.

PRL receptors have not been reported on endothelium or blood vessels and no direct effect of endometrial PRL on menstruation has been substantiated. Nevertheless, vasoactive substances such as vasoactive intestinal peptide appear to be physiological mediators of PRL release, at least in the rat (Abe et al, 1985), and it remains possible that PRL may affect endometrial vasoactive substances in the human. One candidate for a possible effect of endometrial prolactin is endothelin. Endothelin is a potent vasoconstrictor peptide ($EC_{50} = 0.4$ nm) which was first isolated and purified from media conditions by porcine aortic endothelial cells (Yanagisawa et al, 1988). Endothelin is a twenty-one amino acid peptide derived by two proteolytic cleavage steps via a 30 amino acid 'big endothelin' from proendothelin. Endothelin mRNA is synthesized in close proximity to endothelin binding sites in many organs, suggesting a local action (MacCumber et al, 1989). The human endothelin-1 gene was cloned in 1988 (Itoh et al, 1988), and subsequently two additional genes have been identified (Inoue et al, 1989). Endothelin-2 and endothelin-3 differ from endothelin-1 by 2 aminoacids respectively (Inoue et al, 1989). Endothelin-1 exists in many organs, such as the lung and kidney, and a recent support has suggested endothelin production by epithelial cells of the immature rat endometrium (Orlando et al, 1990). Therefore, the endometrium may be an important site for the production of endothelin, not only by endothelial cells but also by epithelial cells, and it is possible that prolactin may regulate these activities.

Prolactin has some effects on blood flow: it can lower blood pressure and increase cardiac output in intact rats. In isolated preparations, PRL concentrations up to 100 ng/ml have no direct effects themselves but have been reported to potentiate responses to pressure agents, such as noradrenaline (Karmazyn et al, 1982). PRL concentrations above 200 ng/ml have been claimed to inhibit vascular responses, including changes in mammary blood flow in lactating animals. These peripheral vascular effects seem to be dependent on the stimulation of prostaglandin synthesis.

PRL receptors have not been found in the heart, although PRL has been demonstrated to stimulate cardiac ornithine decarboxylase, nor have they been reported on endothelium or blood vessels and no direct effect of endometrial PRL on menstruation has been substantiated.

PROLACTIN AND IMMUNOREGULATION

Synthesis of various classic hormones by immunological tissues and cells is now confirmed in a number of species. Such data suggest that endocrine mechanisms may have an immunomodulatory role beyond the activation of the pituitary–adrenocortical axis as a result of stress. Several lines of evidence indicate that PRL may be an important immunoregulatory hormone. In rats, both hypophysectomy and treatment with bromocriptine inhibit the development of delayed cutaneous hypersensitivity and other immunological reactions. Treatment with oxygenous PRL reverses these immunosuppressive effects. Hypopituitary mice develop impaired cellular immunity and this immunodeficiency is prevented by injections of milk, a PRL source.

Replication of cultured nb2 node rat lymphoma cells is specifically stimulated by lactogenic hormones such as PRL and has been used as a PRL bioassay. In these cells, the activity of the enzyme ornithine decarboxylase becomes undetectable when the cells are incubated in PRL-deficient media. This appears to be due to an inhibitor of this enzyme. Addition of PRL blocks synthesis of this inhibitor, increasing ornithine decarboxylase concentrations and promoting growth of these lymphoma cells. In hypoprolactinaemic mice, there is suppression of macrophage activation and T-lymphocyte function (Bernton et al, 1988). Of the multiple events leading to macrophage activation in vivo, the production by T lymphocytes of interferon (IFN) was the most impaired in bromocriptine treated mice.

In mice, lymphocytes appear to constitute an important target tissue for PRL, which seems necessary for the normal production of macrophage activating factors, including IFN. Addition of IFN-α over a dose range 0.5–50 units/ml to human endometrial explants lowers PRL secretion to 69.0 $\pm$ 10.2% of control cultures (Healy et al, 1990). Since human IFN-α has sequence homology to ovine trophoblast protein 1 and is found in high concentration in human pregnancy and fetal tissues, it is possible that human interferon may regulate endometrial and decidual PRL secretion. However, evidence of this interaction between endometrial PRL and the immunological response to implantation is still preliminary and awaits further study.

FUTURE DIRECTIONS

Bioactive PRL is synthesized and released in increasing amounts by decidualized human endometrium from implantation. Endometrial PRL is glycosylated and glycosylated human PRL may have different biological activities to the non-glycosylated forms of this hormone. It is possible that endometrial PRL is a paracrine hormone with local actions influencing implantation or menstruation. Whether endometrial PRL influences the production of endothelin from human endometrium awaits further study.

SUMMARY

The role of prolactin in human implantation and human endometrial function is still unclear. Synthesis of prolactin from human endometrium and decidua was first demonstrated in 1977. Prolactin mRNA isolation from term decidua subsequently confirmed expression of the prolactin gene in human endometrium. More recently, a glycosylated form of prolactin has been isolated from both the human pituitary and human endometrium. It appears that predominately glycosylated prolactin is secreted in the late luteal phase of the menstrual cycle, with increasingly greater amounts of non-glycosylated prolactin secreted as pregnancy advances. The biological significance and regulation of prolactin glycosylation is uncertain, although glycosylated ovine prolactin has only 20–33% of the lactogenic activity of ovine prolactin. Pituitary lactotropes, of ectodermal origin, produce pituitary prolactin and are regulated by dopamine, oestradiol and thyrotropin releasing hormone. Decidual cells, of mesodermal origin, are not influenced by these pituitary secretogogues. Progesterone and calcium both appear to stimulate pituitary and decidual prolactin secretion, while arachidonic acid seems to inhibit decidual prolactin release. More recently, insulin like growth factor-1, a polypeptide growth factor implicated in the oestrogen promoted growth reproductive tissues, has been found in high concentration in the pig uterus and has been shown to stimulate the synthesis and secretion of prolactin from human decidua. Prolactin receptors have not been reported on endothelium of blood vessels and no clear evidence exists that endometrial prolactin may modulate the secretion of endothelin, endothelium derived relaxing factor or other potentially important substances controlling menstruation. Prolactin does appear necessary for the normal production of macrophage activating factors, including interferon, and may have a local immunomodulatory role upon human implantation for this reason. Human α_2-interferon has sequence homology to ovine trophoblast protein-1 and is found in high concentration in human pregnancy and fetal tissues. There is some evidence that interferon may reduce human endometrial prolactin secretion, but whether endometrial or decidual prolactin is critical to human implantation awaits further study.

Acknowledgements

This study is supported by the NH & MRC of Australia. Mrs Marilyn Pfisterer provided secretarial assistance.

REFERENCES

Abe H, Ingler D, Molitch M, Mollinger-Gruber J & Reichlin S (1985) Vasoactive intestinal peptide is a physiological mediator of prolactin release in the rat. *Endocrinology* **116:** 1383–1390.

Bernton EW, Meltzer MS & Holaday JW (1988) Suppression of macrophage activation and T-lymphocyte function in hypoprolactinemic mice. *Science* **239:** 401–404.

Clements RJ, Crooks N, Healy DL, Shine J, Thunder JW & Whitfield P (1983) Expression of the prolactin gene in human decidua chorion. *Endocrinology* **112:** 1133–1134.

Daly DC, Maslar IA, Rosenberg SN, Tohann N & Riddick DH (1981) Prolactin production by luteal phase defect endometrium. *American Journal of Obstetrics and Gynecology* **140:** 587–591.

Golander A, Hurley T, Barrett J, Hizi A & Handwerger S (1978) Prolactin synthesis by human chorion-decidual tissue: a possible source of prolactin in the amniotic fluid. *Science* **202:** 311–313.

Healy DL & Hodgen GD (1983) The endocrinology of human endometrium. *Obstetrics and Gynaecology Survey* **38:** 509–530.

Healy DL, Muller HK & Burger HG (1977) Immunofluorescence localization of prolactin to human amnion. *Nature* **265:** 642–643.

Healy DL, Kimpton WG, Muller HK & Burger HG (1979) The synthesis of immunoreactive prolactin by decidua-chorion. *British Journal of Obstetrics and Gynaecology* **86:** 307–313.

Healy DL, Herrington AC & O'Herlihy C (1985) Chronic polyhydramnios is a syndrome with a lactogen receptor defect in the chorion laeve. *British Journal of Obstetrics and Gynaecology* **92:** 461–467.

Healy DL, Salamonsen L, Moon J, Cameron IT & Findlay JK (1990) Human endometrial prolactin. In D'Arcangues C (ed.) *Contraception and Mechanisms of Endometrial Bleeding*, pp 213–226. Cambridge: Cambridge University Press.

Hwang P, Guyda H & Friesen H (1971) A radioimmunoassay for human prolactin. *Proceedings of the National Academy of Sciences of the USA* **68:** 1092–1096.

Inoue A, Yanagisawa M, Kimura S et al (1989) The human endothelin family: three structurally and pharmacologically distinct isopeptides predicted by three separate genes. *Proceedings of the National Academy of Sciences of the USA* **86:** 2863–2867.

Itoh Y, Yanagisiwa M, Ohkuvo S et al (1988) Cloning and sequence analysis of cDNA in coding the precursor of a human endothelium-derived vasoconstrictor peptide, endothelin: identity of human and porcine endothelin. *FEBS Letters* **231:** 440–444.

Karmazyn M, Daly MJ, Moffat MP & Dhalla NS (1982) A possible mechanism of inotropic action of prolactin on rat heart. *American Journal of Physiology* **243:** E458–E463.

Knazek RA, Cristy RJ, Watson KC et al (1981) Prolactin modifies follicle-stimulating hormone-induced prostaglandin synthesis by the rat granulosa cell. *Endocrinology* **109:** 1566–1572.

Lewis UJ, Singh RN, Lewis LJ, Seavey BK & Sinha YN (1984) Glycosylated ovine prolactin. *Proceedings of the National Academy of Sciences of the USA* **81:** 385–389.

MacCumber MW, Ross CA, Glaser BM & Snider SH (1989) Endothelin: visualization of mRNAs by DNA hybridization provides evidence for local action. *Proceedings of the National Academy of Sciences of the USA* **86:** 7285–7289.

Markoff E & Lee DW (1987) Glycosylated prolactin is a major circulating variant in human serum. *Journal of Clinical Endocrinology and Metabolism* **65:** 1102–1106.

Markoff E, Barry S & Handwerger S (1982) Influence of osmolality and ionic environment on the secretion of prolactin by human decidua in vitro. *Journal of Endocrinology* **92:** 103–110.

Markoff E, Lee DW & Hollingsworth DR (1988) Glycosylated and non-glycosylated prolactin in serum during pregnancy. *Journal of Clinical Endocrinology and Metabolism* **67:** 519–523.

Maslar IA & Riddick DH (1979) Prolactin production by human endometrium in the normal menstrual cycle. *American Journal of Obstetrics and Gynecology* **135:** 751–754.

Maslar IA, Kaplan BM, Luciano AA & Riddick DH (1980) Prolactin production by the endometrium of early human pregnancy. *Journal of Clinical Endocrinology and Metabolism* **51:** 78–83.

Mills DE, Buchman MT & Peake GT (1982) Neonatal treatment with anti-serum to prolactin lowers blood pressure in rats. *Science* **217**: 162–164.

Orlando C, Brandi ML, Peri A et al (1990) Neurohypophyseal hormonal regulation of endothelin secretion from rabbit endometrial cells in primary culture. *Endocrinology* **126**: 1780–1793.

Rein MS, Friedman AJ & Heffner LJ (1990) Decreased prolactin secretion by explant cultures of fibroids from women treated with gonadotrophin releasing hormone agonist. *Journal of Clinical Endocrinology and Metabolism* **70**: 1554–1558.

Rogers PAW & Murphy CR (1989) Uterine receptivity for implantation: human studies. In Yoshinaga K (ed.) *Blastocyst Implantation*, Serono Symposia, USA, 1989, pp 231–238 Boston: Adams Publishing Group.

Rogers PAW, Milne BJ & Trounson AO (1986) A model to show human uterine receptivity and embryo viability following ovarian stimulation for in vitro fertilization. *Journal of In Vitro Fertilization and Embryo Transfer* **3**: 93–98.

Shome B & Parlow AF (1977) Human pituitary prolactin: the entire linea amino acid sequence. *Journal of Clinical Endocrinology and Metabolism* **45**: 1112–1115.

Thrailkill KM, Golander A, Underwood LE & Handwertger S (1988) Insulin-like growth factor 1 stimulates the synthesis and release of prolactin from human decidual cells. *Endocrinology* **123**: 2930–2934.

Tyson JE, McCoshen JA & Dubin NH (1985) Inhibition of fetal membrane prostaglandin production by prolactin: relative importance in the initiation of labor. *American Journal of Obstetrics and Gynecology* **151**: 1032–1038.

Walters CA, Daly DC, Chapitis J & Riddick DH (1983) Human endometrium: a new potential source of prolactin. *American Journal of Obstetrics and Gynecology* **147**: 639–644.

Williams RF, Barber DL, Cowan BD, Lynch A, Marut EL & Hodgen GD (1981) Hyper-prolactinemia in monkeys: induction by an oestrogen–progesterone synergy. *Steroids* **38**: 321–331.

Yanagisawa SL, Kurihara H, Kimura S, Tomboe Y et al (1988) A novel potent vasoconstrictor peptide produced by vascular endothelial cells. *Nature* **332**: 411–415.

Ying YK, Walters CA, Cuslas S, Lin JT, Daly DC & Riddick DH (1985) Prolactin production by decidual cells of normal luteal phase defective and corrected luteal phase defective late secretory endometrium. *American Journal of Obstetrics and Gynecology* **151**: 801–804.

Zhou JP, Fraser IS, Cateoson I et al (1989) Reproductive hormones in menstrual blood. *Journal of Clinical Endocrinology and Metabolism* **69**: 338–342.

7

Immunocytochemical localization of oestradiol and progesterone receptors in human endometrium: a tool to assess endometrial maturation

Ph. BOUCHARD
J. MARRAOUI
M. R. MASSAI
D. A. MEDALIE
D. DE ZIEGLER
M. PERROT-APPLANAT
R. FRYDMAN
C. BERGERON

Implantation is determined by the adequacy of endometrium maturation. Appreciation of the endometrial status is therefore mandatory in order to assess infertile women and to determine the quality of the endometrium after therapeutic induction of ovulation or during hormonal therapy. The classic histological changes described by Noyes et al (1950) have been widely used for histological dating of the human endometrium. Such criteria, however, are unable to provide useful information on the preovulatory phase of the cycle and have generated some controversy, especially with regard to assessing the luteal phase defects (Tin-Chiu et al, 1988). Endometrial morphology is strongly influenced by sex steroids. The steroid control of the endometrium is mediated by oestradiol and progesterone via their respective intracellular (intranuclear) receptors. In addition endometrial oestrogen (ER) and progesterone (PR) receptors are regulated by oestradiol and progesterone in the endometrium (Bayard et al, 1978). Variations in endometrial ER and PR levels during the menstrual cycle have been described by the binding technique using radioactive steroids which does not take into account the differences in receptor content of the various cell types and is prone to error due to receptor occupancy (Vu Hai et al, 1977; Savouret et al, 1989).

Endometrial oestrogen and progesterone receptor staining by immunocytochemical techniques, therefore, may provide useful information on the hormonal status and on the interactions between epithelial and stromal cells in the endometrium. We have studied the distribution of endometrial ER and

Baillière's Clinical Obstetrics and Gynaecology—
Vol. 5, No. 1, March 1991
ISBN 0–7020–1533–4

107

PR using monoclonal antibodies against ER and PR during the normal menstrual cycle as well as in endometrial samples obtained from anovulatory women or women with inactive ovaries receiving various hormonal treatments.

METHODS

Biopsies were performed with Novak's cannula or Cornier's aspiration pipette (Laboratoire CCD, Paris, France). Each sample was divided in two parts: one part was frozen in isopentane precooled in liquid nitrogen and stored in liquid nitrogen until processing; the second half was fixed in Bouin's solution and processed for histology.

Endometrial samples were sectioned (4 μm thick) at −24°C and thaw-mounted on gelatin-coated glass slides. The peroxidase-antiperoxidase method was used on frozen sections after fixation with picric acid formaldehyde. The slides were blocked with normal goat or rabbit serum for 10 min before exposure to the first antibody. The antiprogesterone antibody LET 126 (25 μg ml^{-1}) was used (Perrot-Applanat et al, 1987; Lorenzo et al, 1988). ER immunostaining was performed with a kit from Abbott Laboratories (North Chicago Il, USA). Details of the procedure have been described elsewhere (Perrot-Applanat et al, 1987; Garcia et al, 1988).

Controls included immunostaining with mouse receptors unrelated monoclonal antibody and rat normal immunoglobulins. In addition, monoclonal anti PR antibody was presaturated with highly purified PR (Logeat et

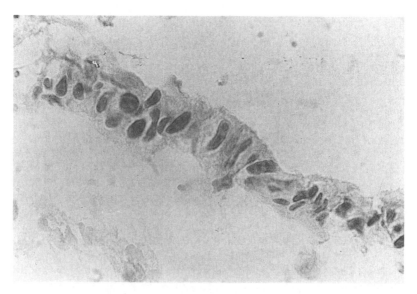

Figure 1. Nuclear localization of PR in glandular cells on day 17 of a normal cycle (× 400, reproduced at 70% of original).

al, 1985). The staining patterns were similar when other monoclonal anti PR antibodies directed against different epitopes of the receptor were used (Lorenzo et al, 1988).

The intensity of specific staining was characterized as absent (0), +, ++ or +++, and the number of stained cells was estimated as absent (0), 25%, 50% or 75%.

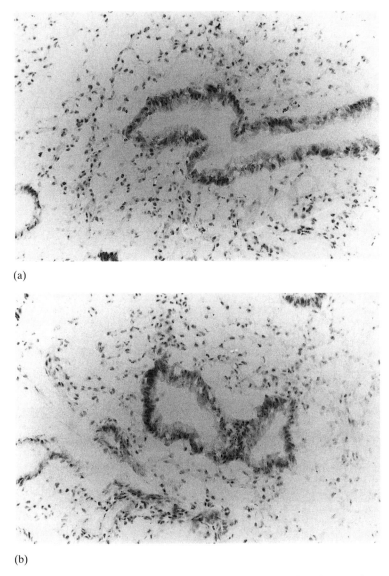

(a)

(b)

Figure 2. Immunostaining of PR and ER during the periovulatory period of a normal menstrual cycle. Glands and stroma are visible in all sections. (a) staining for PR (×250, reproduced at 70% of original); (b) staining for ER (×250, reproduced at 70% of original).

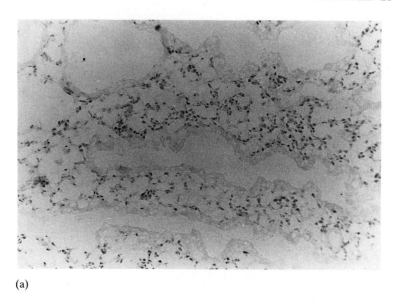

(a)

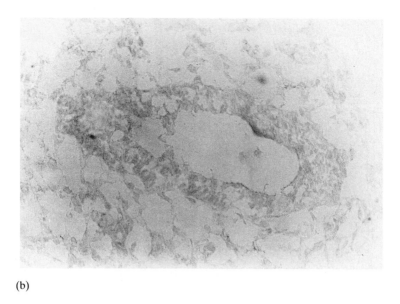

(b)

Figure 3. Immunocytochemical staining for PR (a) and ER (b) on day 24 of a normal cycle (×250, reproduced at 70% of original).

IMMUNOSTAINING OF NORMAL ENDOMETRIUM DURING THE MENSTRUAL CYCLE

Endometrial tissue samples were obtained from 30 normal women aged (18–40 years) participating in an in vitro fertilization programme for male infertility (Garcia et al, 1988). All women had a regular cycle and had not had any hormonal therapy for the previous 6 months.

The specific staining was always localized in cell nuclei throughout the menstrual cycle (Figure 1).

Follicular phase

In the mid-follicular phase, stromal and glandular cells were equally marked for ER and PR. During the late follicular phase, glandular cells were more heavily stained and ER staining was less intense than PR staining (Figure 2).

Luteal phase

Endometrial oestrogen receptors

Glandular cell staining decreased on day 21 and disappeared thereafter (Figure 3b).

Progesterone receptors

In the mid and late luteal phase, the intensity of staining and percentage of stained glandular cells decreased markedly, although PR staining in glandular cells persisted longer than that of ER (day 22 versus day 21). After day 22, no stained glandular cells were seen in virtually all the women. Staining of stromal cells remained quasi identical to the late follicular phase pattern (Figure 3a).

IMMUNOSTAINING OF THE ENDOMETRIUM FROM ANOVULATORY WOMEN

Immunostaining of endometrial biopsies obtained from women with anovulation due to polycystic ovary syndrome was studied (Garcia et al, 1988). All biopsies showed a typical mid-cycle pattern with a moderate staining for ER and a strong staining for PR (data not shown).

EFFECT OF OESTROGEN AND PROGESTERONE THERAPY ON THE ENDOMETRIUM OF WOMEN WITH OVARIAN FAILURE

In patients with ovarian failure, endometrial tissue can be receptive to embryonic implantation after substitution therapy with oestrogens and progesterone (Kretmann et al, 1979).

We studied the effect of increasing exogenous oral oestradiol and progesterone replacement therapy (300 mg/day by the vaginal route) in 16 women undergoing an ovocyte donation programme. Immunocytochemical analysis showed a typical late luteal phase aspect 6 days after commencing treatment with progesterone (Figure 4).

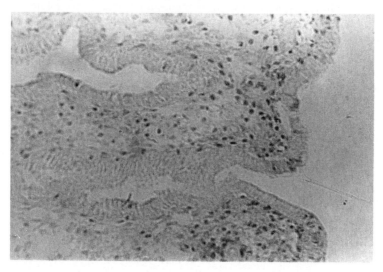

Figure 4. Typical PR staining on day 24 of a treatment regimen of oral oestradiol from day 1 to 28 followed by vaginal progesterone from day 15 to 28 in a woman with inactive ovaries (× 250, reproduced at 75% of original).

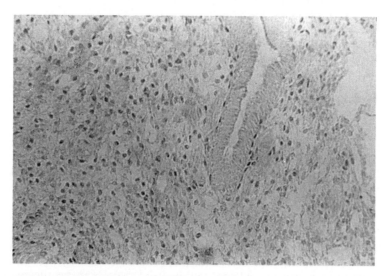

Figure 5. Typical staining on day 24 of a treatment regimen of oral oestradiol from day 1 to 14, followed by vaginal progesterone from day 15 to 28 in a woman with inactive ovaries (× 250, reproduced at 75% of original).

ROLE OF OESTRADIOL AND PROGESTERONE IN THE LUTEAL PHASE

In women with inactive ovaries we administered a treatment regimen of transdermal oestradiol from day 1 to 14 followed by vaginal progesterone from day 15 to 28. The immunocytochemical study of endometrial fragments obtained on day 24 showed the receptor distribution seen on day 24 of a normal menstrual cycle, i.e. ER and PR disappearance in the glands (Figure 5).

ER AND PR IN HUMAN UTERINE ARTERIES

The presence of ER and PR in spiral arteries of the human uterus was observed in endometrial biopsies (functionalis endometrium) at the end of the luteal phase (Figure 6) (Perrot-Applanat et al, 1988). Specific staining occurred in smooth muscle cells.

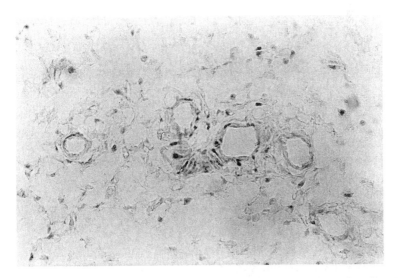

Figure 6. PR immunostaining of human uterine arteries on day 27 of a normal cycle ($\times 400$, reproduced at 70% of original).

DISCUSSION

Oestradiol and progesterone regulate endometrial growth via their intranuclear high affinity receptors. Classical binding studies indicate that receptor concentrations are highest in the late follicular phase and decrease thereafter due to progesterone secretion (Kretmann et al, 1979). Our studies allowed us to analyse the distribution of ER and PR in stromal and epithelial cells. The intense ER and PR staining during the midcycle period is likely to be correlated with the increased oestradiol secretion while the decrease and disappearance of ER and PR from glandular cells during the late luteal phase is probably due to the effect of progesterone. Our observations in anovulatory women confirm this hypothesis by showing a moderate labelling of glandular cells for ER and PR. Furthermore, endo-metrial fragments obtained from women with inactive ovaries treated with high doses of oestrogens and progesterone show a typical late luteal phase aspect, i.e. a disappearance of ER and PR in glandular cells following progesterone therapy. In addition, preliminary studies in women with inactive ovaries showed that treatment with progesterone alone (without oestradiol) during the luteal phase can reproduce the receptor distribution observed in the luteal phase of normal menstrual cycles. This suggests that progesterone plays a role in the disappearance of receptors in the glands during the luteal phase and may support the hypothesis that oestradiol may not be required for the secretory transformation of the endometrium.

The results obtained in normal endometrium as well as the data collected in anovulatory women and women treated for ovocyte donation suggest that receptor immunocytochemistry is useful for evaluating endometrial maturation by showing receptor increase due to the effect of oestradiol, while receptor disappearance in glandular cells is an index of the cumulative activity of progesterone. In addition, the presence of ER and PR in rabbit and human uterine arteries suggests that physiological uterine vascular changes, such as those observed during the menstrual cycle or during pregnancy, may be directly modulated by steroid hormones.

SUMMARY

Uterine oestrogen (ER) and progesterone (PR) receptors are subject to fine hormonal control by oestradiol and progesterone. In order to assess the role of ER and PR measurement in the evaluation of endometrial maturation, both receptors were studied by immunocytochemical techniques using monoclonal antibodies during the menstrual cycle, and in women with inactive ovaries treated by different regimens of hormonal substitution with oestradiol and progesterone.

During the normal menstrual cycle, the concentrations and distribution of ER and PR changed markedly. During the mid follicular period (days 7–8), a small proportion of stromal and glandular cells stained positively for PR while staining for ER was more intense and more frequent. During the late follicular phase and early luteal period (days 9–19), the staining for PR increased markedly in glandular cells. During the mid and late luteal phase (days 21–27), ER and PR staining disappeared in glandular cells. Thus, while oestradiol increases the staining for ER and PR in both glands and stroma, progesterone decreases ER and PR staining in the glands in a dramatic fashion. These variations, especially the disappearance of PR under the effect of progesterone, are potentially useful for studying the cumulative effect of progesterone on endometrial maturation. This was confirmed in anovulatory women, where a late luteal phase aspect was observed, i.e. the absence of a reduction in ER and PR in glandular cells. In women with ovarian failure, the disappearance of ER and PR in glandular cells is correlated with the duration of progesterone therapy. In addition, we observed a staining for PR in muscular cells of human uterine arteries suggesting a role for steroid hormones in uterine vascular changes during the menstrual cycle. Preliminary observations in women with ovarian failure suggest that oestradiol may not be necessary during the luteal phase to induce normal secretory transformations of the endometrium.

REFERENCES

Bayard F, Damilano S, Robel P & Baulieu EE (1978) Cytoplasmic and nuclear estradiol and progesterone receptors in human endometrium. *Journal of Clinical Endocrinology and Metabolism* **46**: 635–648.

Garcia E, Bouchard P, De Brux J et al (1988) Use of immunocytochemistry of progesterone and estrogen receptors for endometrial dating. *Journal of Clinical Endocrinology and Metabolism* **67**: 80–87.

Kretmann B, Bugat R & Bayard F (1979) Estrogen and progestin regulation of the progesterone receptor concentration in human endometrium. *Journal of Clinical Endocrinology and Metabolism* **49**: 926–929.

Logeat F, Pamphile R, Loosfelt H et al (1985) One step immunoaffinity purification of active progesterone receptors. Further evidence in favor of the existence of a single steroid binding subunit. *Biochemistry* **24**: 1029–1035.

Lorenzo F, Jolivet A, Loosfelt A et al (1988) A rapid method of epitope mapping. Application to the immunogenic domains and to the characterization of various forms of rabbit progesterone receptor. *European Journal of Biochemistry* **176**: 53–60.

Noyes RW, Hertig DT & Rock J (1950) Dating the endometrial biopsy. *Fertility and Sterility* **1**: 3–25.

Perrot-Applanat M, Groyer-Picard MT, Lorenzo F et al (1987) Immunocytochemical study with monoclonal antibodies to progesterone receptors in human breast tumors. *Cancer Research* **47**: 2652–2661.

Perrot-Applanat M, Groyer-Picart MT, Garcia E et al (1988) Immunocytochemical demonstration of estrogen and progesterone receptors in muscle cells of uterine arteries in rabbits and humans. *Endocrinology* **123**: 1511–1519.

Savouret JF, Misrahi M, Loosfelt H et al (1989) Molecular and cellular biology of mammalian progesterone receptors. *Recent Progress in Hormone Research* **45**: 65–120.

Tin-Chiu LI, Rogers WA, Dockery P et al (1988) A new method of histologic dating of human endometrium in the luteal phase. *Fertility and Sterility* **50**: 52–62.

Vu Hai MT, Logeat F, Warembourg M & Milgrom E (1977) Hormonal control of progesterone receptors. *Annals of the New York Academy of Sciences* **286**: 199–209.

8

Paracrine regulation of implantation and uterine function

J. K. FINDLAY
L. A. SALAMONSEN

Cells within an organ can communicate through the actions of local regulators, a concept which has received particular attention from those studying malignant transformation of cells (Sporn and Todaro, 1980). The speculation that local regulators may be involved in the processes of attachment, implantation, nutrition and growth of the conceptus was first made nearly 70 years ago (Corner, 1921). The uterine secretions or histotrophe were thought to carry the factors responsible (Amoroso, 1952). It is now appreciated that the communication may not just be from the endometrium to the conceptus but also vice versa and that it may also exist between cells within the endometrium itself. In addition to the major cell types (epithelial, stromal and decidual), endothelial cells of the blood vessels, transiently resident cells (macrophages, lymphocytes, mast cells) and even local regulators stored in the extracellular matrix may have paracrine functions (Figure 1). However, the factors responsible for local regulation and the mechanisms involved are only now being described. What is particularly interesting is the fact that many of the substances are chemically identical to or very similar to local regulators described for other tissues and physiological systems, such as those involved in the immune system and the control of cellular growth and differentiation.

It is convenient to define regulators according to their origin and site of action. Paracrine regulators are secreted by one or more groups of cells and move through the interstitial spaces to act on neighbouring target cells, whereas autocrine regulators act on the same cells which produce them. Local regulators can be factors which mediate or modulate the response of a tissue to stimulation by an endocrine hormone (originating in another organ), leading to localized differentiation and function of cells within that tissue. They can also co-ordinate other functions of cells, such as growth, which may or may not be endocrine dependent.

Based on the definitions of autocrine and paracrine regulation there are at least three criteria which should be satisfied in order to define a substance in one or other of these categories. They are:

1. Evidence of local production of the factor in a tissue, for example by

Baillière's Clinical Obstetrics and Gynaecology—
Vol. 5, No. 1, March 1991
ISBN 0–7020–1533–4

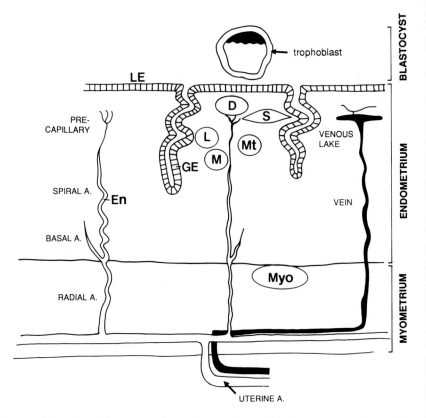

Figure 1. Potential cellular sources of paracrine regulators within the embryo–uterine unit. LE, luminal epithelium; GE, glandular epithelium; D, decidual cell; S, stromal cell; Mt, mast cell; Myo, myometrial cell; En, endothelial cell; M, macrophage; L, lymphocyte.

detection of the substances in the tissue, synthesis of its mRNA, and synthesis of the molecule itself both in vitro and, if possible, in vivo.
2. Evidence that endogenous production of the factor is hormonally and/or locally regulated.
3. Evidence that the factor has a biological effect via receptors on cells within the same tissue at physiologically meaningful concentrations.

Based on some or all of these criteria, the factors listed in Table 1 can be considered as potential para- or autocrine regulators within the uterus. The list includes data from a number of species, mostly laboratory or domestic experimental animals but including the human uterus and conceptus.

Regulation of implantation and uterine function by paracrine or autocrine factors could be very important for the following reasons. Their presence may add precision and local specificity to an otherwise indiscriminate stimulation of the tissue by a peripheral hormone. This would allow different cell types within the same tissue to have separate but co-ordinated growth and

Table 1. Potential local regulators in the endometrium and conceptus.

Epidermal growth factor (EGF)
Transforming growth factor α (TGF-α)
Insulin-like growth factor-1 (IGF-1)
Insulin-like growth factor-1 binding proteins (IGFBPs)
Colony stimulating factor-1 (CSF-1)
Granulocyte–macrophage colony stimulating factor (GM-CSF)
Tumour necrosis factor (TNF)
Transforming growth factor β (TGF-β)
Interleukins-1 and 6 (IL-1, IL-6)
Activin and inhibin (ACT-INH)
Interferon-α and γ (IFN-α, γ)
Platelet activating factor (PAF)
Prostaglandin (E and $F_{2\alpha}$) (PG)
Leukotrienes (LT)
Early pregnancy factor (EPF)
Histamine (Hist)
Oestromedins (OM)
Heparin binding growth factors (fibroblast growth factors, FGFs)
Platelet derived growth factor (PDGF)
Endothelin (ET)
Endothelium derived relaxing factor (EDRF)

From Bell and Smith (1988), Brigstock et al (1989), Pollard (1990), Findlay et al (1990) and Salamonsen and Findlay (1990a).

Table 2. Examples of uterine processes possibly under autocrine or paracrine regulation.

Process	Factor(s) involved
Endometrial cell proliferation	EGF, TGF-α, IGF-1, IGFBP, IL-1
Angiogenesis	FGF
Endometrial bleeding and haemostasis	EDRF, endothelin, PGs
Decidualization	PGs, histamine (?)
Immune suppression	IFN, TNF, IL
Conceptus and placental growth	CSF-1, EGF

differentiation under continued stimulation by the same peripheral hormone or hormones. The local regulators could also mediate the embryonic–maternal interactions necessary for ensuring a nutritional supply for the growing conceptus, the adjustment of the maternal immune system to prevent rejection and allow implantation, and the adaptation of the maternal endocrine system to maintain the function of the corpus luteum on the ovary and to make the other endocrine adjustments necessary for the establishment of pregnancy.

The purpose of this review is to provide examples of instances in which local regulation by paracrine or autocrine factors may be involved in the processes of implantation and uterine function (Table 2). Rather than trying to cover the whole field, specific examples will be described to illustrate the principles. The reader is referred to several recent reviews covering this subject in more detail (Bell and Smith, 1988; Brigstock et al, 1989; Findlay et al, 1990; Pollard, 1990; Salamonsen and Findlay, 1990a).

PROLIFERATION OF ENDOMETRIAL CELLS

The normal endometrium consists of a columnar epithelial layer surrounding the central uterine lumen, branching into glands which penetrate the
underlying stromal matrix with its vascular bed. These epithelial and stromal
cells are steroid responsive and undergo cyclical periods of proliferation and
differentiation, during the follicular and luteal phases respectively. During
the luteal phase of the human menstrual cycle, differentiation of the
glandular compartment occurs during the first week, whereas the stromal
cells differentiate to predecidual cells during the second week of the luteal
phase. The differentiation of the stroma is not uniform and appears initially
as cuffs around spiral arterioles and laterally as sheets underlying the
luminal epithelium.

     Until recently, it was thought that these steroid hormone-dependent
changes would be reflected by the presence of specific steroid receptors in
the respective cell types. However, this has not always proved to be the
case (Brenner et al, 1990). Experiments in female macaque monkeys have
shown that there are instances where both oestrogen and progesterone
receptors are present only in stromal cells, while the adjacent mucosal
epithelium undergoes dramatic oestrogen and progesterone-dependent
differentiation (Figure 2). This supports the hypothesis, originally proposed
by Cunha et al (1983), that stromal cells can mediate the effect of steroids on
epithelial cells, and that in this case, oestrogen may act on receptors in

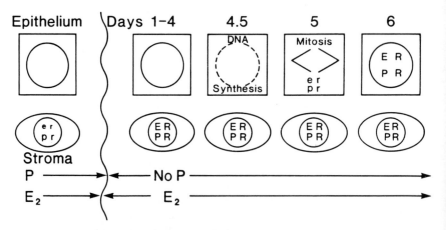

Figure 2. Endometrial receptors during the luteal–follicular transition (LFT) in the macaque
monkey. The figure correlates changes in oestrogen receptor (ER), progesterone receptor
(PR), DNA synthesis, and mitosis during an induced LFT. At the end of the cycle 1, ER and PR
are undetectable in the glandular epithelium. In the stroma, ER is barely detectable and PR
clearly is present, though reduced from previously high levels. After progesterone (P) withdrawal, ER and PR increase in the stroma, but remain undetectable until day 5 in the
epithelium. Oestrogen-dependent DNA synthesis begins in the epithelium on day 4.5, when
ER is only detectable in the stroma. Treatment with P on days 3–4 prevents epithelial DNA
synthesis, even though PR is only detectable in the stroma. E_2, oestradiol 17β. From Brenner et
al (1990) with permission.

stromal cells which, in turn, provoke epithelial proliferation. It implies that stromal cells can secrete epithelial mitogens. However, it is also likely that the extracellular matrix laid down by the stromal cells may be important for the differentiation and function of the epithelial cells, as it is for the mammary epithelial cells (Bissell et al, 1982). Overall, the data suggests that the actions of oestrogen and progesterone on epithelial cells in the endometrium are mediated in paracrine fashion by factors secreted by the neighbouring stromal cells. The nature of these local regulators have not been properly elucidated, although there are a number of strong candidates from among the polypeptide growth factors.

Epidermal growth factor (EGF)

There is substantial evidence that EGF could be involved in mediating oestrogen-induced uterine growth (Brigstock et al, 1989; Pollard, 1990). EGF is a small polypeptide (53 amino acids) with well-documented mitogenic and differentiating effects. Both the growth factor and its receptor have been identified in the uterus at the RNA and protein level and EGF stimulation of proliferation of cultured mouse and rabbit endometrial cells has been demonstrated. There is evidence to suggest that oestradiol acts by causing the cleavage of the EGF precursor to mature EGF and by stimulating synthesis of the EGF receptor resulting in an autocrine loop for epithelial cells (Di Augustine et al, 1988; Lingham et al, 1988). More recent evidence suggests that oestrogen can regulate the expression of the EGF gene specifically in uterine epithelial cells of the mouse, and that the increased expression of this gene results in an increase in the relative rate of synthesis of precursor protein and the accumulation of mature EGF (Huet-Hudson et al, 1990). There are binding sites for EGF in the human uterine tissues (Hofmann et al, 1984) but little is known so far about the mechanisms controlling the expression of the EGF receptor. Taken together, however, the data suggests an important role for EGF in mediating oestrogen-induced proliferation of the endometrium, but how this relates to stromal influences on epithelial cells is not known.

Transforming growth factor-α (TGF-α)

TGF-α is a 50 residue polypeptide which shows 30% sequence homology with EGF and exerts its biological effects by binding to the EGF receptor (see Brigstock et al, 1989). However, there is very little data about the presence of TGF-α in the uterus of the cycle or early pregnancy (see below). There are reports that the mouse embryo can express TGF-α (Twardzik, 1985) and TGF-α expression also occurs in the maternal decidua of rats (but not in the embryo or placenta) (Han et al, 1987).

Insulin-like growth factor-1 (IGF-1) and its binding proteins (IGFBP)

IGF-1 is a mitogen known for its ability to potentiate the activity of other mitogens such as EGF and platelet derived growth factor (PDGF). It is a 70 residue polypeptide which has approximately 45% sequence homology with insulin and was first identified as a principal cell mediator for the stimulatory action of growth hormone (see Ooi and Herington, 1988). Murphy et al (1987a) showed that expression of the mRNA for IGF is higher in the uterus than in any other tissue tested, apart from the liver, and that oestradiol stimulated expression of IGF-1 mRNA (Murphy et al, 1987b). The cell type responsible for producing IGF-1 in the uterus has not yet been defined. It is interesting to note, however, that a recent paper described the presence of receptors for growth hormone on the endometrial glands and epithelium in the rat (Lobie et al, 1990), suggesting that, in addition to oestradiol, growth hormone may be important in regulating the production of IGF-1 by uterine cells.

The actions of IGF-1 are now known to be modulated by the presence of a family of binding proteins (BP) (Ooi and Herington, 1988). It is proposed that IGF-1 acts principally in an autocrine/paracrine manner and that the IGFBPs prevent its action at distal sites. It is of interest, therefore, that decidual cells of the human endometrium produce a protein originally called PP12, but now known to be an IGFBP (Koistinen et al, 1986; Bell and Smith, 1988). The production of this binding protein by the decidua appears to be relatively small during the luteal phase of the conception cycle. Nevertheless, it may be important for regulating the actions of IGF-1 in its role in the regulation of uterine growth.

REGULATION OF GROWTH OF THE TROPHOBLAST AND PLACENTA

The extent of the growth of the trophoblast prior to and during implantation varies considerably between species; for example, in ruminants there is extensive growth of the conceptus during a relatively long preimplantation period, when the glandular secretions of the endometrium are essential for the survival and growth of the conceptus (Findlay, 1983). In contrast, there is relatively little growth of the conceptus prior to implantation in rodents and primates, which have relatively short preimplantation periods. Nevertheless, during this time the conceptus is dependent upon the endometrium for its supply of nutrients and growth factors. In addition to growth of the conceptus there are also changes in the endometrium in relation to implantation, particularly in those species exhibiting haemochorial placentation, such as rodents and primates. In these species the conceptus tissue penetrates the endometrial stroma, which undergoes decidualization. This is followed by the formation and growth of the placenta. There is indirect evidence that growth of the conceptus and the early stages of placentation may be under the control of autocrine and paracrine regulators.

There are binding sites for EGF in placental and fetal membranes (Hofmann et al, 1988). However, there is only one report of EGF receptors in preimplantation trophoblast, that of the rabbit (Hofmann and Anderson, 1990). Given the fact that EGF is a product of uterine epithelial cells (see above), it is possible that uterine EGF may be important for the growth and proliferation of trophoblast cells and placental and fetal membranes. There are reports that the mouse embryo can express TGF-α (Twardzik, 1985) and that TGF expression also occurs in the maternal decidua of rats (but not in the embryo or placenta) (Han et al, 1987). In view of the localization of EGF/TGF-α receptors in the placenta and preimplantation trophoblast (see above), it is possible that TGF-α produced by the decidua may have a paracrine action on these tissues to induce growth and differentiation. The decidual cells of the human endometrium produce IGFBP (Koistinen et al, 1986; Bell and Smith, 1988), which could be important in modulating the action of endometrial IGF-1 on the decidua and possibly the trophoblast tissue.

According to Pollard (1990), the colony stimulating factors (CSFs) are among the best candidates as uterine factors which influence the growth of the conceptus. The majority of the activity of colony stimulating factor found in the pregnant uterus is CSF-1, a homodimeric glycoprotein growth factor which was originally purified as a lineage specific growth factor for mononuclear phagocytes, promoting their survival, differentiation and proliferation. The data available (see Pollard, 1990) suggests that steroid hormones (oestradiol and progesterone) regulate uterine CSF-1 synthesis through the induction of CSF-1 mRNA in epithelial cells. This production is relatively low early in pregnancy but increases as the pregnancy advances. CSF-1 mRNA is certainly present on day 3 of pregnancy in mice, which is in the preimplantation period at the time when the epithelium is first noticeably progestational. The CSF-1 receptor is a transmembrane glycoprotein tyrosine kinase identified as a product of the c-*fms* proto-oncogene. The CSF-1 receptor has been identified in the placenta and in human trophoblast, as well as in the uterus before placentation. In mice there is a high level of CSF-1 receptor mRNA detectable in the decidua starting on day 6, which persists in the decidua basalis during formation of the placenta but declines once the mature placenta is formed. The CSF-1 receptor mRNA expression has also been detected coincidentally in the trophectoderm of mice. The temporal relationship of the uterine CSF-1 synthesis with both decidual and trophoblast cell expression of the CSF-1 receptor and placental growth suggests a role for CSF-1 in placental growth and development. If the patterns of expression of CSF-1 and its receptor are the same during gestation in humans as found in the mouse, and if a definitive role of CSF-1 can be demonstrated in placental growth, then it could be concluded that CSF-1 is a key substance regulating growth and development of the placenta in the human.

ANGIOGENESIS

Angiogenesis is the process of generating new capillaries and therefore leads to vascularization of tissues. The endometrium is characterized by cyclical changes in angiogenesis, which are under steroid hormonal control (Findlay, 1986). In the human the radial arteries cross the myoendometrial junction to give rise to the steroid-sensitive spiral arteries which supply the stratum functionale and the steroid-insensitive basal arteries which supply the stratum basale (see Figure 1). Spiral arteries extend little further than the stratum basale early in the proliferative phase when oestradiol levels are low and they are connected to the subepithelial capillary plexus by long straight precapillaries. Oestradiol induces thickening and coiling of these precapillaries, with the convolution being most intense around midcycle. Growth continues in the secretory phase under the influence of oestradiol and progesterone and is correlated with increased DNA synthesis of vascular cells.

Angiogenesis is a very complex process which has been shown to involve tissue disruption and reorganization, cellular growth and changes in the composition of the fluid environment and extracellular matrix (Folkman, 1985). New capillaries originate from pre-existing microvasculature rather than from the large vessels which have layers of smooth muscle. It is likely that a family of angiogenic agents rather than one single substance is responsible for the angiogenic steps of exocytosis, chemotaxis, cell division and production of extracellular matrix (Findlay, 1986). Known angiogenic agents include the fibroblast growth factors (FGFs).

The nature of the angiogenic stimuli in the endometrium is not known. FGF-like activity has been demonstrated in bovine epithelial endometrial cells (Fujii and Lee, 1987) and in pig uterine tissues and uterine flushings from early pregnant gilts (Brigstock et al, 1989). As pointed out by Brigstock et al (1989), the secretion of FGF is somewhat controversial because neither the basic nor acidic forms of FGF contain the classical signal peptides which are thought necessary to facilitate the secretion of peptides by cells. Nevertheless, FGFs appear to become deposited in the extracellular matrix, particularly that produced by cultured endothelial cells (Baird and Ling, 1987). It is believed that the FGFs are maintained in a stable but functionally inactive state in the extracellular matrix by binding to the heparan sulphate component. Mobilization of FGFs from the matrix can be effected by the action of heparan sulphate degrading enzymes such as heparinase or heparitinase. Obviously, if FGF is involved in angiogenesis, regulation of the activities of these respective enzymes within the endometrium would be an important determinant of the angiogenic process. If FGFs can be found in the human endometrium, then a role for these factors in the control of endometrial angiogenesis would presuppose an endothelial–epithelial cell or endothelial–stromal cell interaction as part of the angiogenic stimulus.

Because angiogenesis in the endometrium is partly steroid dependent, it would be important to examine the effect of oestradiol and progesterone on expression of FGF and other angiogenic activities by the different endometrial cell types. Macqueo (1980) concluded that steroidal contraceptives, which commonly cause problems of menstrual bleeding, were associated with underdevelopment of the arterioles, degenerative changes in the venules and even lesions in the vascular endothelium. One possibility is that the progestagens are interfering with the stimulatory action of oestradiol by suppressing the synthesis of steroid receptors. It is of interest in this regard that McClellan et al (1986) found no evidence for the presence of oestrogen receptors in endothelial cells of macaque endometrium during the luteal–

follicular transition. Immediately prior to progesterone withdrawal, there was evidence of oestrogen receptors in stromal fibroblasts and smooth muscle cells associated with the walls of spiral arteries. This suggests that paracrine regulation could be responsible for the influence of oestradiol on endothelial cell function in the primate endometrium.

HAEMOSTASIS AND UTERINE BLEEDING

Disturbances of normal menstrual rhythm remain one of the major gynaeco-logical complications, particularly in women who are taking steroidal contraceptives (Gray, 1980). Not only do we know very little about the factors controlling the onset and extent of menstruation in the normal endometrium, we know even less about the mechanisms by which steroidal contraceptives and other factors cause disturbances in this normal rhythm. These disturbances range from amenorrhoea to prolonged breakthrough bleeding and are most prominent in women who use long-acting progestagen-only contraceptives. We consider that the haemostasis and uterine bleeding in the endometrium at the time of menstruation is under paracrine regulation. Two very different factors which may be involved in this process are the prostaglandins and endothelin.

Prostaglandins (PGs) are well recognized as agents controlling vasocon-striction and vasodilatation and the endometrium is a major site of production and release of PGs. The onset of menstruation has been linked to the increase in $PGF_{2\alpha}$ levels in the luteal phase of the menstrual cycle (Poyser, 1981), either through enhanced synthesis (Abel and Baird, 1980) or decreased metabolism (Casey et al, 1980). In a recent review, Bell and Smith (1988) provided data supporting an interaction between different cell types, and even between myometrium and endometrium, to explain the mechanisms controlling PG production in the endometrium. It would appear that epithelial cells are the major source of endometrial $PGF_{2\alpha}$ and its metabolites and that steroids can influence the synthesis and metabolism of $PGF_{2\alpha}$ by these cells. In contrast, studies on a number of species suggests that PGE is produced primarily by stromal cells (e.g. sheep: Cherny and Findlay, 1990) and may not be regulated by steroids (Salamonsen and Findlay, 1990a). Progesterone withdrawal at the end of the cycle is hypothesized to allow expression by epithelial cells of $PGF_{2\alpha}$ synthesis, which in turn has a paracrine influence initially by vasoconstriction of the spiral arterioles. The role of stromal cells and the sites of action of ovarian steroids modulating PG production by epithelial cells remain subjects for further study. It is hypothesized that a balance in the synthesis and/or metabolism of PGs may be associated with menstrual disorders such as primary dysmenorrhoea or menorrhagia (Baird et al, 1981; Smith, 1986).

The vascular endothelium is now recognized as an important functional unit involved in the regulation of a vascular smooth muscle tonus. A short-lived, endothelial cell derived relaxing factor (EDRF), made in response to vasoactive agents such as acetylcholine and recently identified as nitric oxide or a closely related substance (Palmer et al, 1987), is thought to act on the neighbouring vascular smooth muscle cells to bring about relaxation. A potent vasoconstrictor peptide, endothelin, has now been isolated and purified from media conditioned by porcine aortic endothelial cells, and its cDNA has been cloned and sequenced (Yanagisawa et al, 1988). Endothelin is a 21 amino acid peptide derived by two proteolytic cleavage steps via 39 amino acid 'big endothelin' from proendothelin. Endothelin mRNA has also been shown to be expressed in endothelial cells. Endothelin is related to a peptide family called sarafotoxins which are found in snake venom and act as voltage dependent sodium channel regulators. Of particular interest has been the demonstration of endothelin in the epithelial cells of the rabbit endometrium (Orlando et al, 1990) and of its receptors in human endometrium (Cameron et al, 1989). Endothelin may be able to act as a growth regulator under certain circumstances (Brown and Littlewood, 1989; Bobik et al, 1990). Whereas EDRF would appear to be involved in rapid local control of vascular tonus, endothelin is a very potent, long-lasting vasoconstrictor. An investigation of these activities in the endometrium and the influence of steroids on their expression and action is warranted, particularly in relation to menstruation and to the establishment of the haemochorial placenta.

CONCEPTUS DERIVED FACTORS IN PARACRINE REGULATION

The ability of the conceptus to influence endometrial function has been well established (Findlay, 1983; Clark and Chaouat, 1989; Salamonsen and Findlay, 1990a). These actions of the conceptus on the endometrium include alterations in endometrial protein and prostaglandin production as well as modification of the local immune response. Platelet activating factor (PAF) (Harper, 1989; O'Neill et al, 1990) and interferons (IFNs) (Roberts et al, 1989) are two conceptus-derived factors recently identified as responsible for some of these changes. The blastocysts of some species are also known to make prostaglandins and steroid hormones (Findlay, 1983). In this review we will concentrate on the blastocyst IFN.

The identification of IFNs as major products of the sheep and cow preimplantation conceptuses has been a major advance in our understanding of conceptus–endometrial interactions in early pregnancy (Roberts et al, 1989). Ovine trophoblast protein-1 (oTP-1) and bovine trophoblast protein-1 (bTP-1) are members of the IFN-α_{11} subfamily. There is a 55–65% base sequence homology between the DNA coding for oTP-1 and IFN-α_1 but a greater than 80% identity with the gene for bovine IFN-α_{11}. Like other IFN-α, oTP-1 has potent antiviral activity and antiproliferative activities, inhibiting both the growth of bovine kidney epithelial cells in culture and the incorporation of [^{3}H]thymidine into mitogen stimulated ovine lymphocytes. Antiviral activity has recently been detected in medium following culture of pig and goat conceptuses (Cross and Roberts, 1989; Gnatek et al, 1989; Godkin et al, 1989).

There are as yet no reports of the production or release of IFN-like activity by preimplantation human conceptuses. This may reflect the differences in the forms of implantation and placentation between ruminants and humans, and particularly the stage of development of the conceptus at the time of implantation. IFN activity has been detected in the fetoplacental unit later in pregnancy, and its association with placental tissue and amniotic fluid has been widely reported (human: Chard et al, 1986; Howatson et al, 1988; mouse: Fowler et al, 1980; hamster: Green and Ts'o, 1986).

In addition to its antiviral and antiproliferative properties, oTP-1 also has the capacity to modulate prostaglandin production by endometrial cells both in vivo and in vitro. For example, we have shown that oTP-1 and recombinant human IFN-α cause a dose-dependent inhibition of the production of PGE and $PGF_{2\alpha}$ by cultured ovine endometrial cells (mainly epithelial cells) (Salamonsen et al, 1988). Both interferons were highly potent, with IC_{50} values of 10^{-11} M and 10^{-13} M for oTP-1 and HuIFN, respectively (Salamonsen et al, 1989). Activity at such low concentrations suggests that these IFNs are potent local regulatory factors and that their actions on eicosanoid release may be a fundamental property of the IFN family. Indeed IFNs have previously been demonstrated to decrease PG release from other cell types, such as human peripheral monocytes and mononuclear cells (Browning and Ribolini, 1987). In subsequent studies, we have attempted to elucidate the mechanism of action of oTP-1 on endometrial release (Salamonsen et al, 1989). We were unable to demonstrate any effects of IFN on the uptake of arachidonic acid (the major precursor of PG) by endometrial cells, neither did it change the incorporation of arachidonic acid into cellular lipid. The addition of arachidonic acid increased the overall release of both PGE and $PGF_{2\alpha}$ from the cell cultures, which was inhibited by oTP-1. Thus it is likely that oTP-1/IFN is acting either directly or indirectly on the prostaglandin synthetase enzyme (PGS), although an additional effect on other enzymes such as phospholipase A_2 cannot be discounted. More recently, we have shown by immunocytochemical analysis of PGs that the immunoactive levels of this enzyme protein in endometrial epithelial cells do not differ between pregnant and non-pregnant ewes, suggesting that it is the activity of the PGs which is being modified in some way by the oTP-1 (Salamonsen and Findlay, 1990b). This could involve the production of a tissue inhibitor of PGS activity (Basu, 1989).

It is now established that oTP-1 is an antiluteolysin in ruminants, in that it prevents the production of PGF and therefore results in maintenance of the corpus luteum (Bazer, 1989). A similar mechanism does not occur in the primate. However, the possibility that IFNs act on human endometrial cells to modify production of prostaglandin and other cellular products remains to be explored. The IFNs may also be involved in regulating the maternal immune response to tolerate the presence of the blastocyst.

CONCLUSIONS

The case has been made for the involvement of local regulators in several of the processes associated with implantation and uterine growth, some of which are known to be dependent on ovarian steroids. It can be concluded that in some cases using experimental animals there is strong circumstantial evidence for the involvement of local regulators in these processes. There are very few instances where the role of a local regulator has been demonstrated directly and, for obvious ethical reasons, very little has been done to establish paracrine regulation of human implantation. More use should be made of primate models (e.g. Brenner et al, 1990) and in vitro systems using human tissues (Kliman et al, 1989). Nevertheless, the involvement of local regulators in the control of implantation and uterine growth does offer logical explanations for many of the phenomena which were difficult to explain simply by the actions of ovarian and placental steroids.

What is the likely clinical significance of these local regulators? Gynaecological problems such as recurrent bleeding, early abortion and inadequate placental growth and function can now be observed in a new light, and tests can be made to discover whether or not an imbalance in production and action of local regulators is involved in their aetiology. The possibility of using local regulators as the basis of diagnosis and treatment of such disorders remains speculative. However, as an example, it may be that treatment with growth hormone could influence endometrial growth via an action on the growth hormone (GH) receptors (Lobie et al, 1990) and consequently IGF-1 production. A similar GH treatment regimen has been found to enhance follicular maturation in the ovary, presumably by the same mechanism. In the case of the uterus, the possibility of treatment with locally acting effectors, probably administered at very low concentrations near their site of action and therefore devoid of generalized side-effects, is a hope for the future.

Acknowledgements

We are grateful to Faye Coates and Sue Panckridge for their help in producing the manuscript, and the National Health and Medical Research Council of Australia and the Buckland Foundation for financial support.

REFERENCES

Abel MH & Baird DT (1980) The effect of 17β oestradiol and progesterone on prostaglandin production by human endometrium maintained in organ culture. *Endocrinology* **106:** 1599–1606.
Amoroso EC (1952) Placentation. In Parks AS (ed.) *Marshall's Physiology of Reproduction*, pp 127–311. London: Longmans.
Baird A & Ling N (1987) Fibroblast growth factors are present in the extracellular matrix produced by endothelial cells in vitro; implications for a role of heparinase-like enzymes in the neovascular response. *Biochemical and Biophysical Research Communications* **142:** 428–435.
Baird DT, Abel MH, Kelly RW & Smith SK (1981) Endocrinology of dysfunctional uterine bleeding: the role of endometrial prostaglandins. In Crosignani PG & Rubin BL (eds) *Endocrinology of Human Infertility: New Aspects Serono Clinical Colliquia on Reproduction 2*, pp 399–417. London: Academic Press.
Basu S (1989) Endogenous inhibition of arachidonic acid metabolism in the endometrium of the sheep. *Prostaglandins, Leukotrienes and Essential Fatty Acids* **35:** 147–152.

Bazer FW (1989) Establishment of pregnancy in sheep and pigs. *Reproduction, Fertility and Development* 1: 237–242.

Bell SC & Smith SK (1988) The endometrium as a paracrine organ. In Chamberlain GVP (ed.) *Contemporary Topics in Obstetrics and Gynaecology*, pp 273–298. London: Butterworths.

Bissell MJ, Hall HG & Parry G (1982) How does the extracellular matrix direct gene expression? *Journal of Theoretical Biology* 99: 31–68.

Bobik A, Grooms A, Millar JA, Mitchell A & Grinpukel S (1990) Growth factor activity of endothelin on vascular smooth muscle. *American Journal of Physiology* 258: C408–C415.

Brenner RM, West NB & McClellan MC (1990) Estrogen and progestin receptors in the reproductive tract of male and female primates. *Biology of Reproduction* 42: 11–19.

Brigstock DR, Heap RB & Brown KD (1989) Polypeptide growth factors in uterine tissues and secretions. *Journal of Reproduction and Fertility* 85: 747–758.

Brown KD & Littlewood CJ (1989) Endothelin stimulates DNA synthesis in Swiss 3T3 cells. Synergy with polypeptide growth factors. *Biochemical Journal* 263: 977–980.

Browning JL & Ribolini A (1987) Interferon blocks interleukin-1 induced prostaglandin release from human peripheral monocytes. *Journal of Immunology* 138: 2857–2863.

Cameron IT, Davenport AP, Brown MJ & Smith SK (1989) Autoradiographical localization of binding sites for endothelin in the human uterus. *Journal of Reproduction and Fertility. Abstract Series* 4: 27.

Casey ML, Hemsell DL, MacDonald PC & Johnston JM (1980) NAD+-dependent 15-hydroxy prostaglandin dehydrogenase activity in human endometrium. *Prostaglandins* 19: 115–122.

Chard T, Craig PH, Menabawey M & Lee C (1986) Alpha interferon in human pregnancy. *British Journal of Obstetrics and Gynaecology* 93: 1145–1149.

Cherny RA & Findlay JK (1990) Separation and culture of ovine endometrial epithelial and stromal cells: evidence of morphological and functional polarity. *Biology of Reproduction* 43: 241–250.

Clark DA & Chaouat G (1989) Determinants of embryo survival in the peri- and post-implantation period. In Yoshinaga K (ed.) *Blastocyst Implantation*, pp 171–178. Boston, MA: Adams Publishing.

Corner GW (1921) Cyclic changes in the ovaries and uterus of the sow and their relation to the mechanism of implantation. *Contributions to Embryology. (Carnegie Institute of Washington)* 13: 119–146.

Cross JC & Roberts RM (1989) Porcine conceptuses secrete an interferon during the pre-attachment period of early pregnancy. *Biology of Reproduction* 40: 1109–1118.

Cunha GR, Chung LWK, Shannon JM, Taguchi O & Fujii H (1983) Hormone-induced morphogenesis and growth: role of mesenchymal-epithelial interactions. *Recent Progress in Hormone Research* 39: 559–598.

Di Augustine RP, Petrusz P, Bell GI et al (1988) Influence of estrogens on mouse uterine epidermal growth factor precursor protein and messenger ribonucleic acid. *Endocrinology* 122: 2355–2363.

Findlay JK (1983) The endocrinology of the preimplantation period. In Martini L & James VHT (eds) *The Endocrinology of Pregnancy and Parturition*, pp 35–67. London: Academic Press.

Findlay JK (1986) Angiogenesis in reproductive tissues. *Journal of Endocrinology* 111: 357–366.

Findlay JK, Cherny RA & Salamonsen LA (1990) Paracrine interactions amongst cells of the endometrium. In d'Arcangues C, Fraser IS, Newton JR & Odlind V (eds) *Contraception and Mechanisms of Endometrial Bleeding*, pp 253–265. Cambridge: Cambridge University Press.

Folkman J (1985) Tumour angiogenesis. *Advances in Cancer Research* 43: 175–203.

Fowler AK, Reed CD & Giron DJ (1980) Identification of an interferon in murine placentas. *Nature* 286: 266–267.

Fujii DK & Lee E (1987) Growth and hormonal responsiveness of cultured bovine uterine epithelium. *Abstracts of the Proceedings of the Endocrine Society of the USA* 69: 127.

Gnatek GG, Smith LD, Duby RT & Godkin JD (1989) Maternal recognition of pregnancy in the goat: effects of conceptus removal on interestrus intervals and characterization of conceptus protein production during early pregnancy. *Biology of Reproduction* 41: 655–663.

Godkin JD, Baumbach GA & Duby RT (1989) Characterization of caprine trophoblast protein-1 (cTP-1). *Biology of Reproduction* **40** (supplement 1): 115.

Gray R (1980) Patterns of bleeding associated with the use of steroidal contraceptives. In Diczfalusy E, Fraser IS & Webb FTG (eds) *Endometrial Bleeding and Steroidal Contraception*, pp 14–49. Bath: Pitman Press.

Greene JJ & Ts'o POP (1986) Preferential modulation of embryonic cell proliferation and differentiation by embryonic interferon. *Experimental Cell Research* **167**: 400–406.

Han VKM, Hunter ES, Pratt RM, Zendegui JG & Lee DC (1987) Expression of rat transforming growth factor alpha mRNA during development occurs predominantly in maternal decidua. *Molecular and Cellular Biology* **7**: 2335–2343.

Harper MJK (1989) Platelet-activating factor: a paracrine factor in preimplantation stages of reproduction? *Biology of Reproduction* **40**: 907–913.

Hofmann GE & Anderson TL (1990) Immunohistochemical localization of epidermal growth factor receptor during implantation in the rabbit. *American Journal of Obstetrics and Gynecology* **162**: 837–841.

Hofmann GE, Rao CV, Barrows GH, Schultz GS & Sanfilippo JS (1984) Binding sites for epidermal growth factor in human uterine tissues and leiomyomas. *Journal of Clinical Endocrinology and Metabolism* **58**: 880–884.

Hofmann GE, Rao CV, Carmen FR Jr & Siddiqi TA (1988) [125]I human epidermal growth factor binding to placentas and fetal membranes from various pregnancy states. *Acta Endocrinologica* **117**: 5239–5334.

Howatson AG, Farquharson M, Meager A, McNichol AM & Foulis AK (1988) Localization of α-interferon in the human feto-placental unit. *Journal of Endocrinology* **119**: 531–534.

Huet-Hudson YM, Chakraborty C, De Swapan K et al (1990) Estrogen regulates the synthesis of epidermal growth factor in mouse uterine epithelial cells. *Molecular Endocrinology* **4**: 510–523.

Kliman HJ, Coutifaris C, Feinberg RF, Strauss JF III & Haimowitz JE (1989) Implantation: in vitro models utilizing human tissues. In Yoshinaga K (ed.) *Blastocyst Implantation*, pp 83–91. Boston, MA: Adams Publishing.

Koistinen R, Kalkkinen N, Huhtala M.-L et al (1986) Placental protein 12 is a decidual protein that binds somatomedin and has an identical N-terminal amino acid sequence with somatomedin-binding protein from human amniotic fluid. *Endocrinology* **118**: 1375–1378.

Lingham RB, Stancel GM & Loose-Mitchell DS (1988) Estrogen regulation of epidermal growth factor receptor messenger ribonucleic acid. *Molecular Endocrinology* **2**: 230–235.

Lobie PE, Breipohl W, Garcia Aragon J & Waters MJ (1990) Cellular localization of the growth hormone receptor/binding protein in the male and female reproductive systems. *Endocrinology* **126**: 2214–2221.

McClellan M, West NB & Brenner RM (1986) Immunocytochemical localization of estrogen receptors in the Macaque endometrium during the luteal-follicular transition. *Endocrinology* **119**: 2467–2675.

Macqueo M (1980) Vascular and perivascular changes in the endometrium of women using steroidal contraceptives. In Diczfalusy E, Fraser IS & Webb FTG (eds) *Endometrial Bleeding and Steroidal Contraception*, pp 138–152. Bath: Pitman Press.

Murphy LJ, Bell GI & Friesen HG (1987a) Tissue distribution of insulin-like growth factor 1 and 2 messenger ribonucleic acid in the adult rat. *Endocrinology* **120**: 1279–1282.

Murphy LJ, Murphy LC & Friesen HG (1987b) Estrogen induces insulin-like growth factor-1 expression in the rat uterus. *Molecular Endocrinology* **1**: 445–450.

O'Neill C, Wells X & Battye K (1990) Embryo-derived platelet activating factor: interactions with the arachidonic acid cascade and the establishment and maintenance of pregnancy. *Reproduction, Fertility and Development* **2**: 423–441.

Ooi GT & Herington AC (1988) The biological and structural characterization of specific serum-binding proteins for the insulin-like growth factors. *Journal of Endocrinology* **118**: 7–18.

Orlando C, Brandi ML, Peri A et al (1990) Neurohypophyseal hormone regulation of endothelin secretion from rabbit endometrial cells in primary culture. *Endocrinology* **126**: 1780–1785.

Palmer RMJ, Ferridge AG & Moncada S (1987) Nitric oxide release accounts for the biological activity of endothelium-derived relaxing factor. *Nature* **327**: 524–526.

Pollard JW (1990) Regulation of polypeptide growth factor synthesis and growth factor-related gene expression in the rat and mouse uterus before and after implantation. *Journal of Reproduction and Fertility* **88:** 721–731.

Poyser NL (1981) *Prostaglandins in Reproduction*, 127 pp. Chichester: John Wiley & Sons.

Roberts RM, Imakawa K, Niwano Y et al (1989) Interferon production by the preimplantation sheep embryo. *Journal of Interferon Research* **9:** 171–183.

Salamonsen LA & Findlay JK (1990a) Regulation of endometrial prostaglandins during the menstrual cycle and in early pregnancy. *Reproduction, Fertility and Development* **2:** 443–457.

Salamonsen LA & Findlay JK (1990b) Immunocytochemical localization of prostaglandin synthase in the ovine uterus during the oestrous cycle and in early pregnancy. *Reproduction, Fertility and Development* **2:** 311–319.

Salamonsen LA, Stuchbery SJ, O'Grady CM, Godkin JD & Findlay JK (1988) Interferon mimics the in vitro bioactivity of ovine trophoblast antiluteolytic protein. *Journal of Endocrinology* **117:** R1–R4.

Salamonsen LA, Manikhot J, Healy DL & Findlay JK (1989) Ovine trophoblast protein-1 and human interferon alpha reduce prostaglandin synthesis by ovine endometrial cells. *Prostaglandins* **38:** 289–306.

Smith SK (1986) Aetiology of menstrual disorders. *Prostaglandin Perspectives* **2:** 8–9.

Sporn MB & Todaro GJ (1980) Autocrine secretion and malignant transforming of cells. *New England Journal of Medicine* **303:** 878–880.

Twardzik DR (1985) Differential expression of transforming growth factor α during prenatal development of the mouse. *Cancer Research* **45:** 5413–5416.

Yanagisawa M, Kurihara H, Kimura S et al (1988) A novel potent vasoconstrictor peptide produced by vascular endothelial cells. *Nature* **332:** 411–415.

9

Role of embryonic factors in implantation: recent developments

GERALDINE M. HARTSHORNE
ROBERT G. EDWARDS

Human implantation is particularly difficult to study, due to technical and ethical considerations, although some information is emerging on the earliest stages of embryonic development and the embryo–maternal dialogue, which are essential for implantation. Knowledge about embryonic factors influencing implantation in non-human primates is also limited. Many different strategies of implantation have evolved among various species to protect both mother and fetus during pregnancy, so extrapolations of data are unreliable. Fortunately, there is much more information about implantation in laboratory and domestic mammals, which is already of benefit in animal husbandry and the preservation of rare breeds.

Implantation is a dialogue, involving interactions between the embryo and the mother. Intrinsic features of the embryo and its ability to communicate with the mother modify the metabolism of the uterus and other organs during implantation and pregnancy. Human fecundity is low in comparison with many animal species, the chances of pregnancy in a fertile couple during the midcycle being at most 30%. This low fecundity is apparently partly due to a high degree of embryonic wastage, and specifically to genetic abnormalities in the embryos, but implantation can fail for other reasons, many unknown.

Information about implantation has arisen from various sources. Human implantation has been achieved in an isolated perfused uterus (Bulletti et al, 1988), which questions the need for extrauterine factors and implies that the process is more robust than previously believed. Moreover, 0.4–3.5% (depending upon ethnic origin) of naturally occurring human pregnancies are extrauterine, where implantation presumably occurs in suboptimal conditions. Ectopic implantation shows that the uterus is not essential for embryonic survival and indicates the intrinsic ability of embryos to implant. The embryo might be more invasive in ectopic sites, suggesting that the endometrium could control and limit trophoblastic invasion.

Some forms of human implantation are highly unusual. The hydatidiform mole is of special interest, since it has a high capacity to transform into a choriocarcinoma, an invasive and potentially life-threatening tumour. Its androgenetic origin (most arising from a single spermatozoon) raises

Baillière's Clinical Obstetrics and Gynaecology—
Vol. 5, No. 1, March 1991
ISBN 0–7020–1533–4

questions about the role of maternal and paternal factors and the effect of genomic imprinting on embryonic growth and implantation (Kajii and Ohama, 1977). Likewise, genetically identical twins and higher order pregnancies show that the embryo can divide into totipotential parts, and raises questions about how this occurs and whether such twin embryos with varying amounts of trophectoderm or inner cell mass have an equal ability to implant.

Many clues to understanding human implantation will be found within the embryo. Several detailed reviews have covered early discoveries in this field (Heap et al, 1979; Edwards, 1980; Weitlauf, 1988) and the blastocyst–endometrial relationship has also been reviewed by Glasser et al (1990). This chapter will identify recent advances relating to the role of the embryo in implantation, especially those made possible by modern techniques in molecular biology and human reproductive medicine.

INTRINSIC FEATURES OF THE EMBRYO

Genetic constitution

Few human zygotes, perhaps about 20% (Buster et al, 1985), reach the blastocyst stage of development at which implantation may occur. The others either do not fertilize, display fragmentation of blastomeres, or fail to compact and degenerate before becoming blastocysts. Many human oocytes, perhaps as many as 30%, are genetically abnormal (Plachot et al, 1987; Veiga et al, 1987; Wramsby et al, 1987). Spermatozoa have a lower incidence of genetic defects, approximately 8%, of which more than half are balanced translocations and deletions (Martin et al, 1983).

Many embryos fertilized in vivo or in vitro inherit some form of chromosomal imbalance from the gametes, and others can arise during fertilization and cleavage. About 20% of human embryos growing in vitro are genetically abnormal, but this level increases by a factor of 2 or 3 if fertilization is delayed or if the embryos have fragmented blastomeres during early growth (Plachot et al, 1987). The observed defects include mosaicism, haploidy, triploidy (and higher levels of euploidy) originating from either polyspermy or digyny, trisomies, monosomies and chromosome fragmentation (Angell et al, 1983; Plachot et al, 1987; Veiga et al, 1987). A delay between extrusion of the first polar body and fertilization increases not only the risk of chromosomal errors but also the chances of parthenogenetic activation, polyspermy and polar body retention. Many embryos with specific forms of chromosomal monosomy and trisomy arise from meiotic non-disjunction during oocyte or sperm formation, and rarely at the first cleavage division, whereas mosaic forms arise during a later cleavage division. Many of these embryos are capable of implantation, as are some triploid and tetraploid embryos. Some astonishing forms have been identified, e.g. complex haploid mosaics arising from the movements of multiple pronuclei in a fertilized oocyte (Michelmann et al, 1986). The majority of chromosomally abnormal embryos fail to implant, or are lost as early abortions.

Similar anomalies arise in vivo. This has been shown by the identification of many chromosomally imbalanced abortuses, which comprise almost 80% of embryos lost soon after implantation (Brambati, 1990). Many pregnancies are also lost before implantation, as 'biochemical' or 'preclinical' pregnancies, identified by a transient rise in plasma β-human chorionic gonadotrophin (β-hCG). It is highly probable that many of these early deaths arise from chromosomal imbalance.

Some embryos develop abnormally through other genetic causes, e.g. the inheritance of genes which impair early embryonic growth. It is difficult to identify such situations in human embryos, but some have been well described in mice, e.g. the T series, in which different alleles impose an arrest or a malformation at a specific embryonic stage. Genomic imprinting might also play a role, for several human genes determining various conditions in man are inherited from one parent or the other and not in a mendelian fashion (Nicholls et al, 1989). The androgenetic hydatidiform mole is the classic example of genomic imprinting (Surani et al, 1990) and it is possible that such disturbances influence the chances of implantation by stimulating an overgrowth of trophectoderm (determined primarily by the action of paternal genes) or perhaps induce unusual immune responses in the mother during implantation (Loke and King, 1989).

Gene transcription for implantation in oocyte and embryo

During oocyte growth and maturation, and for a few days in the embryo after fertilization, protein synthesis is encoded by 'maternal' mRNA synthesized and stored during the growth of the oocyte in the ovary. The transcription of this mRNA results in the synthesis of many proteins of fundamental importance for oocyte maturation, fertilization, the early cleavage divisions of the embryo and for implantation itself. Such proteins include those present in the zona pellucida and those synthesized during oocyte maturation, including the *mos* proteins which are possibly involved in meiotic arrest at metaphase II in *Xenopus*, and the enzyme calpain which destroys the *mos* protein after fertilization has begun (Watanabe et al, 1990). Many of these proteins are essential for normal development through the initial cleavage divisions, blastocyst formation and perhaps even extending to the early stages of implantation.

Following fertilization, the early blastomeres are totipotent, a property which is gradually lost as differentiation proceeds. In mouse embryos, totipotency is apparently maintained by the activity of the gene *oct*-3, which contains homeodomains and encodes a nuclear factor specific for a regulatory DNA octamer (Rosner et al, 1990). This gene remains active in inner cell mass, but not in trophectoderm, and persists in ectoderm until differentiation has begun. Differentiation itself involves various growth factors as shown below.

The embryonic genome becomes active soon after fertilization, transcription beginning at the 2-cell stage in mice and about the 4- to 8-cell stage in humans (Braude et al, 1988; Tesarik et al, 1988). The gene *oct*-3, for example, is first transcribed from maternal RNA and then embryonic RNA

(Rosner et al, 1990) whereon β-hCG transcripts appear to be embryonic, first appearing at the 8-cell stage (Bonduelle et al, 1988). In contrast, the increasing activity in blastocysts of enzymes involved in N-linked glyco-protein synthesis is independent of newly synthesized RNA (Armant et al, 1986). A failure of genome activation may be one cause of early embryonic demise, since some embryos arrest in their early growth without obvious cause.

This combination of maternal and embryonic transcription is an essential phase of early embryonic growth, although the extent of their respective contributions at any particular time is still unknown. Once fertilization has occurred, maternally inherited factors have a declining role as development proceeds.

The embryonic genome is evidently active in regulating several other factors involved in implantation. Transcripts for β-hCG are found in human embryos at the 8-cell stage (Bonduelle et al, 1988). There is no formal evidence to show that these transcripts are embryonic, for there are no known isohormones of hCG which could act as markers differentiating maternal versus embryonic transcription. As human development proceeds to the blastocyst, more novel transcripts essential for growth and implantation have been identified in mammalian embryos, including those encoding growth factors (Rappollee et al, 1988).

For normal development, both maternal and paternal genomes must contribute to the embryo. Neither gynogenetic nor androgenetic embryos can develop normally, because each lacks a genetic component from the other parent, and this is an example of genomic imprinting (Surani et al, 1990). Selective effects apparently arise through the variable degrees of methylation of some genes in the ovary or testis, which introduce functional differences between the parental genomes. Some genes remain inactive, and apparently methylated, for a considerable period—often for years—if they are inherited from one of the two parents. The genes responsible for Prader–Willi syndrome in man are inherited from the father only, and the condition is not evident if inherited from the mother (Nicholls et al, 1989). Angelman syndrome displays the opposite effect, being inherited from the mother but remaining unexpressed when inherited from the father (Nicholls et al, 1989).

Genomic imprinting is therefore effective at the level of individual genes and also on a larger genetic scale. Parthenogenetic embryos have no paternal complement and under these circumstances the embryo can proceed along its 'embryonic' lineage, but inadequate trophoblast develop-ment occurs (Surani et al, 1990). Their impaired growth in mammals could arise from the consequential deficiencies in placental formation (Surani et al, 1990). Conversely, the hydatidiform mole arises androgenetically and contains only paternally imprinted genes and maternal mitochondria. This displays considerable growth of trophoblast but cannot sustain the growth of the embryonic line. Similar situations arise in mice following the transfer of male and female pronuclei between fertilized eggs, indicating that the inheritance of maternal and paternal complements is essential for normal growth to proceed.

Finally, some genes influence differentiation of the embryo. The best-characterized is undoubtedly the t-locus in mice, where a series of alleles can impair growth at specific stages from the morula onwards (Sherman and Wudl, 1977). So far, no similar examples have been found in human embryos, but they must exist to regulate the formation of the blastocyst, the differentiation of trophectoderm and the chorion, and perhaps specific situations, such as the production of hCG or growth factors.

Morphology of preimplantation embryos

A great deal of information on the morphology of embryos has arisen from in vitro fertilization. Experience has been gained on the developmental fate of embryos according to their morphology, and the appearance of embryos is often used to choose which should be replaced in the mother or cryopreserved. This approach is highly subjective and relies on visual estimates of fragmentation and the evenness of blastomeres; alternatively, semi-computerized scanning videos can be used to automate the calculation of these parameters (Cohen et al, 1989a). Nevertheless, some value is gained by typing embryos visually, even though the results of replacing various grades of embryos into the uterus are not greatly different unless substantial fragmentation has occurred (Claman et al, 1987). Some forms of fragmentation may be a means by which embryos can shed genetically abnormal cells (Tesarik, 1988), the localized fragmentation of a few cells permitting or enhancing repair or compensatory mechanisms. Some fragmentation might also result from cell death during morphogenesis, which is known to occur from the earliest stages of mammalian development. Fragmentation and misshapen blastomeres are not consequences of growth in vitro, for all the different grades of embryos observed in vitro have also been found in embryos recovered by uterine lavage (Buster et al, 1985).

The relative unimportance of some degree of fragmentation has also been shown by studies on cleaving embryos considered too abnormal morphologically for cryopreservation. When cultured for a longer period, only a small proportion ($<5\%$) of these embryos developed into blastocysts. When the blastocysts were cryopreserved and then thawed for replacement, there was no difference in the incidence of implantation, whatever their earlier morphology (Hartshorne et al, in press). This is further evidence that some forms of abnormal embryonic morphology during cleavage have little relationship to subsequent developmental capacity.

Hatching and the zona pellucida

The zona pellucida plays an essential role in early mammalian development. It is essential for monospermic fertilization; it must be formed normally to permit embryonic growth, when the blastomeres must remain in close contact. By the time the blastocyst has formed, it has become an obstacle to further growth and the embryo must 'hatch' from it if implantation and continued growth are to occur (Figure 1).

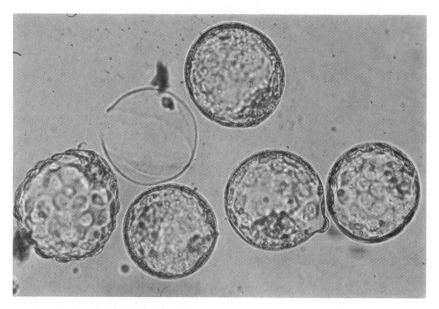

Figure 1. Five preimplantation mouse blastocysts, of which one has hatched (bottom left) and one has initiating hatching ($\times$ 320). Note the empty zona pellucida, centre left.

Formation of the zona pellucida can be impaired under certain circumstances. In some animals, it can become prematurely hardened in the ovulatory follicle, evidently due to oximes and other free radicals. Hardening may be a consequence of superovulation protocols, when the zona pellucida shows increasing resistance to proteolytic digestion. Some hardening also occurs during the growth of human embryos in vitro to the blastocyst (De Felici et al, 1985). The resulting problems for the embryos during hatching might be the cause of human identical twinning, which is much more frequent in women who have undergone ovarian stimulation (Edwards et al, 1986; Derom et al, 1987).

The appearance of the zona pellucida around human embryos might indicate the potential of an embryo for implantation. An uneven zona with thinning areas is a good prognosis, whereas a regular, thick zona is a barrier to hatching (Chan, 1987; Cohen et al, 1989b). Hatching apparently takes different forms in human and mouse embryos, since the enzyme strypsin, which digests the mouse zona pellucida to facilitate hatching, is produced in specific cells of the mural trophectoderm and not over the whole surface of the embryo (Perona and Wassarman, 1986). Bovine embryos might also have their own specific means of hatching, for the blastocyst expands until the zona splits (Massip and Mulnard, 1980), whereas periodic contractions are seen in mouse blastocysts (Cole, 1967). Hatching may be an insurmountable problem for some human embryos growing in vitro, and may prevent their further development. Some hatch incompletely, remaining partly trapped inside the zona pellucida. The severance of the two halves of the embryo might be a mechanism leading to the formation of identical twins (Edwards et al, 1986). Blastocysts might sometimes contain two inner cell masses, as in mice, although this is very rare and few examples have been reported in human embryos (Hardy et al, 1989). This condition might also result in the formation of identical twins.

Hatching is a prerequisite to successful implantation, and embryos which cannot hatch will not implant. It is possible that small incisions in the zona pellucida during cleavage might improve the overall chances of implantation (Cohen et al, 1989b).

INTRINSIC SIGNALS

There is a well-defined sequence of events in embryonic growth which must be achieved if a fertilized oocyte is to become a blastocyst competent to implant (see Table 1). Some of the events essential for normal fertilization and inheritance have been described earlier in this article. The cleaving embryo

Table 1. Stages of human embryo development in preparation for implantation.

Days post-fertilization	Carnegie stage[1]	Stage[2-4]	Event
1	1	Pronucleate/2-cell	
2⎫ 3⎭	2	2- to 6-cell ⎫ 8- to 12-cell ⎭	⎧Activation of embryonic DNA[5] ⎩hCG mRNA transcripts[6]
4⎫ 5⎬ 6⎭	3	Morula/early blastocyst Expanding blastocyst Fully expanding blastocyst/hatching	
7		Hatching	hCG secretion Initiation of twinning?[7]
8⎫ 9⎭	4–5	Hatched/enlarging Enlarging	Increasing hCG secretion Increasing hCG secretion
10⎫ 11⎭	5	Amniogenesis	

[1] O'Rahilly (1973).
[2] Edwards (1980).
[3] Edwards (1989).
[4] Lopata and Hay (1989).
[5] Braude et al (1988).
[6] Bonduelle et al (1988).
[7] Edwards et al (1986).

and blastocyst must then respond to intrinsic and extrinsic signals for differentiation to begin. The initiating signal for embryonic transcription and differentiation has not been identified, although the selective methylation of specific genes might exert some control over these processes (Surani et al, 1990). In mouse embryos, blastomeres in late cleavage stages begin to polarize and subsequently divide into 'inside' and 'outside' cells, according to the distribution of cytoskeletal and cytoplasmic constituents (Johnson et al, 1988). Polarity of the 'outside' cells is maintained during the formation of the mature trophectoderm (Fleming, 1987; Johnson, 1989), although the acquisition of polarity, and allocation to the inner cell mass or trophectoderm lineages are not irreversible in mouse embryos (Dyce et al, 1987; Winkel and Pedersen, 1988). There are no data available on human embryos to indicate whether a similar situation exists.

When the primary step leading to different cell types in the embryo has been taken, inductive influences between them might govern their subsequent differentiation (Gurdon et al, 1990). Communication between blastomeres occurs directly via gap junctions (Lehtonen, 1980) and also by interactions between surface molecules and local autocrine and paracrine signals. Cytokeratin-type intermediate filament proteins are involved in the formation of intercellular junctions, particularly between trophectoderm cells, which are required for compaction and cavitation of mouse morulae (Iwakura and Nozaki, 1989). Other components mediating communication between mouse blastomeres include $\beta 1,4$-galactosyl transferase (Gal Tase), a membrane protein involved in maintaining cell–cell contacts and securing the compaction of morulae (Bayna et al, 1988). Cell adhesion may be predictive of the potential of an embryo to establish pregnancy (Cohen et al, 1989a). Gal Tase may also be involved in the migrations of various cell types in the embryo, and interference with this system during differentiation induces teratological effects on mesodermal tissues in mice (Shur, 1977). Cavitation and fluid accumulation require the active pumping of ions in trophectoderm cells by Na^+/K^+ ATPase, a transmembrane protein which is synthesized at a great rate during the formation of rabbit blastocysts (Overstrom et al, 1989).

By the blastocyst stage, differentiation has produced a distinct trophectoderm and an inner cell mass providing the cellular basis for differentiation of the embryo and some placental elements (Gardner and Rossant, 1976). Some cytodifferentiation has occurred, as shown by the presence of large secretory cells adjacent to the blastocoelic cavity in human embryos and distinct from the thin trophectoderm layer (Edwards, 1980). Similar cells are found in mouse embryos, although they seem to be smaller in size. A human blastocyst is shown in Figure 2, together with a conjoined degenerating oocyte. The two oocytes forming this pair were believed to originate from a binovular follicle (Hartshorne et al, 1990).

The differentiation of trophectoderm into mural and polar regions, with their own distinctive properties, has also begun. In the mouse, polar trophectoderm is active in cell division, under the inductive influence of the inner cell mass, and some of its descendent cells populate the mural trophoblast (Gardner and Rossant, 1976). Differences between these tissues also exist in the distribution of some receptors, sugar incorporation, DNA synthesis and protein secretion (Perona and Wassarman, 1986). Components synthesized by specific regions of the blastocyst include: strypsin, which was described earlier; actin, which is restricted particularly to the boundary between the inner cell mass and trophectoderm in the pig spherical blastocyst (Albertini et al, 1987); and proteinases, which may locally degrade the uterine extracellular matrix (Glass et al, 1983). Positional information relative to the blastocoelic cavity is responsible for the differentiation of the primary endoderm and ectoderm (Tesarik, 1988) and, when this occurs, the radial

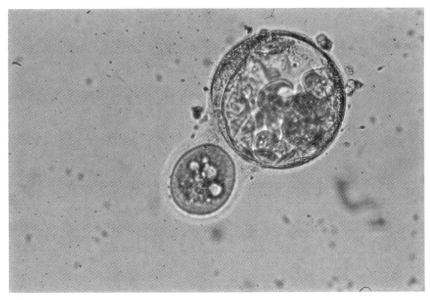

Figure 2. Human blastocyst and degenerating oocyte, originating from two conjoined oocytes, believed to have originated from a binovular follicle ($\times 250$). This embryo failed to hatch in vitro, after showing early signs of hatching on day 7. From Hartshorne et al (1990) with permission.

symmetry of the blastocyst is lost (Gardner, 1990).

Numerous biochemical and ultrastructural changes arise in the maturing blastocyst (Enders, 1989). There is some migration of cells between various lineages in mice (Winkel and Pedersen, 1988), and this residual fluidity in cytodifferentiation might help embryos to withstand damage or overcome abnormalities. Mouse embryos have a great capacity to recovery from various forms of trauma or exposure to chemicals and adverse environmental factors. Compensatory mechanisms may account for the recovery of embryos after the loss of or damage to cells of a certain lineage (Johnson, 1989). The inner cell mass and trophectoderm are closely associated in the mouse blastocyst, without an intervening basal lamina, which might confer a potential to compensate for damage to the trophectoderm (Enders, 1989).

The required ratio of inner cell mass to trophectoderm cells in mice is achieved during the two groups of cell divisions between the 8-cell and 32-cell stages (Fleming, 1987). Whether similar systems are operational in the human has not yet been determined but they could be of great significance for the cryopreservation of embryos, for the continued growth of those with fragments or other irregularities, and those deficient in trophectoderm cells. Such compensatory mechanisms could explain how some frozen–thawed human blastocysts with abnormal features, such as multiple cavities or dark areas, can implant and give pregnancies (Hartshorne et al, 1991). There is some evidence to suggest that removal of small pieces of trophectoderm from marmoset embryos might be detrimental to continued survival unless hCG support is given to maintain the pregnancy

Table 2. The occurrence and actions of growth regulating factors in mammalian tissue.

Gene/GF	Initial expression	Tissue expression	Oncogenic effect	Mode of action	Reference
Oct-3	Primordial germ cells. Totipotent/pluripotent stem cells	Inner cell mass, undifferentiated EC cells	?	Required for totipotential development	Rosner et al (1990)
IGF-2	Postimplantation	Widespread in fetus, suppressed in mature tissues	Probable association with Wilms' and other developmental tumours	Associated with tissue maturation + cytotrophoblast invasion	Brice et al (1989)
TGF-β family	Induction of mesoderm	Ubiquitous differentiated EC cells	Increased in most malignant tumours and transformed cells in vitro	Anchorage-independent growth via extracellular matrix. Influences responses to other GF	Rizzino (1988)
EGF family	No embryonic expression before implantation	TGF-α found in mid/late gestation. Differentiated EC cells	EGF has homology with products of *Notch* and *lin-12* proto-oncogenes. Receptor for EGF coded by *c-erb B* proto-oncogene	Precursors are membrane proteins and affect cell-cell interactions. Stimulates protein synthesis at compaction and differentiation of trophoblast. Receptors are tyr-specific protein kinases	Mercola and Stiles (1988) Wood and Kaye (1989)
PDGF family	Maternal mRNA in egg. Mouse embryos at cavitation	Undifferentiated EC cells	?	Receptors are tyr-specific protein kinases	Mercola and Stiles (1988) Rappolee et al (1988)
FGF	No embryonic expression of bFGF before implantation	Undifferentiated EC cells. Most normal tissues	Putative oncogenes *hst* and *int-2* and Kaposi's sarcoma. Found in tumours associated with endothelial cell growth and angiogenesis	Level reduced after differentiation. Acts with TGF in transformation and mesoderm induction. Tissue repair	Rizzino et al (1988) Mercola and Stiles (1988)

EC = embryonal carcinoma.

(Summers et al, 1988). The situation in human embryos remains to be clarified, although pregnancies arising from frozen–thawed blastocysts have satisfactory levels of β-hCG, regardless of damage to the embryos.

The two major components of the blastocyst, the inner cell mass and trophectoderm, have been examined in mice and display many differences in their fundamental properties. Human trophectoderm cells, isolated from the blastocyst, can survive for a short period of time in vitro as monolayers. They form cell clusters or trophoblastic vesicles in marmosets (Summers et al, 1988), and extensive cell monolayers supporting the differentiation of overlying inner cell mass in rabbits (Cole et al, 1966). Nevertheless, the trophoblast in primates is presumed to be regulated by the inductive actions of the inner cell mass, as it is in rodents (Gardner and Rossant, 1977).

Growth factors

The fundamental importance of growth factors in embryogenesis has been demonstrated during the last decade. Several growth factors have now been identified as having essential roles in early embryonic growth, some secreted by particular tissues of the embryo, and others from the maternal organism. A summary of the location and actions of some of the growth factors is given in Table 2. Receptors for several growth factors have been identified on embryos or on embryonic cell lines growing in vitro. The interrelationships between various embryonic tissues have begun to emerge, based on such evidence, and clearly indicate that embryonic tissues and the uterus communicate continuously during the peri-implantation period. Growth factors and their receptors are controlled by complex interregulatory influences. Several growth factors exist in multiple related forms, some of which may be inactive, and various receptors with variable affinities have been identified. The receptor profiles expressed may be related primarily to cell density (Rizzino, 1988).

Receptors for epidermal growth factor (EGF) are found in mouse embryos during the transition between morula and blastocyst. They become restricted to the trophectoderm, at a time when EGF stimulates protein synthesis, possibly relating to the concurrent increase in Na^+/K^+ ATPase (Wood and Kaye, 1989). EGF enhances the growth of mouse embryos in vitro, affecting their action between the 8-cell and blastocyst stages (Paria and Dey, 1990). EGF receptors on human syncytiotrophoblast cells are believed to promote differentiation, possibly also stimulating the production of hCG (Maruo and Mochizuki, 1987).

Mouse blastocysts contain transcripts for several growth factors (GFs) including platelet derived (PD)GF and transforming (T)GF-α and -$β_1$. TGF-$β_1$ was not detected in the unfertilized oocyte, implying that it is synthesized during embryogenesis. EGF, basic fibroblast GF (FGF), nerve GF-β and granulocyte colony stimulating factor were not found in mouse embryos (Rappolee et al, 1988). TGF-α binds efficiently to EGF receptors and might therefore act in an autocrine manner within the blastocyst. FGF may also be produced by mouse blastocysts (Rizzino, 1988). TGF-β, perhaps in combination with FGF, induces mesoderm formation in *Xenopus*

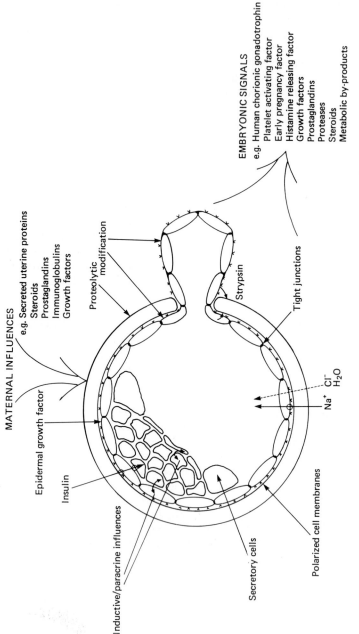

Figure 3. Embryonic factors and the embryo–maternal dialogue in the implanting mammalian blastocyst.

(Kimelman and Kirschner, 1987) and, in the mouse, the product of the *T* gene is essential for mesoderm formation (Herrmann et al, 1990). TGFs may also have a role in the local stimulation of angiogenesis at the implantation site (Folkman and Klagsbrun, 1987), possibly acting in addition to factors mentioned below. TGF-β is almost universally produced by most cells, but with variable levels of expression. TGF-$β_1$ has been temporally and spatially linked by immunohistochemistry to mouse embryonic tissues during morphogenesis, possibly suggesting a regulatory role in differentiation (Rizzino, 1988). Both inhibitory and stimulatory effects of TGF-β have been observed, dependent upon cell type (Rizzino, 1988). The effects of TGF-β on differentiation may be exerted via effects on extracellular matrix which can influence mRNA formation and translation and change cell shape. Conversely, the responsiveness of cells in vitro to growth factors depends upon the extracellular matrix used for cell culture (Rizzino, 1988).

Transcripts of insulin-like growth factor-2 (IGF-2) have been identified in preimplantation mouse embryos, although IGF-1 and insulin have not been detected (Rappolee et al, 1989). Transcripts for insulin and IGF-1 and -2 receptors have been found in mouse preimplantation embryos (see Smith et al, 1987; Graham et al, 1990). Insulin is actively transported into mouse embryos from the morula stage and is passed through the trophectoderm to the inner cell mass (Heyner et al, 1989). Its functions at this time are to generally promote the synthesis of various macromolecules, including, DNA, RNA and proteins, and to support cell division (see Graham et al, 1990). These experiments have been performed in mice; the potential actions of the insulin family in human embryos remain to be assessed.

Growth factors are present in the uterine secretions (Brigstock et al, 1989) and growth factors of maternal origin may have paracrine effects on embryos (Heyner et al, 1989). Most information on growth factors and related proteins in mammalian embryos has come from studies of laboratory animals (Mercola and Stiles, 1988) and detailed studies are just beginning on human embryos (Brice et al, 1989; Ohlson et al, 1989).

It is clear that growth factors include some of the molecules previously classified as inducers of mesoderm and endoderm. TGF is almost certainly equivalent to mesodermal inducer, and must be active as connective and vascular tissues differentiate in the late blastocyst.

PREIMPLANTATION SIGNALS

Platelet activating factor

The earliest event in implantation is the expression by a competent preimplantation embryo of some factor which signals its presence to the mother. A diagrammatic summary of some of the intrinsic and extrinsic factors involved in implantation is given in Figure 3. At the time of writing, a likely candidate for the first signal is platelet activating factor (PAF, 1-0-alkyl-2-sn-glycero-3-phosphocholine).

PAF is an intercellular messenger, having specific receptors linked to the membrane phospholipase C and calcium ion transport systems. Its effects on calcium ions link PAF with the prostaglandin synthase system (Parr et al, 1988). In addition to the activation of platelets suggested by its name, PAF has various physiological effects, including an increase in vascular permeability. However, the rabbit and human endometrium also produce PAF and have PAF receptors (Harper et al, 1989), hampering the study of interactions between the endometrium and the blastocyst.

To date, the earliest reliable maternal sign of implantation has been the locally increased vascular permeability around the implantation site. In mice, PAF acether is detected in the maternal circulation within 6 h of fertilization (Heap et al, 1988). The local vascular effects might be due to PAF, since PAF antagonists inhibit this reaction in mice, a result that is eliminated by concomitant administration of PAF acether (Spinks and O'Neill, 1988). Similar observations have not yet been made in other species.

Human embryos in vitro secrete significant but variable quantities of PAF within 48 h of oocyte insemination, and PAF production has been related to embryo quality (Collier et al, 1988). There are clear indications of an early reduction in circulating blood platelets in mice, but this effect is more variable in primates (O'Neill et al, 1985; Hearn et al, 1988). Other vasoactive products of the embryo, such as histamine, prostaglandins or oestrogen, might also contribute to the local increase in the capillary permeability of the uterus and other maternal signs of the presence of an embryo, or may be mediators in these processes.

The addition of PAF to media used to culture human embryos has been reported to improve their subsequent chances of implantation (O'Neill et al, 1989), but the reported rates of implantation were low. Moreover, since PAF is secreted very soon after fertilization, and before the embryonic genome is activated, it is difficult to explain how PAF production could reflect other than an event preprogrammed within the oocyte, nor is it easy to understand how the addition of PAF to culture medium could, without carry-over, modify the later maternal response to this putative embryonic signal. Nevertheless, evidence is building up that PAF may be of importance as one, if not the earliest, embryonic signal.

In mice, PAF has also been suggested to stimulate the production of early pregnancy factor (EPF) (Orozco et al, 1986). Similar EPF-like activity also exists in humans (Morton et al, 1977) and other species and may represent a common maternal response to early embryonic PAF. EPF has also been credited with immunosuppressive properties (Bose et al, 1989). A major drawback to studies on EPF concerns the failure to introduce a simple and reliable assay, which has raised doubts about its role in embryogenesis and implantation, although it has now been partly purified (Sueoka et al, 1989).

Prostaglandins

The increased vascular permeability at the implantation site, which occurs even before hatching of the blastocyst has led to searches for other active compounds. In addition to PAF, various vasoactive factors have been proposed to have a role in implantation, including the prostaglandins (PGs). PAF at high doses might indirectly stimulate local oedema and vaso-dilatation by promoting PGE_2 production by the endometrium (Smith, 1989). Prostaglandins of the E and F series are synthesized by peri-implantation embryos of many species (Bazer et al, 1986; Parr et al, 1988), although there is no evidence yet that human embryos produce prosta-glandins.

It is not easy to demonstrate any effect of these molecules since the endometrium also produces prostaglandins (Parr et al, 1988), especially at menstruation. Nevertheless, such a paracrine effect has been proposed in pigs (Jones et al, 1986). The prostaglandins may also have other effects equally important for implantation, e.g. in mice, embryonic prostaglandin E is probably involved in blastocyst expansion, since antagonists reduce the incidence of hatching in vitro (Biggers et al, 1978).

Prostaglandin synthesis may also be stimulated by histamine, a factor associated with implantation because of the close similarity of some aspects of inflammation and implantation (Shelesnyak, 1957). Mast cells are present in the uterus, and in maximal numbers around the time of implantation (Finn, 1986). In addition, the preimplantation embryo may secrete histamine or a histamine releasing factor (HRF) (Cocchiara et al, 1987), and oestrogens may be implicated in the formation or release of histamine (Smith, 1989), which may act directly or indirectly on either the embryo, via specific receptors, or the endometrium (Weitlauf, 1988). However, the role of histamine has been contentious and there are many conflicting data.

Uterine prostaglandin formation may be suppressed by progesterone (Smith, 1989) and also by interferons and related proteins, such as ovine/bovine trophoblast protein-1 (oTP-1, bTP-1) (Salamonsen et al, 1988).

Steroids

Steroids are the sole means of exogenous support required to obtain a functional endometrium in primary ovarian failure, but preimplantation embryos also possess enzymes concerned with steroid metabolism. Studies to date have demonstrated *de novo* synthesis from acetate, and substrates including progesterone, pregnenolone and 17α-hydroxypregnenolone may be converted to other steroids (Huff and Eik-Nes, 1966; Wu, 1987). The ability of embryos from various species to make oestradiol-17β from an androgen substrate via the aromatase pathway has also been documented (e.g. rabbit: Tandon et al, 1983; pig: Bate and King, 1988), though not yet in humans, and a role for embryonic oestrogen in implantation has been suggested (Dickmann and Dey, 1973). However, oestrogens may be pro-duced by embryos even in species where there is no known requirement for oestrogen in implantation (Glasser et al, 1990). It is unclear whether the production of small quantities of oestrogen or other steroids by the embryo may influence the endometrium locally.

High levels of circulating oestrogens are detrimental to implantation in both animals and man. Stimulation protocols which include agonists of gonadotrophin releasing hormone (GnRHa) are associated with lower circulating levels of total oestrogens and have been related to increased pregnancy rates in couples undergoing in vitro fertilization (Macnamee et al, 1989). Oestradiol can inhibit the attachment of rat blastocysts to polarized monolayers of uterine epithelial cells, although it has no effect on the receptivity of uterine stromal cells in vitro (Glasser et al, 1990). This may represent a mechanism for maintaining the non-receptive state under oestrogenic conditions in this species.

Although oestradiol is known to modify blood vessels and might cause oedema, either directly or via an effect on uterine mast cells, the high circulating concentrations of ovarian steroids during the peri-implantation period make a role for small quantities of embryonic steroids questionable. However, the progesterone : oestradiol ($P:E_2$) ratio is known to be important for implantation and the presence of an embryo might exert a local influence. The $P:E_2$ ratio also controls blastocyst arrest in animals with delayed implantation.

Implanting mouse embryos may metabolize progesterone (Wu, 1987). This steroid hormone is essential to maintain implantation and reduces the endometrial production of prostaglandins associated with menstruation (Smith, 1989), although this is unlikely to be a local embryonic effect. A progesterone antagonist, RU 486, has recently been introduced for clinical use and is a potent abortifacient. The effects of this inhibitor upon embryonic function have not yet been examined, although antibodies against progesterone arrest the development of mouse embryos prior to cavitation (Wang et al, 1984).

Embryonic secretory proteins

Various stage-specific proteins have been detected in supernatant media from preimplantation embryos (Nieder et al, 1987; Godkin et al, 1988). Perhaps the most important in primates is the glycoprotein chorionic gonadotrophin (CG). Messenger RNA for hCG has been detected at the 8-cell stage (Bonduelle et al, 1988) and is believed to be among the first products of the embryonic genome, later becoming restricted to the trophoblast. Large quantities of hCG are produced by the embryo and are detectable within the maternal circulation at around the time of implantation or shortly after, reflecting this hormone's activity as a systemic effector. Measurements of hCG can discriminate between normal and pathological implantations and the multiplicity of the pregnancy can also be discerned. The effects of hCG in rescuing and supporting corpus luteum function are well known but it has recently been reported to exert local effects within the endometrium (Levin et al, 1990).

Proteases are also of great importance in peri-implantation development, for example, in permitting hatching from the zona pellucida (Perona and Wassarman, 1986) and in trophoblast invasion (Glass et al, 1983). Proteases are present in uterine secretions, but observations of embryos cultured in vitro in serum-free medium suggest that the uterine proteases are not strictly necessary for hatching, though they may have a facilitatory effect.

Major secretory products of ovine and bovine blastocysts respectively are trophoblast proteins (oTP-1, bTP-1) with a variable degree of glycosylation. These proteins are believed to be the major embryonic signal in these species, preventing luteal regression and causing significant changes in endometrial protein production (Nieder et al, 1987; Salamonsen et al, 1988). Recently, oTP and bTP have been shown to have homology with human and bovine α-interferon and to share their characteristic antiviral and antiproliferative effects (Imakawa and Roberts, 1989). Both oTP and interferon reduce prostaglandin production in ovine endometrial cells (Salamonsen et al, 1988). Culture media from human blastocysts cultured in vitro contained no interferon-like antiviral activity (Roberts et al, 1990) and it seems that there is no such role for these compounds in human implantation as exists in ruminants.

Metabolic products

Secondary secretions of the embryo, such as metabolic by-products of respiration, might also be involved in implantation. The early human embryo utilizes pyruvate as an energy source, but after about 3 days in vitro, increases its utilization of glucose (Hardy et al, 1989). Respiration gives rise to carbon dioxide, which might reduce the local pH and influence the endometrium. Lactate is also a product of the developing preimplantation embryo, and might conceivably affect other nearby cells, though no studies have reported any effect on embryonic or endometrial cells of minute changes in the concentration of lactate.

Immune-active factors

Blastocysts usually differ in their HLA types from the mother and such histoincompatibility has been considered essential in sustaining implantation and even regulating some forms of abortion. There has been a long debate about the expression of HLA class I antigens on trophoblast, or of H-2 antigens in mice, and there have been both positive and negative findings.

There must be some doubt about the expression of such highly polymorphic antigens on trophoblast, with the attendant risk of stimulating immune responses in the mother. Nor can such antigenic differences play any role when a highly inbred embryo implants in a mother of the same strain. Human trophoblast expresses the 'neutral' HLA class I molecule HLA-G, which is not polymorphic in man although it is in other species (Ellis et al, 1990). However, there are some data which suggest that the maternal immune response is influenced by pregnancy.

Following fertilization, the zygote plasma membrane has been reported to express both maternal transplantation antigens (Edidin et al, 1975) and sperm antigens (mouse: Webb et al, 1977), and during cleavage, stage specific antigens are expressed (e.g. SSEA-1, F9: Solter and Knowles, 1978). The maternal immune response to the embryo begins rapidly after fertilization. The lack of rejection of the early embryo may be due in part to protection by the surrounding cumulus and zona pellucida, which become non-specifically coated with maternal proteins and immune cells such as immunoglobulin (Ig)A-secreting plasma cells, uterine T cells and peritoneal macrophages (Bernard et al, 1977). These may protect the embryo, provided the zona pellucida is intact (Willadsen, 1979).

Selective suppression of the maternal immune response during pregnancy has been suggested. TGF-β, discussed above, may inhibit the immune system (Rizzino, 1988) and α-fetoprotein (AFP) may suppress primary and secondary immunoglobulin responses in vitro (Murgita and Tomasi, 1975). Human AFP may also inhibit lymphocyte proliferation (Yachnin and Lester, 1976), and natural killer cells are less active during pregnancy (Nicholas and Panayi, 1985).

Certain maternal antibodies may protect the embryo from attack by the maternal immune system. This phenomenon has been exploited by deliberate immunization with paternal antigens to evoke protective antibodies, a procedure known as enhancement. This method has been used to treat couples with repeated spontaneous abortions, although the precise mechanism is currently unknown.

The issue of immune factors in early pregnancy has been contentious for many years. While immune-active factors undoubtedly exist and are involved in pregnancy, the nature of their involvement is still unclear.

IMPLANTATION

The process of bringing together the blastocyst and the uterine epithelium is complex and, although considerable progress has been made in rodents (Glasser et al, 1990), there are only minimal data available in primates, including man. The stages of implantation are often classified as apposition, attachment and invasion, and different processes are almost certainly involved in each stage. It is known that the blastocyst and endometrium become increasingly close and approach each other, their membranes interdigitating, but it is far from clear how such events are controlled. The two tissues presumably contain complementary binding proteins which attach and eventually fuse the two systems together (Yoshinaga, 1989).

In rodents, attachment occurs at specific sites within the uterus, with distribution probably achieved by uterine muscle activity. Orientation in rodents is controlled by the asymmetry of the blastocyst, where attachment occurs via the mural trophectoderm. This contrasts with the situation in humans where the polar trophoblast is first to attach and implantation sites are more variable (Gardner, 1990). Most implantation sites are found in the upper regions of the human uterus and commonly on the posterior wall. How the blastocyst becomes located for implantation within the human uterus is unknown and may be complicated in the presence of more that one embryo (Gardner, 1990). Interactions leading to orientation clearly require adequate previous differentiation as far as the asymmetric stage, together with the appropriate cell surface expression mediating implantation (Enders and Schlafke, 1974). The blastocyst surface may also require proteolytic modification to enhance adhesion (see Perona and Wassarman, 1986).

It is, of course, equally important that the implantation site should be competent to receive the blastocyst. The expression of complementary surface molecules, biochemical markers, local proteins, etc. should be in a suitable state of organization, particularly when using in vitro models of implantation where the maintenance of cell polarity is essential to observe physiological functions (Glasser et al, 1990). For example, laminin is secreted by early mouse embryos (Cooper and MacQueen, 1983) and is also found in a pericellular distribution around human decidual cells in the secretory and pregnant endometrium (Loke et al, 1989).

Trophoblast cells from first-trimester pregnancies preferentially attach to laminin coated dishes (Loke et al, 1989), indicating that this compound might have a role in adhesion and invasion by the trophoblast. Other factors produced by the implanting embryo, such as a collagenase-like activity, may also be important in trophoblast invasion (Puistola et al, 1989). Glyco-protein synthesis increases in amount and complexity as the mouse embryo becomes a blastocyst, when glycosylation is also enhanced (Armant et al, 1986). These proteins are essential for blastocoele formation, hatching and the adhesion of the trophectoderm. Glycosidases and proteases, present in trophoblast and uterine secretions, seem to play a role in attachment and implantation, and proteinase inhibitors will impair implantation when applied via the uterus (Denker, 1977).

The degree of invasion is highly variable between species, but the initial stages of attachment and incipient penetration have been observed in vitro, using monolayers of endometrial cells and homologous embryos (Linden-berg et al, 1989; Glasser et al, 1990). The profile of expression of various uterine proteins such as α_2-PEG and 24K protein could be markers of endometrial competence (Manners, 1990), as may other, as yet unidenti-fied, glycoprotein secretory products (Smith et al, 1989). The levels of these proteins vary throughout the menstrual cycle and the 'window' of implan-tation may be regulated by compounds such as these. The expression of endometrial competence may not be a prerequisite for implantation, which can occur in various ectopic sites, and the endometrium or decidua might contain the invasiveness of the trophoblast.

Deciduomata in the rat endometrium may in some instances be elicited by non-specific stimuli, such as oil droplets or trauma, not requiring the presence of an embryo (see Weitlauf, 1988) but in other situations local endometrial responses are conditional on the presence of an embryo, as in the locally increased uterine perfusion which depends on embryos competent to secrete prostaglandins (Jones et al, 1986).

It is clearly easier to gain information on the human endometrium rather than the implanting embryo, and markers of endometrial function are being characterized. Most research is currently conducted in infertile couples using assisted conception techniques, which may bias the results.

SUMMARY

The embryonic factors influencing implantation have been studied extensively in laboratory and domestic animals, but not in primates, including humans. Species differences make extrapolation inadvisable.

Embryonic factors affecting implantation include intrinsic features of the embryo, such as its genetic constitution, morphology and hatching. Abnormal genetic constitutions or unsuccessful transitions from maternal to embryonic transcription could account for many failures of early embryonic growth and implantation. Morphology *per se* does not greatly influence implantation, except when it reflects an abnormal genetic constitution, e.g. in severe fragmentation, although subtle effects may be detected as experimental techniques are refined. The initiation of differentiation and intra-embryonic communication between cells and cell types has been studied in animal embryos.

Signals must be exchanged between the embryo and the mother to ensure satisfactory implantation. These could include platelet activating factor, prostaglandins, histamine related factors, steroids, proteins, metabolic products and immune-active factors. No one factor seems to be totally responsible for alerting the mother to the presence of an embryo, and a concerted action of these and other agents is probably responsible.

The process of implantation itself is poorly understood because of a lack of adequate experimental models. The expression of complementary proteins and the role of specific enzymes and markers of endometrial and embryonic competence are factors well worthy of further study.

Knowledge about human implantation is increasing because of recent developments in assisted reproductive technology, and concepts arising from many years of research in animals should find clinical applications in understanding and controlling human reproduction.

Acknowledgements

The authors wish to thank Dr D Dillon for his contribution to this manuscript.

REFERENCES

Albertini DF, Overstrom EW & Ebert KM (1987) Changes in the organization of the actin cytoskeleton during preimplantation development of the pig embryo. *Biology of Reproduction* 37: 441–451.

Angell RR, Aitken RJ, Van Look PFA, Lumsden MA & Templeton AA (1983) Chromosome abnormalities in human embryos after in vitro fertilization. *Nature* 303: 336–338.

Armant DK, Kaplan HA & Lennarz WJ (1986) N-linked glycoprotein biosynthesis in the developing mouse embryo. *Development* 113: 228–237.

Bate LA & King GJ (1988) Production of oestrone and oestradiol-17β by different regions of the filamentous pig blastocyst. *Journal of Reproduction and Fertility* 84: 163–169.

Bayna EM, Shaper JH & Shur BD (1988) Temporally specific involvement of cell surface galactosyl transferase during mouse embryos morula compaction. *Cell* 53: 145–147.

Bazer FW, Vallet JL, Roberts RM, Sharp DC & Thatcher WW (1986) Role of conceptus secretory products in establishment of pregnancy. *Journal of Reproduction and Fertility* 76: 841–850.

Bernard O, Bennett D & Ripoche M (1977) Distribution of maternal immunoglobulins in the mouse uterus and embryo in the days after implantation. *Journal of Experimental Medicine* 145: 58–75.

Biggers JD, Leonov BV, Baskar JF & Fried J (1978) Inhibition of hatching of mouse blastocysts in vitro by prostaglandin antagonists. *Biology of Reproduction* **19**: 519–533.

Bonduelle ML, Dodd R, Liebaers I, Van Steirteghem A, Williamson R & Akhurst R (1988) Chorionic gonadotrophin-β mRNA, a trophoblast marker, is expressed in human 8-cell embryos derived from tripronucleate zygotes. *Human Reproduction* **3**: 909–914.

Bose R, Cheng H, Sabbadini E, McCoshen J, Mahadevan MM & Fleetham J (1989) Purified human early pregnancy factor possesses immunosuppressive properties. *American Journal of Obstetrics and Gynecology* **160**: 954–960.

Brambati B (1990) Fate of human pregnancies. In Edwards RG (ed.) *Establishing a Successful Human Pregnancy*, Serono Symposia Publications, vol. 66, pp 269–281. Rome: Raven Press.

Braude P, Bolton V & Moore S (1988) Human gene expression first occurs between the four- and eight-cell stages of preimplantation development. *Nature* **332**: 459–462.

Brice AL, Cheetham JE, Bolton VN, Hill NCW & Schofield PN (1989) Temporal changes in the expression of the insulin-like growth factor II gene associated with tissue maturation in the human fetus. *Development* **106**: 543–554.

Brigstock DR, Heap RB & Brown KD (1989) Polypeptide growth factors in uterine tissues and secretions. *Journal of Reproduction and Fertility* **55**: 267–275.

Bulletti C, Jasonni VM, Tabanelli S et al (1988) Early human pregnancy in vitro utilizing an artificially perfused uterus. *Fertility and Sterility* **49**: 991–996.

Buster JE, Bustillo M, Rodi IA et al (1985) Biologic and morphologic development of donated human ova recovered by nonsurgical uterine lavage. *American Journal of Obstetrics and Gynecology* **153**: 211–217.

Chan PJ (1987) Developmental potential of human oocytes according to zona pellucida thickness. *Journal of In Vitro Fertilization and Embryo Transfer* **4**: 237–241.

Claman P, Armant DR, Seibel MM, Wang TA, Oskowitz SP & Taynor ML (1987) The impact of embryo quality and quantity on implantation and the establishment of viable pregnancies. *Journal of In Vitro Fertilization and Embryo Transfer* **4**: 218–222.

Cocchiara R, Di Trapani G, Azzolina A et al (1987) Isolation of a histamine releasing factor from human embryo culture medium after in vitro fertilization. *Human Reproduction* **2**: 341–344.

Cohen J, Inge KL, Suzman N & Wright G (1989a) Videocinematography of fresh and cryo-preserved embryos: a retrospective analysis of embryonic morphology and implantation. *Fertility and Sterility* **51**: 820–827.

Cohen J, Elsner C, Kort H et al (1989b) Impairment of the hatching process following IVF in the human and improvement of implantation by assisting hatching using micro-manipulation. *Human Reproduction* **5**: 7–13.

Cole RJ (1967) Cinematographic observations on the trophoblast and zona pellucida of the mouse blastocyst. *Journal of Embryology and Experimental Morphology* **17**: 481–490.

Cole RJ, Edwards RG & Paul J (1966) Cytodifferentiation and embryogenesis in cell colonies and tissue cultures derived from ova and blastocysts of the rabbit. *Developmental Biology* **13**: 385–407.

Collier M, O'Neill C, Ammit AJ & Saunders DM (1988) Biochemical and pharmacological characterization of human embryo-derived platelet activating factor. *Human Reproduction* **3**: 993–998.

Cooper AR & MacQueen HA (1983) Subunits of laminin are differentially synthesised in mouse eggs and early embryos. *Developmental Biology* **96**: 467–471.

De Felici M, Salustri A & Siracusa G (1985) Spontaneous hardening of the zona pellucida of mouse oocytes during in vitro culture. II. The effect of follicular fluid and glycosamino-glycans. *Gamete Research* **12**: 227–235.

Denker HW (1977) Implantation. *Advances in Anatomy, Embryology and Cell Biology* **53**: 1–123.

Derom C, Derom R, Vlietinck R, Van den Berghe H & Thiery M (1987) Increased mono-zygotic twinning rate after ovulation induction. *Lancet* **i**: 1236–1238.

Dickmann Z & Dey SK (1973) Two theories: the preimplantation embryo is a source of steroid hormones controlling (1) morula-blastocyst transformation and (2) implantation. *Journal of Reproduction and Fertility* **35**: 615–617.

Dyce J, George MA, Goodall H & Fleming TP (1987) Do cells belonging to trophectoderm and inner cell mass in the mouse blastocyst maintain discrete lineages? *Development* **100**: 685–698.

Edidin M, Gooding LR & Johnson MI (1975) Surface antigens of normal early embryos and a tumor model system useful for their further study. *Acta Endocrinologica* (Supplement) 78: 336–356.

Edwards RG (ed.) (1980) Implantation. In *Conception in the Human Female*, pp 767–826. London: Academic Press.

Edwards RG (1989) Tribute to Patrick Steptoe: beginnings of laparoscopy. *Human Reproduction* **4** (supplement 1): 1–9.

Edwards RG, Mettler L & Walters DE (1986) Identical twins and in vitro fertilization. *Journal of In Vitro Fertilization and Embryo Transfer* **3**: 114–117.

Ellis SA, Palmer MS & McMichael AJ (1990) Human trophoblast and the choriocarcinoma cell line BeWo express a truncated HLA class 1 molecule. *Journal of Immunology* **144**: 731–735.

Enders AC (1989) Morphological manifestations of maturation of the blastocyst. *Progress in Clinical and Biological Research* **294**: 151–170.

Enders AC & Schlafke S (1974) Surface coats of the mouse blastocyst and uterus during the preimplantation period. *Anatomical Record* **180**: 31–46.

Finn CA (1986) Implantation, menstruation and inflammation. *Biological Reviews of the Cambridge Philosophical Society* **61**: 313–328.

Fleming TP (1987) A quantitative analysis of cell allocation to trophectoderm and inner cell mass in the mouse blastocyst. *Developmental Biology* **119**: 520–531.

Folkman J & Klagsbrun M (1987) Angiogenic Factors. *Science* **235**: 442–447.

Gardner RL (1990) Location and orientation of implantation. In Edwards RG (ed.) *Establishing a Successful Human Pregnancy*, Serono Symposia Publications, vol. 66, pp 225–238. Rome: Raven Press.

Gardner RL & Rossant J (1976) Determination during embryogenesis. In Elliott K & O'Connor M (eds) *Embryogenesis in Mammals*, pp 15–25. Amsterdam: Associated Scientific Publishers.

Glass RH, Aggeler J, Spindle A, Pedersen RA & Werb Z (1983) Degradation of extracellular matrix by mouse trophoblast outgrowths: a model for implantation. *Journal of Cell Biology* **96**: 1108–1116.

Glasser SR, Julian J, Mani SK et al (1990) Blastocyst–endometrial relationships: reciprocal interaction between uterine epithelial and stromal cells and blastocysts. *Trophoblast Research* **5** (in press).

Godkin JD, Lifsey BJ Jr & Gillespie BE (1988) Characterization of bovine conceptus proteins produced during the peri- and postattachment periods of early pregnancy. *Biology of Reproduction* **38**: 703–711.

Graham CF, Elliss CJ, Brice AL, Richardson LJ, Marshall H & Schofield PN (1990) Growth factors and early mammalian development. In Edwards RG (ed.) *Establishing a Successful Human Pregnancy*, Serono Symposia Publications, vol. 66, pp 239–254. Rome: Raven Press.

Gurdon JB, Mohun TJ, Sharpe CR & Taylor MV (1990) Induction, gene activation and embryonic differentiation. In Edwards RG (ed.) *Establishing a Successful Human Pregnancy*, Serono Symposia Publications, vol. 66, pp 155–169. Rome: Raven Press.

Hardy K, Hooper MAK, Handyside AH, Rutherford AJ, Winston RML & Leese HJ (1989) Non-invasive measurement of glucose and pyruvate uptake by individual human oocytes and preimplantation embryos. *Human Reproduction* **4**: 188–191.

Harper MJK, Kudolo GB, Alecozay AA & Jones MA (1989) Platelet-activating factor (PAF) and blastocyst–endometrial interactions. *Progress in Clinical and Biological Research* **294**: 305–315.

Hartshorne GM, Blayney M, Dyson H & Elder K (1990) Case Report: in vitro fertilization and development of one of two human oocytes with fused zonae pellucidae. *Fertility and Sterility* **54**: 947–949.

Hartshorne GM, Elder K, Crow J, Dyson H & Edwards RG (1991) The influence of in vitro development upon post-thaw survival and implantation of cryopreserved human blastocysts. *Human Reproduction* (in press).

Heap RB, Flint AP & Gadsby JG (1979) Role of embryonic signals in the establishment of pregnancy. *British Medical Bulletin* **35**: 129–135.

Heap RB, Fleet IR, Finn C et al (1988) Maternal reactions affecting early embryogenesis and implantation. *Journal of Reproduction and Fertility* **36** (supplement): 83–97.

Hearn JP, Gidley-Baird AA, Hodges JK, Summers PM & Webley GE (1988) Embryonic signals during the peri-implantation period in primates. *Journal of Reproduction and Fertility* **36** (supplement): 49–58.

Herrmann BG, Labeit S, Poustka A, King TR & Lehrach H (1990) Cloning of the T gene required in mesoderm formation in the mouse. *Nature* **343**: 617–622.

Heyner S, Rao LV, Jarett L & Smith RM (1989) Preimplantation mouse embryos internalise maternal insulin via receptor-mediated endocytosis: pattern of uptake and functional correlations. *Developmental Biology* **134**: 48–58.

Huff RL & Eik-Nes KB (1966) Metabolism in vitro of acetate and certain steroids by six-day-old rabbit blastocysts. *Journal of Reproduction and Fertility* **11**: 57–63.

Imakawa K & Roberts RM (1989) Interferons and maternal recognition of pregnancy. *Progress in Clinical and Biological Research* **294**: 347–358.

Iwakura Y & Nozaki M (1989) Role of cell surface glycoproteins in the early development of the mouse embryo. *Progress in Clinical and Biological Research* **294**: 199–210.

Johnson MH (1989) How are two lineages established in early mouse development? *Progress in Clinical and Biological Research* **294**: 189–198.

Johnson MH, Pickering SJ, Dhiman A, Radcliffe GS & Maro B (1988) Cytocortical organisation during natural and prolonged mitosis of mouse 8-cell blastomeres. *Development* **102**: 143–158.

Jones MA, De Cao Z, Anderson W, Norris C & Harper JK (1986) Capillary permeability changes in the uteri of recipient rabbits after transfer of blastocysts from indomethacin-treated donors. *Journal of Reproduction and Fertility* **78**: 261–273.

Kajii T & Ohama K (1977) Androgenetic origin of the hydatidiform mole. *Nature* **268**: 633–634.

Kimelman D & Kirschner M (1987) Synergistic induction of mesoderm by FGF and TGF-β and the identification of an mRNA coding for FGF in the early *Xenopus* embryo. *Cell* **51**: 869–877.

Lehtonen E (1980) Changes in cell dimensions and intracellular contacts during cleavage stage cell cycles in mouse embryonic cells. *Journal of Embryology and Experimental Morphology* **58**: 231–249.

Levin JH, Tonetta SA & Lobo RA (1990) Human chorionic gonadotropin (hCG) enhances progestin stimulation of prolactin (PRL) production by human endometrial stromal cells in culture: evidence for trophoblast–endometrial paracrine interaction. *38th Annual Meeting of the Pacific Coast Fertility Society*, Programme Supplement, abstract 7.

Lindenberg S, Hyttel P, Sjogren A & Greve T (1989) A comparative study of attachment of human, bovine and mouse blastocysts to uterine epithelial monolayer. *Human Reproduction* **4**: 446–456.

Loke YW & King A (1989) Immunology of pregnancy: quo vadis? *Human Reproduction* **4**: 613–615.

Loke YW, Gardner L, Burland K & King A (1989) Laminin in human trophoblast–decidua interaction. *Human Reproduction* **4**: 457–463.

Lopata A & Hay DL (1989) The potential of early human embryos to form blastocysts, hatch from their zona and secrete hCG in culture. *Human Reproduction* **4** (supplement 1): 87–94.

Macnamee MC, Howles CM, Edwards RG & Taylor PJ (1989) Short term LHRH agonist treatment: a novel ovarian stimulation regimen for in vitro fertilization. *Fertility and Sterility* **52**: 264–269.

Manners CV (1990) Endometrial assessment in a group of infertile women on stimulated cycles for IVF: immunohistochemical findings. *Human Reproduction* **5**: 128–132.

Martin RH, Balkan W, Burns K, Rademaker AW, Lin CC & Rudd NL (1983) The chromosome constitution of 1000 human spermatozoa. *Human Genetics* **63**: 305–309.

Maruo T & Mochizuki M (1987) Immunohistochemical localization of epidermal growth factor receptor and *myc* oncogene product in human placenta: implication for trophoblast proliferation and differentiation. *American Journal of Obstetrics and Gynecology* **156**: 721–727.

Massip A & Mulnard J (1980) Time lapse cinematographic analysis of hatching of normal and frozen-thawed cow blastocysts. *Journal of Reproduction and Fertility* **58**: 475–478.

Mercola M & Stiles CD (1988) Growth factor superfamilies and mammalian embryogenesis. *Development* **102**: 451–460.

Michelmann HW, Bonhoff A & Mettler L (1986) Chromosome analysis in polyploid human embryos. *Human Reproduction* **1**: 243–246.

Morton H, Rolfe B, Clunie GJA, Anderson MJ & Morrison J (1977) An early pregnancy factor detected in human serum by the rosette inhibition test. *Lancet* **i:** 394–397.

Murgita RA & Tomasi TB (1975) Suppression of the immune response by α-fetoprotein I and II. *Journal of Experimental Medicine* **141:** 269, 440.

Nicholas NS & Panayi GS (1985) Inhibition of interleukin-2 production by retroplacental sera: a possible mechanism for human fetal allograft survival. *American Journal of Reproductive Immunology and Microbiology* **9:** 6–12.

Nicholls RD, Knoll JHM, Butler MG, Karam S & Lalande M (1989) Genetic imprinting suggested by maternal heterodisomy in non-deletion Prader–Willi syndrome. *Nature* **342:** 281–285.

Nieder GL, Weitlauf HM & Suda-Hartman M (1987) Synthesis and secretion of stage specific proteins by peri-implantation mouse embryos. *Biology of Reproduction* **36:** 687–699.

Ohlson R, Larsson E, Nilsson O, Wahlstrom T & Sundstrom P (1989) Blastocyst implantation precedes induction of insulin-like growth factor II gene expression in human trophoblast. *Development* **106:** 555–559.

O'Neill C, Gidley-Baird AA, Pike IL, Porter RN, Sinosich MJ & Saunders DM (1985) Maternal blood platelet physiology and luteal phase endocrinology as a means of monitoring preimplantation embryo viability following in vitro fertilization. *Journal of In Vitro Fertilization and Embryo Transfer* **2:** 87–93.

O'Neill C, Collier M, Ammit AJ, Ryan JP, Saunders DM & Pike IL (1989) Supplementation of in-vitro fertilisation culture medium with platelet activating factor. *Lancet* **ii:** 769–772.

O'Rahilly R (1973) *Developmental Stages in Human Embryos*, Part A. Washington: Carnegie Institute.

Orozco C, Perkins F & Clark FN (1986) Platelet activating factor induces the expression of early pregnancy factor activity in female mice. *Journal of Reproduction and Fertility* **78:** 549–555.

Overstrom EW, Benos DJ & Biggers JD (1989) Synthesis of Na^+/K^+ ATPase by the pre-implantation rabbit blastocyst. *Journal of Reproduction and Fertility* **85:** 283–295.

Paria SC & Dey SK (1990) Preimplantation embryo development in vitro: cooperative interactions among embryos and role of growth factors. *Proceedings of the National Academy of Sciences of the USA* **87:** 4756–4760.

Parr MB, Parr EL, Munaretto K, Clark MR & Dey SK (1988) Immunohistochemical localization of prostaglandin synthase in the rat uterus and embryo during the peri-implantation period. *Biology of Reproduction* **38:** 333–343.

Perona RM & Wassarman PM (1986) Mouse blastocysts hatch in vitro by using a trypsin-like proteinase associated with cells of mural trophectoderm. *Developmental Biology* **114:** 42–52.

Plachot M, DeGrouchy J, Junca A-M et al (1987) From oocyte to embryo: a model, deduced from in vitro fertilization for natural selection against chromosome abnormalities. *Annals de Génétique* **30:** 22–32.

Puistola U, Ronnberg L, Martikainen H & Turpeenniemi-Hujanen T (1989) The human embryo produces basement membrane collagen (type IV collagen)-degrading protease activity. *Human Reproduction* **4:** 309–311.

Rappolee DA, Brenner CA, Schultz R, Mark D & Werb Z (1988) Developmental expression of PDGF, TGF-α, and TGF-β genes in preimplantation mouse embryos. *Science* **241:** 1823–1825.

Rappolee DA, Sturm KS, Schultz GA, Pedersen RA & Werb Z (1989) Early embryonic development and paracrine relationships. In Heyner S & Wiley L (eds) *UCLA Symposia on Molecular and Cellular Biology, News Series 117*. New York: Alan R Liss.

Rizzino A (1988) Transforming growth factor-β: multiple effects on cell differentiation and extracellular matrices. *Developmental Biology* **130:** 411–422.

Rizzino A, Kuszynski C, Ruff E & Tiesman J (1988) Production and utilization of growth factors related to fibroblast growth factor by embryonal carcinoma cells and their differentiated cells. *Developmental Biology* **129:** 61–71.

Roberts RM, Cross JC, Farin CF, Kramer K, Schalve Francis T & Hansen TR (1990) Trophoblast interferons and anti-luteolysins. In Edwards RG (ed.) *Establishing a Successful Human Pregnancy*, Serono Symposia Publications, vol. 66, pp 257–268. Rome: Raven Press.

Rosner MH, Vigano MA, Ozato K et al (1990) A POU-domain transcription factor in early stem cells and germ cells of the mammalian embryo. *Nature* **345**: 686–692.

Salamonsen LA, Stuchbery SJ, O'Grady CM, Godkin JD & Findlay JK (1988) Interferon-α mimics effects of ovine trophoblast protein 1 on prostaglandin and protein secretion by ovine endometrial cells in vitro. *Journal of Endocrinology* **117**: R1–R4.

Shelesnyak MC (1957) Some experimental studies on the mechanism of ovo-implantation in the rat. *Recent Progress in Hormone Research* **13**: 269–322.

Sherman MI & Wudl LR (1977) T-complex mutants and their effects. In Sherman MC (ed.) *Concepts in Mammalian Embryogenesis*, p 136. Cambridge, MA: MIT Press.

Shur BD (1977) Cell surface glycosyltransferases in gastrulating chick embryos. I. Temporally and spatially specific patterns of four endogenous glycosyltransferase activities. *Developmental Biology* **58**: 23–39.

Smith EP, Sadler TW & D'Ercole AJ (1987) Somatomedins/insulin-like growth factors, their receptors and binding proteins are present during mouse embryogenesis. *Development* **101**: 73–82.

Smith RA, Seif MW, Rogers AW et al (1989) The endometrial cycle: the expression of a secretory component correlated with the luteinizing hormone peak. *Human Reproduction* **4**: 236–242.

Smith SK (1989) Prostaglandins and growth factors in the endometrium. *Baillière's Clinical Obstetrics and Gynaecology* **3**: 249–270.

Solter D & Knowles BB (1978) Monoclonal antibody defining a stage-specific mouse embryonic antigen (SSEA-1). *Proceedings of the National Academy of Sciences of the USA* **75**: 5565–5569.

Spinks NR & O'Neill C (1988) Antagonists of embryo-derived platelet-activating factor prevent implantation of mouse embryos. *Journal of Reproduction and Fertility* **84**: 89–98.

Sueoka K, Kusama T, Baba J, Wallach EE & Iizuka R (1989) Biochemical consideration of human early pregnancy factor (EPF). *Progress in Clinical and Biological Research* **294**: 317–329.

Summers PM, Campbell JM & Miller MW (1988) Normal in-vivo development of marmoset monkey embryos after trophectoderm biopsy. *Human Reproduction* **3**: 389–393.

Surani MA, Allen ND, Barton SC et al (1990) Developmental consequences of imprinting of parental chromosomes by DNA methylation. *Philosophical Transactions of the Royal Society of London; B: Biological Sciences* **326**: 313–327.

Tandon A, Singh MM & Kamboj VP (1983) Steroid metabolism by rabbit embryos: time of onset of steroidogenic activity. *Experimental and Clinical Endocrinology* **82**: 285–290.

Tesarik J (1988) Developmental control of human preimplantation embryos: a comparative approach. *Journal of In Vitro Fertilization and Embryo Transfer* **5**: 347–362.

Tesarik J, Kopecny V, Plachot M & Mandelbaum J (1988) Early morphological signs of embryonic genome expression in human preimplantation development as revealed by quantitative electron microscopy. *Developmental Biology* **128**: 15–20.

Veiga A, Calderon G, Santalo J, Barri PN & Egozcue J (1987) Chromosome studies in oocytes and zygotes from an IVF programme. *Human Reproduction* **2**: 425–430.

Wang M-Y, Rider V, Heap RB & Feinstein A (1984) Action of anti-progesterone monoclonal antibody in blocking pregnancy after post-coital administration in mice. *Journal of Endocrinology* **101**: 95–100.

Watanabe N, VandeWoude GF, Ikawa Y & Sagata N (1990) Specific proteolysis of the c-*mos* proto-oncogene product by calpain on fertilization of *Xenopus* eggs. *Nature* **342**: 505–511.

Webb CG, Gall WE & Edelmann GM (1977) Synthesis and distribution of H-2 antigens in preimplantation mouse embryos. *Journal of Experimental Medicine* **146**: 923–932.

Weitlauf HM (1988) Biology of implantation. In Knobil E, Neill J et al (eds) *The Physiology of Reproduction*, pp 231–262. New York: Raven Press.

Willadsen S (1979) A method for culture of micromanipulated sheep embryos and its use to produce monozygotic twins. *Nature* **277**: 298.

Winkel GK & Pedersen RA (1988) Fate of the inner cell mass in mouse embryos as studied by microinjection of lineage markers. *Developmental Biology* **127**: 143–156.

Wood SA & Kaye PL (1989) Effects of epidermal growth factor on preimplantation mouse embryos. *Journal of Reproduction and Fertility* **85**: 575–582.

Wramsby H, Fredga K & Liedholm P (1987) Chromosome analysis of human oocytes recovered from preovulatory follicles in stimulated cycles. *New England Journal of Medicine* **316**: 121–124.

Wu JT (1987) Metabolism of progesterone by preimplantation mouse blastocysts in culture. *Biology of Reproduction* **36:** 549–556.
Yachnin S & Lester E (1976) Inhibition of human lymphocyte transformation by human alpha fetoprotein (HAFP). Comparison of foetal and hepatoma HAFP and kinetic studies of in vitro immunosuppression. *Clinical and Experimental Immunology* **26:** 484.
Yoshinaga K (1989) Receptor concept in implantation research. *Progress in Clinical and Biological Research* **294:** 379–387.

10

A consideration of the factors which influence and control the viability and developmental potential of the preimplantation embryo

CHRIS O'NEILL

While almost every aspect of assisted reproduction is far from optimal, there is one area where these techniques cause a considerable limitation to fertility: that is the failure of embryo implantation. For the majority of couples presenting for in vitro fertilization (IVF), oocyte retrieval is achieved and, except in severe male factor infertility, fertilization in vitro and subsequent first and second cleavage of the embryo are highly efficient. However, judging by the reports of the National Perinatal Statistics Unit (1989), more than 90% of embryos transferred to the uterus fail to result in the establishment of pregnancy.

This high failure rate is perplexing and is clearly a major barrier to the optimization of these procedures. There are certainly many contributing factors to this poor embryo viability. In an extensive study of the chromosomal integrity of morphologically normal human pre-embryos produced by IVF it was found that 20% had gross abnormalities (Plachot et al, 1988). While this is high, it is probably not substantially higher than occurs following natural conception. It is certainly not sufficient to explain the failure of over 90% of pre-embryos to implant.

The poor pregnancy potential of embryos after IVF is reflected by their poor developmental capacity in vitro. In a study of 317 embryos produced by IVF, only 17% of zygotes developed to the blastocyst stage (Bolton et al, 1989). Of importance, most developed successfully to the 4-cell stage but rapidly ceased development thereafter, so that the greatest loss in developmental capacity occurred from the 4-cell to the 8-cell stage.

The developmental potential of embryos fertilized in vitro is limited and shows striking similarity whether subsequent development occurs in vitro or in vivo, suggesting that fertilization and culture in vitro significantly compromise the developmental potential of the embryo. This is confirmed by studies with experimental animals.

CAUSES OF REDUCED EMBRYO VIABILITY

In an elegantly designed study (Vanderhyden et al, 1986), controlled for various aspects of gamete and embryo manipulation (including ovarian stimulation), it was shown that it was the actual process of fertilization of rat ova in vitro which caused a marked reduction in the developmental capacity of the resulting embryos. The zygotes were cultured in vitro for a minimum period of only 16 h, yet a reduction of 80% in the capacity for pregnancy of embryos occurred.

It was subsequently shown (Vanderhyden and Armstrong, 1988) that embryos fertilized in vitro developed more slowly than control embryos and that, at a given development stage, they had fewer cells. This slower development resulted in an asynchrony between the preparation of the embryo and the endometrium for implantation. If embryos were given extra time in vitro to reach a more advanced developmental stage prior to transfer to synchronized recipients, the implantation rate was improved.

This tendency for slower development in vitro is not only due to fertilization in vitro but is a general characteristic of culture of preimplantation embryos in vitro. For the mouse embryo, culture from the 1-cell stage to the blastocyst stage generally takes 24 h longer than similar development in situ. Combined, such studies show us that only brief culture in vitro during fertilization has the capacity to slow subsequent development (even in vivo) and fertilization in vivo but subsequent culture in vitro also retards development. Clearly there are aspects of the maternal environment important for embryonic development which are not normally catered for by culture media.

Genetic influences

The rate at which embryos develop is undoubtedly controlled by many factors, including their genotype. In mice a preimplantation embryo development (*Ped*) gene has been shown to be in the major histocompatibility complex, linked to the H-2 complex (Warner et al, 1987; 1988). This gene has *fast* and *slow* alleles, with *fast* being dominant. It has been suggested that the Qa-2 antigen (expressed on preimplantation mouse embryos) is the *Ped* gene product. Strains of mice which are homozygous for *slow* have embryos which develop more slowly, and mice of this genotype appear to have reduced fertility. If homologues of the *Ped* gene exist in other species, including humans, they may be a cause of reduced embryonic development and perhaps cause heterogeneity in the developmental rates of embryos from the same parents. It would also be of interest to determine the effects of suboptimal growth conditions, such as culture in vitro, on the growth rates of hetero-zygous embryos. Assuming that a similar gene occurs in humans, the fact that the *slow* gene is recessive suggests that the *slow* phenotype is likely to be only a limited cause of poor embryonic development.

In its most extreme form, the detrimental effects of in vitro culture may cause a 'block' to embryonic development. In most species studied to date, there appears to be a developmental stage which is particularly susceptible to culture. The mouse embryo of many strains stops development at the 2-cell stage. In humans this appears to be at the 8-cell stage of development (Bolton et al, 1989), as is the case for ovine and bovine embryos. The hamster, like the mouse, often suffers a '2-cell block' of development. The biochemical cause of the developmental block is not clear. The fact that it is caused by culture in vitro suggests some suboptimal feature of this environment.

Influence of the reproductive tract

Some lines of experimental evidence have suggested that the developmental blocks may be due to the lack of some specific maternal (trophic) factor(s). In particular, it was shown that 1-cell embryos developed to the blastocyst stage at comparable rates to embryos grown in vivo if they were grown with oviduct explants in organ culture (Biggers et al, 1962), and similar results were shown for the hamster (Bavister and Minami, 1986). Whittingham (1968) showed with the mouse that it was the ampulla, but not the isthmus or uterus, which promotes such development. The concept that the oviductal environment provided some specific benefit for embryo development was given impetus by the observation that the 8-cell block of ovine embryos was overcome and the production of viable embryos resulted from their co-culture with oviduct epithelial cells.

It was of particular interest that, while monolayers of fetal fibroblasts also promoted preimplantation development, they did not result in the dramatic increase in embryo viability (as assessed by extensive further development after embryo transfer) (Gandolfi and Moor, 1987). Similar results have been demonstrated in other species. The effect of co-culture is apparently not due to contact between the embryo and oviductal cells, since medium conditioned by oviductal tissue also enhances embryonic development (Eyestone and First, 1989). This conditioning might result in the addition of secretory products to the medium (a number of oviducal secretory products have been reported from various species), the removal (metabolism) of inhibitory substances from the medium (it is not known what these inhibitory factors might be, particularly in a simple chemically defined medium, although for the hamster, at least, glucose can inhibit development), or the dynamic change of the composition of medium to one more suitable for development.

Co-culture with somatic cells in vitro

A number of recent studies have suggested that co-culture of human embryos with somatic cells may be beneficial. Wiemer et al (1989a, 1989b) reported the use of fetal bovine uterine fibroblast cells in co-culture. They claimed that in such co-culture the incidence of blastomere fragmentation is reduced, while implantation was increased from 17 to 35% ($P < 0.05$). The same group reported elsewhere that co-culture with fetal bovine uterine fibroblasts resulted in a 19% implantation rate, compared with 13% ($P > 0.05$) for controls, while the ongoing pregnancy rate for patients receiving embryos from co-culture doubled to 35% (Wiemer et al, 1989b). Another group has examined the use of human ampullary epithelial cells obtained from fertile women undergoing hysterectomy. Using T6 + 15% patient serum as control medium, Bongso et al (1989) found that 60% of human embryos underwent cavitation in co-culture with human ampullary cells, compared with 33% for controls ($P < 0.01$). However, an equivalent proportion of control and co-cultured embryos underwent hatching from their zona pellucida. Examined ultrastructurally (Sathananthan et al, 1990), the co-culture embryos were similar to those cultured in T6 medium.

These preliminary studies show that the human preimplantation embryo, like other species, may benefit from co-culture with oviductal material. The use of heterologous cellular materials is, however, fraught with many difficulties, not least of which is the possibility of viral contamination. Clearly the way ahead is to understand the mechanisms by which co-culture exerts its apparently beneficial effect and develop means of mimicking these in a chemically defined medium.

Towards a defined, optimum embryo culture medium

Some recent studies have suggested that the role of the oviduct may not be specific. In sheep it was found that co-culture with oviductal epithelial cells was not essential for good preimplantation development (Walker et al, 1988). A medium based on the ionic composition of sheep oviduct fluid (Tervit et al, 1972), with a high serum content and partially buffered with Hepes, supported development (Walker et al, 1988). The authors concluded that factors within human serum, and rigorous control of the medium's pH, eliminated the need for somatic cell support. Similarly, in mice, modifications to the media composition has resulted in overcoming the 1-cell block in development. It was found that increasing the lactate:pyruvate ratio, exchanging glutamine (1 mM) for glucose and the addition of the metal chelating agent ethylenediaminetetraacetic acid (EDTA) (0.1 mM) stimulated normal development in a strain of mice which exhibits the 2-cell block in conventional embryo culture media (Poueymirou et al, 1989).

The role of these media additives is not defined. Clearly glutamine is likely to have an important role as both an energy substrate and a donor of nitrogen. The altered lactate:pyruvate ratio may be important for maintaining the redox potential of the cells. The beneficial effect of EDTA is less clear: perhaps it serves to sequester toxic metal ions from the medium, or it may dampen intracellular Ca^{2+} concentrations. This is an important issue to be resolved. It clearly affects embryonic metabolism, since absence of EDTA from two media resulted in a marked delay in the expression of transcription dependent proteins by embryos (Poueymirou et al, 1989).

GENOMIC CONTROL OF EMBRYONIC DEVELOPMENT

This general issue of transcription of the embryonic genome may be critically related to the effect of culture in vitro on embryo development. In each of the species studied in detail, the developmental stage most sensitive to culture conditions is that stage when the embryonic genome is first activated and, as noted above, in the mouse at least, the rate of embryo development may be under genetic control. In the mouse, this is the 2-cell stage (Flach et al, 1982; Bensaude et al, 1983) and mouse embryos exhibit a 2-cell block. For humans, genome activation occurs at the 4–8-cell stage

(Braude et al, 1988) and this is the stage where most developmental arrest occurs (Bolton et al, 1989). This temporal correlation between the activation of the zygotic genome and developmental arrest has led to the widespread speculation that culture in vitro results in the failure of, or only partial activation of, the embryonic genome, with resulting developmental deprivation. The observation that injection of cytoplasm from the blastomeres of 2-cell embryos that do not exhibit 2-cell blockage into embryos that do, rescues the injected embryos and allows normal development (Muggleton-Harris et al, 1982) is consistent with the possibility that the absence of some specific gene products is the cause of this developmental failure. It is relevant that retardation of development may be a result of fertilization in vitro in the rat, even when subsequent development is in vivo (Vanderhyden et al, 1986). It will be of considerable interest to understand how the process of fertilization in vitro exerts these downstream developmental effects, particularly if they are exerted at the level of activation of the embryonic genome.

In view of the possibility that the detrimental effects of culture in vitro are due to partial or complete failure of embryonic genome activation, it is worthwhile briefly considering the current understanding of this process.

Activation of the embryo genome

The transition from maternal to embryonic genetic control of development is best studied in the mouse. Much of the work to date has utilized the pharmacological agent α-amanitin. This drug inhibits preferentially the synthesis of new mRNA, compared with rRNA and tRNA. Egg activation and first cleavage of the zygote can proceed in the presence of α-amanitin and the proteins synthesized by the embryo at this time are not markedly affected by the presence of the drug (Johnson et al, 1976). By the 2-cell stage, however, proteins which are sensitive to α-amanitin appear. The first of these is a set of proteins of approximately 67 kDa (Flach et al, 1982) to 70 kDa (Bensaude et al, 1983), which are claimed to be homologous to the mouse heat shock proteins, HSP-68 and HSP-70 (Bensaude et al, 1983). Flach et al (1982) showed that addition of α-amanitin 18–21 h postinsemination reduced or prevented the synthesis of these proteins. At around the same time, many of the pre-existing species of proteins, presumably resulting from maternal mRNA, begin to disappear. Bolton et al (1984) showed that two rounds of transcription occurred in 2-cell embryos. One occurred immediately before and the other immediately after DNA replication, but DNA replication was not dependent upon the transcription products. It was also noted that by the late 2-cell stage there were numerous new polypeptide products apart from the putative HSPs.

It is of interest to note that at concentrations of α-amanitin that specifically block transcription, 2-cell development is not blocked but development is gradually retarded, with significantly fewer embryos developing to morulae and blastocysts (Johnson et al, 1976). Thus, inhibition of the activation of the embryonic genome appears not to have direct involvement in the proximal developmental fate of embryos (and as such seems less likely to be the primary cause of the 2-cell block in mice) but does have essential downstream developmental sequelae. Thus, pharmacological inhibition of the activation of the embryonic genome mimics some of the developmental consequences of suboptimal culture conditions, and since suboptimal culture conditions have been shown to delay the activation of the embryonic genome (Poueymirou et al, 1989), it seems likely that this is a major cause of poor embryonic development and viability associated with manipulation of embryos and gametes in vitro.

Homeobox genes

The control of the activation of transcription is currently an area of vigorous investigation and no satisfactory summary of its status can be given here. There are, however, a number of recent developments which warrant highlighting for consideration. A range of proteins and peptides have been shown to be transcriptional regulators. Perhaps the most important of these with respect to embryonic development are the products of the homeobox genes (see Holland and Hogan, 1988, for review). The homeobox is a relatively short sequence of DNA, coding for peptides that act as sequence-specific DNA binding proteins regulating gene expression. Many of the homeobox genes have been identified in *Drosophila melanogaster* and have been found to have homologues in vertebrate species; in particular, they are important for pattern formation in the embryo (see De Robertis et al, 1990, for review).

It has recently been speculated that homeodomains of maternal origin may positively autoregulate the expression of a zygotic transcriptional activator (Rosner et al, 1990). In this regard some homeobox products were recently described in the early mouse embryo. The DNA sequence ATTTGCAT (an octamer), or its complementary inverse, is a highly conserved promoter region for gene transcription. A number of cellular proteins bind in a sequence-specific manner to this motif and are termed the *Oct* proteins. It is now clear that the *Oct* proteins are derived from a subfamily of homeobox genes. The *Oct* genes are members of the subfamily which contains two independent DNA binding protein-encoding domains: the POU domain (named because of its presence in the *Pit-1*, *Oct* and *Unc-86* genes) and a homeobox domain. Recently, a member of the *Oct* family, *Oct-3*, was found to be expressed in totipotent and pluripotent stem cells derived from embryos (Rosner et al, 1990). Using northern blotting, messenger RNA (mRNA) was found in undifferentiated embryonal carcinoma and embryonic stem cells. The mRNA for *Oct-3* was detected in oocytes and fertilized ova. It was then lost and reappeared in the morula and blastocyst stages. Induction of differentiation of embryonic stem cells resulted in loss of *Oct-3*, while it was no longer present in the trophectoderm of hatched blastocysts. *Oct-3* codes for a protein of 42 kDa (Rosner et al, 1990).

Unlike most homeobox genes that are expressed later in development and are involved in pattern formation in the embryo, *Oct-3* appears to be restricted to undifferentiated cells which maintain a capacity for differentiation into more committed cell types, suggesting a relationship between

Oct-3 expression and pluripotency (Rosner et al, 1990). If this hypothesis is correct, the implication is that compromising the expression of *Oct-3* may interfere with the pluripotency of the early embryo and hence its capacity for continued development and implantation. The role of *Oct-3* as a positive transcriptional regulator in undifferentiated cells makes it an attractive candidate for involvement in the activation of the embryonic genome. Should *Oct-3* be involved in its own positive autoregulation (and since expression is correlated with the maintenance of the undifferentiated state), factors which influence the expression of *Oct-3* will greatly affect embryonic development. It is now important to examine experimentally the effects of embryo culture and manipulation in vitro on the expression of *Oct-3*. It is of course possible that other transcriptional regulators are also present and active in the early embryo.

Heat shock proteins

Since the HSP-70-like proteins are the earliest signs of transcriptional activity by the embryo, it will be of considerable relevance to consider the effect of the POU domain transcription factors on HSP-70 class transcription and also the role of HSP-70 in POU domain containing homeobox protein expression. Current evidence suggests that, at least for heat shock induced synthesis of HSP-70, the promoter region is not related to the POU homeobox domain (Amin et al, 1988). It seems unlikely, however, that constitutive expression of the cognate proteins, as apparently occurs in the early embryo, would be under the same control as shock induced expression.

With respect to HSP-70-related proteins, apparently the first products of the embryonic genome, there is now an extensive literature on their likely roles in cell physiology. The HSP-70 class of proteins have, among their roles, the property of 'chaperone' molecules (see Flaherty et al, 1990, for review). This function includes facilitating the correct assembly or disassembly of some oligomeric protein complexes and targeting of certain proteins to their membrane sites. These HSPs are highly conserved phylogenetically, suggesting a fairly fundamental role. Structural analysis of HSP-70 indicates that it has a highly conserved N terminal 44 kDa ATPase and a more variable substrate recognition domain on the C terminal (Flaherty et al, 1990). It is suggested that this structure and the active ATPase activity of the molecule allow it to transfer conformation change to its target substrates (Flaherty et al, 1990). Its specific activities include ATP-dependent disassembly of clatherin coated internalized vesicles, the assembly of oligomeric proteins in the endoplasmic reticulum and the import of proteins into the mitochondria (Murakami et al, 1988). Many of the important proteins for mitochondrial function are of nuclear origin. Uptake of the proteins by the mitochondria requires them to be of relatively simple tertiary structure, and it is argued that HSP-70 acts as an energy dependent 'unfoldase' to facilitate protein import. This diverse range of important functions makes it very tempting to mount a teleological argument for the role of embryonic HSPs. This is made even more attractive by the recent demonstration (Muggleton-Harris and Brown, 1988) that embryo culture conditions which result in the '2-cell block' in mice are associated with aggregation of mitochondria and their localization to the perinuclear region, compared with non-arrested embryos in which the mitochondria tend to be homogeneously distributed throughout the cytoplasm. Furthermore, reactivation of blocked embryos by injection of cytoplasm from cycling embryos resulted in redistribution of the aggregated mitochondria (Muggleton-Harris and Brown, 1988). Clearly there is much exciting research for the future to determine whether it is the reduced production of embryonic HSP 'chaperones' which leads to this aberrant mitochondrial behaviour, and to discover which features of the culture environment led to this.

ASSESSMENT OF EMBRYONIC VIABILITY

These issues have been discussed in an attempt to give a summary of the theoretical groundwork for an understanding of the development of the early embryo. They do not of course offer immediate solutions to the practical problem of improving the viability and pregnancy potential of preimplantation embryos. The current limitations of embryo culture arise from the fact that the media in current use are derived from the early studies of embryology which were directed to defining the 'minimal essential media' for preimplantation growth. Minimal essential media are designed to be the minimal, not the optimal requirements for development. The next issue is the definition of development: with few exceptions the embryo culture media were designed for the support of embryo development from the 1–2-cell stage through to the blastocyst stage. Clearly, for clinical practice, the definition of development is the production of viable fetuses resulting in live young. For any species, the task of testing different media and their influence on the production of viable fetuses is a daunting logistical exercise. For the human it is practically impossible. The demonstration that a single change in culture conditions has a significant effect on pregnancy rates requires a minimum of several hundred treatment cycles. Thus an empirical approach is not practical. What is required is a parameter of preimplantation development in vitro which is known to be highly correlated with the capacity of the embryo to develop into a viable fetus after transfer. The effect of alterations to culture media upon this parameter may then be a means of systematically assessing changes to the protocols and procedures of reproductive technology on embryo viability. Such a parameter should ideally be non-destructive and not compromise the viability of the embryo, be readily able to be assayed, and be quantitative.

That such a parameter exists remains to be proven beyond doubt. It is now clear that the morphology of the embryo or its cleavage rate in vitro are only relatively poor predictive indicators of embryo viability (Cummins et al, 1986). The assessment of carbohydrate metabolism has been shown to be correlated with embryo viability and developmental potential in some species, including humans. Gardner and Leese (1987) demonstrated that the uptake of glucose by mouse blastocysts was indicative of their ability to implant following transfer. Human embryos at different developmental stages consumed different amounts of pyruvate (Leese, 1987), with embryos undergoing developmental arrest consuming less pyruvate than those which developed to blastocysts (Hardy et al, 1989). These results suggest that carbohydrate metabolism may be a parameter correlated with the long-term developmental potential of the embryo (and such a concept is intuitively attractive). The logistics and safety of carrying out such tests in the clinical setting is in doubt, however, and obtaining sufficient human zygotes for 'research only' purposes to prove the power of such a correlation is fraught with difficulties and concern.

Embryo-derived platelet activating factor

Over the last few years it has been reported that the preimplantation embryo of a number of species, including humans, produces and secretes a soluble ether phospholipid, known as embryo-derived platelet activating factor (PAF). This occurs soon after fertilization and at least until the time of implantation, and perhaps thereafter. PAF secretion appears to be essential for embryo development and implantation and its secretion in vitro appears to be related to the developmental potential of embryos following transfer. The evidence for a role of embryo-derived PAF in the establishment of pregnancy and for its potential as a predictive parameter of an embryo's developmental potential is discussed below.

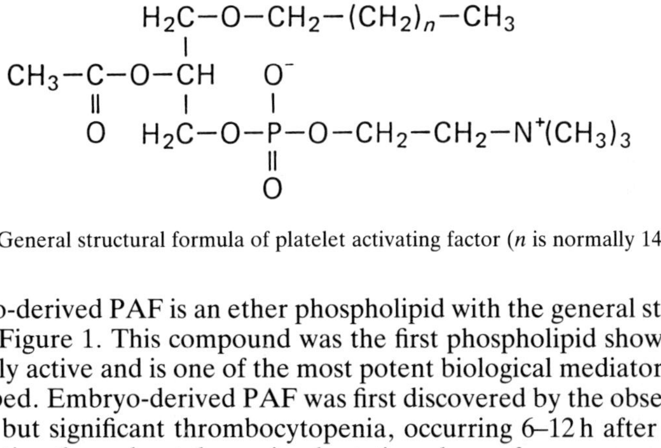

$$H_2C-O-CH_2-(CH_2)_n-CH_3$$
$$CH_3-\underset{\underset{O}{\|}}{C}-O-\underset{\underset{H_2C-O-\underset{\underset{O}{\|}}{P}-O-CH_2-CH_2-N^+(CH_3)_3}{|}}{CH} \quad O^-$$

Figure 1. General structural formula of platelet activating factor (n is normally 14 or 16).

Embryo-derived PAF is an ether phospholipid with the general structure shown in Figure 1. This compound was the first phospholipid shown to be biologically active and is one of the most potent biological mediators yet to be described. Embryo-derived PAF was first discovered by the observation of a mild but significant thrombocytopenia, occurring 6–12 h after mating and persisting throughout the preimplantation phase of pregnancy, in mice (O'Neill, 1985a). This initial maternal response to conception was solely due to the presence of a viable embryo (O'Neill, 1985b) and resulted from a secretory product. Those findings have been independently confirmed (Roberts et al, 1987) for the mouse, and PAF is apparently produced by the human (O'Neill et al, 1987; Collier et al, 1988, 1990), marmoset monkey (O'Neill, 1987), rat (Acker et al, 1988), ovine (Battye et al, 1990) and bovine (unpublished data) preimplantation embryo. In the mouse, PAF is produced from the 1-cell through at least to the blastocyst stage, as assessed by the onset of thrombocytopenia (O'Neill, 1985a). It is produced by the 2-cell to the blastocyst stage embryos in vitro (Ryan et al, 1989). PAF production by some 1-cell human zygotes was reported (Collier et al, 1988).

The biosynthesis of PAF is complex and has previously been reviewed (general, Lee and Snyder, 1989; embryos, O'Neill et al, 1990a). Its production by embryos appears to be at least partially de novo since feeding mouse 2-cell embryos long-chain alcohols led to the incorporation of the long-chain alkyl group into secreted embryo-derived PAF (O'Neill et al, 1990a), while carbon atoms from the carbohydrate substrates glucose, lactate and pyruvate are readily incorporated into embryo-derived PAF (Wells and O'Neill, 1990). Of these three substrates, pyruvate, the essential

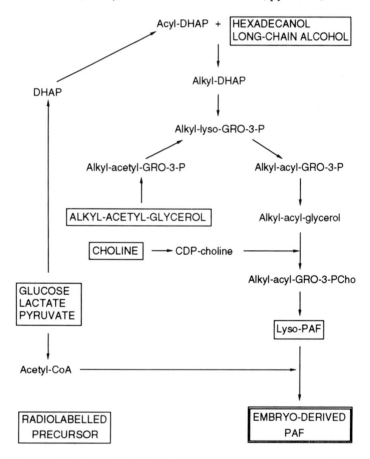

Figure 2. Suggested pathway of PAF biosynthesis in the 2-cell mouse embryo. Embryos were fed various radiolabelled substrates which were considered possible precursors of PAF production. Following incubation for various periods the incubation media were extracted and subjected to high-performance liquid chromatography and radioactivity co-eluting with PAF and lyso-PAF was noted. DHAP, dihydroxyacetone phosphate; GRO, glycero; CoA, coenzyme A; CDP, cytidine diphosphate; PCho, phosphocholine. From Wells and O'Neill (1990).

carbohydrate substrate for the early preimplantation embryo, showed the highest rates of incorporation (Wells and O'Neill, 1990). Exogenous choline is also incorporated in secreted embryo-derived PAF (Wells and O'Neill, 1990). The precise role of the carbohydrate substrates is yet to be defined, but it is likely that they serve as a substrate for both the glyceryl backbone of PAF and the acetyl group on the carbon-2 of glycerol. The possible bio-synthetic pathway for embryo-derived PAF is shown in Figure 2.

It is perhaps not surprising that PAF synthesis should be de novo, since secretion of amounts as high as 385 ng PAF/day in vitro occurs for the human 2–4-cell embryo (Collier et al, 1990). Such secretion rates would clearly place a substantial drain on endogenous stores of phospholipids. It also suggests that careful consideration of substrate requirements of the embryo should not only take into account the energy requirements of the embryo, but also such secretory activity. For instance it has long been held that nitrogen was not an essential nutrient for the preimplantation embryo. Yet Figure 1 shows that choline in PAF requires nitrogen, thus the secretion of PAF observed in vitro would place a significant drain on the choline pool of the embryo in the absence of an exogenous source. Perhaps the recently demonstrated advantage of glutamine as an energy substrate in vitro (Poueymirou et al, 1989) is because of its capacity to donate nitrogen, not only to nucleotides and amino acids, but also the polar head groups of nitrogen-containing phospholipids such as PAF.

PAF as a measure of embryo viability

There is recent evidence that culture in vitro compromises the secretion of PAF by the embryo. O'Neill (1985b) showed that 80% (12/15) of mouse 8–16-cell stage embryo-conditioned cultures produced detectable levels of PAF in the culture medium. Ryan et al (1989), using a similar bioassay, found that PAF activity in embryo culture media increased with increasing time of 2-cell mouse embryos in culture up to 6 h. After 24 h the amount of PAF was not different to that after 6 h, demonstrating no further net increase in PAF secretion. After 72 h in culture the embryos had developed to the blastocyst stage. Over this same period a linear ($P < 0.05$) reduction in PAF activity occurred for the three consecutive 24-h culture periods. This seemed to be a consequence of culture in vitro, since morulae and blasto-cysts collected from the reproductive tract and placed in culture for 24 h produced the same levels of PAF as 2-cell embryos. The declining PAF production with time in vitro might conceivably be due to the down-regulation of PAF production as its concentration in the media increases. The observation that subpassage to two fresh culture media at 24 h intervals resulted in a persistent decline in the secretion of PAF (Ryan et al, 1989) suggests that is not the cause but rather that it is a consequence of culture, perhaps due to starvation of the appropriate substrates for PAF synthesis or due to a general suboptimal environment which reduces the biosynthetic capacity of the embryos.

These results in mice are consistent with the observations of PAF secretion by human embryos produced by IVF and cultured for 24 h in vitro.

In an initial study (O'Neill et al, 1987), all culture media ($n = 12$) known to have definitely resulted in pregnancy contained detectable quantities of embryo-derived PAF. Embryos which were transferred but did not result in pregnancy produced significantly less PAF in vitro with 57% ($n = 85$) of such embryos showing a PAF concentration below the second standard deviation from the mean of results for embryos resulting in pregnancy. The production of PAF was correlated with the size of the follicles from which the oocyte was derived and its oestradiol secretory activity, the form of ovarian stimulation regimen, and the morphology of the embryos in vitro.

These general trends have been confirmed using a quantitative bioassay for PAF. This bioassay was shown to be specific and confirmed the homology of embryo-derived PAF with 1-o-alkyl-2-acetyl-sn-glyceryl-3-phosphorylcholine (Collier et al, 1988). It had a limit of sensitivity of 5.6 nM and intra-assay and inter-assay coefficient of variation generally less than 15% (Collier et al, 1990). For 228 media in which human embryos were cultured for 24 h, the PAF concentration was 1.85–2700 nM, of which 53% had a PAF concentration greater than the corresponding control media. Again, it was confirmed that embryos transferred to women who achieved pregnancies produced significantly more PAF (295 nM) than those who failed to achieve pregnancy (75 nM) ($P < 0.03$). It is important to note in this context that, for both pregnant and non-pregnant women, three embryos were generally transferred, while most pregnancies were only singleton. Since it is impossible to tell which of the embryos cultured in vitro resulted in pregnancy in the case of multiple embryo transfers, the value of 295 nM PAF for 'pregnancy' embryos is likely to be an underestimate of the true value for embryos which resulted in pregnancy.

Recent studies (Battye et al, 1990) have demonstrated that the ovine preimplantation embryo also produces PAF and that the type of culture medium in which the embryos were grown affected the amount of PAF secreted. Embryos were collected from merino ewes on day 2 (2–4 cell), day 4 (8–16 cell) or day 6 (morula/early blastocyst). The embryos were cultured in either Ham's F10 + 4 mg bovine serum albumin (BSA)/ml, synthetic oviduct fluid medium (SOFM) + 20% human serum, human tubule fluid medium (HTF) + 3 mg BSA/ml or HTF + 10% acid-treated fetal calf serum. PAF was produced in 44% (41/94) of cultures. Embryos cultured in Ham's F10–BSA produced the highest concentration of PAF over a 24-h period ($P < 0.05$), being 26.7 ± 7.3 ng/ml (mean $\pm$ s.e.m.), while HTF–BSA was the least effective in this regard (8.0 ± 2.9 ng/ml).

Thus, the results to date show that a variety of species produce PAF, that PAF production in two separate trials was shown to be positively correlated with the pregnancy potential of the embryos following transfer, and that aspects of gamete manipulation and embryo culture conditions affected embryo-derived PAF production. It remains to determine the predictive power of measuring PAF production by embryos. This has not proven possible up until now because of the limitation of measuring PAF by bioassay.

While the bioassay is specific, reliable and quantitative, like all bioassays it is technically difficult to set up and validate. The full assessment of the predictive power of PAF will depend on the development of a robust assay for PAF. This criterion may now have been fulfilled with the recent development of a radioimmunoassay for PAF. It was recently reported (Ammit and O'Neill, 1990) that this radioimmunoassay could successfully detect PAF produced by the murine and human preimplantation embryo. Dose–response curves were generated with authentic PAF standards over a concentration range of 0.3–30 ng/ml. The coefficients of variation at the EC_{50} were 3.35% and 6.77%, intra-assay, and 7.33% and 12.65%, inter-assay, for the radioimmunoassay and bioassay, respectively. Both assays had detection limits of 0.3 ng/ml. For mouse 2-cell embryos the correlation between bioassay and radioimmunoassay was 0.71. For 38 individual culture media tested, ranges of 0.1–141.1 and 0.25–99.15 ng/ml were detected by the bioassay and immunoassay. Culture media from human embryos produced by IVF were also tested. The correlation was 0.994 for 11 culture media, the range being 0.40–78.31 and 2.0–119.10 ng/ml for bioassay and radio-immunoassay, respectively.

The advent of this radioimmunoassay provides the promise of now being able to undertake large-scale screening of embryo culture media for PAF under sufficiently controlled conditions to allow assessment of its predictive power. The likelihood of PAF having some useful predictive power is enhanced if an essential role in the establishment of pregnancy for embryo-derived PAF can be demonstrated. The evidence that this may be the case is steadily accumulating.

Role of PAF in pregnancy

The first evidence to suggest that PAF may have a role in the successful establishment of pregnancy was the observation that inhibitors of PAF's action reduced the capacity of embryos to undergo implantation and the establishment of pregnancy. Two pharmacological approaches have been used to inhibit PAF in early pregnancy (Spinks and O'Neill, 1988). Hoprost (5-(E)-(1S,5S,6R,7R)-7-hydroxy-6-(E)-(3S,4RS)-3-hydroxy-4-methyl-oct-1-en-6-yn-yl-bicylo3.3.0-octano-3-yliden-pentanoic acid; Schering AG, Berlin, Germany) is a stable analogue of prostacyclin which stimulates adenylcyclase activity, leading to increased cellular cyclic adenosine mono-phosphate (cAMP) and reduced cytoplasmic calcium. These effects inhibit the action of PAF in most cells; SRI 63-441 ([cis-(+)-1-[2-hydroxy[tetrahydro-5-[(octadecylaminocarbonyl)oxy]methyl]-furan-2-yl]methoxy-phosphinyl-oxy]ethyl]-quinolinium hydroxide; Sandoz Research Institute, East Hanover NJ, USA) is a specific PAF receptor antagonist with potent pharmacological actions (Spinks and O'Neill, 1988).

Both of these agents, when administered to pregnant mice (on days 1–4 of pregnancy), significantly reduced the number of implantation sites. The specificity of action was suggested by the ability of concomitant administration of synthetic PAF to completely overcome the inhibitory action of the antagonists (Spinks and O'Neill, 1988). They did not act by having gross toxic effects on the embryo either in vitro or in vivo. A similar effect has been shown in the rat (Acker et al, 1988) using a third antagonist, BN 52021 (INH, Le Plessis-Robinson, France). They appear to act by prevention of implantation rather than its subsequent disruption. The earliest sign of implantation is a local increase in the vascular permeability surrounding the site of implantation. This can be visualized by high molecular weight dyes. PAF inhibitors caused significantly fewer dye bands in the uterus on day 4 of pregnancy in mice (Spinks and O'Neill, 1988). There was no evidence of an effect of the antagonists on the early luteal endocrine profile (Spinks and O'Neill, 1988).

In a further study (Spinks et al, 1990), experiments were performed to determine whether the PAF antagonist acted primarily at the maternal or embryonic level. The experiment used reciprocal embryo transfers, in which blastocysts from mice treated with PAF antagonist (SRI 63-441) or saline (controls), from days 1–4 of pregnancy, were transferred to day 4 pseudo-pregnant recipients that were also treated with SRI 63-441 or saline on days 1–4 of pregnancy. The antagonist (40 μg) was administered at 16.00 on day 1 and at 19.00 on days 2–4 of pregnancy. The percentage of the transferred embryos which implanted was determined on day 8 of pregnancy. Treatment of the donor female had a dramatic effect on the implantation rate, resulting in a reduction by 64% (from 40% to 14.3%; $P < 0.04$), while treatment of the recipient female had no significant effect. Experiments with PAF antagonist treated animals show that the antagonists exerted their contragestational effect primarily on the day of implantation (rat, Acker et al, 1988; mouse, C. O'Neill, unpublished data).

The PAF inhibitors, however, rarely completely inhibited implantation. Indeed, as the concentration of drug administered increased past the maximum effective dose (for five structurally different compounds tested), the inhibitory effect was lost (O'Neill et al, 1990b). This pattern of response occurred irrespective of route, time, frequency or formulation of administration and is the type of response expected for partial agonists rather than true antagonists. This effect is confirmed by the study of Milligan and Finn (1990), who also failed to demonstrate a contragestational effect of antagonists when administered at high doses.

Recent studies suggest that the pattern of response is due to an apparent partial agonism rather than true partial agonism at the receptor level. The PAF antagonists and the PAF inhibitor, Iloprost, at high concentration block the metabolism of PAF (O'Neill et al, 1990c). The embryo does not metabolize PAF itself (C. O'Neill et al, unpublished data), but rather embryo derived PAF is most likely to be metabolized by maternal cells, probably the tissues (particularly vascular tissues) of the reproductive tract. We hypothesize that the inhibition of metabolism of embryo-derived PAF would result in a local increase in the concentration of PAF in the reproductive tract and hence overcome the inhibitory effects of the antagonists.

Experimental support for this suggestion of the functional partial agonism of these compounds comes from studies in vitro. A process showing some analogy with implantation occurs in vitro. The provision of a complex culture medium leads to the outgrowth of the trophoblast on to the substrate and differentiation of the inner cell mass. PAF antagonists inhibited trophoblast outgrowth in a dose dependent manner (Spinks et al, 1990), at doses that did not affect development from the 1-cell to blastocyst stage (Spinks and O'Neill, 1988). This occurred at even very high concentrations of PAF antagonist, with no loss of inhibition at these doses. The results of this study are consistent with a pharmacodynamic explanation of the apparent partial agonism of PAF antagonists in vitro and also adds support for an autocrine effect of PAF on the preimplantation embryo itself.

This pharmacological approach was confirmed by observing the effect that PAF had on the metabolism of pre-embryos in vitro. The production of carbon dioxide from radiolabelled lactate or glucose was measured to determine whether PAF had an effect on embryonic metabolism. PAF enhanced the metabolism of lactate by 2-cell, 4-cell, morulae and blastocyst stages (Ryan et al, 1989) and glucose at the 2-cell and blastocyst stage (Ryan et al, 1990a). These effects were dose dependent and were significantly inhibited by the PAF receptor antagonist SRI 63-441. Lyso-PAF had no effect on embryo metabolism and the embryos were not desensitized to PAF. Following culture for 72 h in the presence of PAF, further enhancement of the metabolic response occurred after re-exposure to PAF. Culture of embryos in medium supplemented with PAF did not significantly increase the proportion of embryos developing to the expanded blastocyst stage; however, there was a modest ($P < 0.05$) increase in the number of cells in each embryo (Ryan et al, 1990b).

The effects of PAF on the anabolic metabolism of preimplantation mouse embryos were also examined in order to elucidate its apparent autocrine role in early embryo development. Mouse morulae and blastocysts were incubated in bicarbonate-buffered HFT medium in droplets under oil with concentrations of PAF from 0.186–18.6 μM for periods of 3–5 h. After this time, the blastocysts were either pulsed for 1 h with radiolabelled amino acids, uridine or thymidine, or transferred to colchicine for mitotic index determination. Total uptake and radioactivity incorporated into the protein, DNA and RNA were measured. No effect was found on protein or RNA synthesis (L. C. Wright and C. O'Neill, unpublished data). In contrast, both thymidine uptake and incorporation into DNA were elevated by around 30% with PAF. The mitotic index increased in a dose dependent manner (Roberts and O'Neill, 1990). Thus, PAF appears to act as an autocrine growth factor for the preimplantation embryo.

A clinical role for PAF in enhancing embryo viability

This evidence for the action of PAF as an autocrine growth factor, together with the demonstration that its synthesis by embryos is reduced following in vitro culture, suggested that the addition of PAF to embryo culture media as a supplement would enhance the pregnancy potential and viability of pre-embryos. This has proven to be the case. The effect of PAF on the pregnancy potential of embryos cultured in vitro was assessed (Ryan et al, 1990b). Expanded mouse blastocysts cultured from the 2-cell stage in medium with or without PAF were transferred to pseudopregnant mice and implantation rates were assessed on day 8 or day 17 of pregnancy. Supplementation of medium with 0.1 μg PAF/ml resulted in a substantial increase in the implantation rate above control levels. By taking into account the between animal variation, the observed effect could be considered to be due solely to enhanced viability of embryos rather than to any maternal effects following transfer (Ryan et al, 1990b).

This direct autocrine action was not restricted to the mouse. Supplementation of culture media with PAF enhanced the metabolism of human polyploid embryos in vitro and also substantially increased the pregnancy potential of human embryos produced by IVF (O'Neill et al, 1989). Embryo culture medium was supplemented with 0 (control), 0.186, 0.93 or 1.49 μmol PAF. Embryos were transferred to PAF-containing medium 15–17 h after insemination (i.e. just before syngamy) for 24 h and then transferred to the uterus. For 185 women receiving control pre-embryos, the pregnancy rate (positive β-human chorionic gonadotrophin per oocyte retrieval) was 10.2%, whereas 166 women who received PAF-treated pre-embryos (all concentrations combined) achieved a pregnancy rate of 17.5%. This difference was significant ($P < 0.05$). The pregnancy rates per pre-embryo transferred were 6.1% and 9.4% for the control and PAF groups, respectively. The percentage of positive pregnancy tests that resulted in a viable pregnancy (presence of fetal heart at 8 weeks) was 79% in the controls and 76% in the PAF group. The observations that PAF is secreted by the early embryo of a variety of species suggests that it may have a general role as a mitogenic autocrine growth factor for the preimplantation mammalian embryo.

These experimental findings provide good preliminary evidence for an essential role for PAF in pregnancy. They provide a sound theoretical basis for the use of PAF, or (in the future) structural analogues, to enhance fertility (both in vitro and in vivo) and for the use of PAF measurements as a marker for the implantation and developmental potential of preimplantation embryos.

CONCLUSIONS

Our knowledge of the basic physiology of the preimplantation embryo and its response to its environment is still in its infancy. The recent development of amplification techniques in molecular biology will open doors to the understanding of control of gene action in early development, but the demonstration of a relationship of this activation to development potential will be a daunting task. The preliminary demonstration that the production of embryo-derived PAF may serve as an essential embryonic mediator suggests that its measurement may eventually prove to be a useful prognostic tool for measuring the embryo's developmental potential.

The relative state of our ignorance in the general area of embryo development and the likely great complexity of the issues involved suggests that an empirical systematic modification of the culture environment in the clinical setting has only limited potential for success. What is required in the first instance is a detailed fundamental understanding of the principle of pre-implantation embryo physiology and biochemistry and its interactions and interdependencies with the maternal reproductive tract. Much of this fundamental work can be performed in experimental animals.

SUMMARY

The advent of the new reproductive technologies (including in vitro fertilization) has led to a revolution in the treatment of infertility. It has not yet led to a marked improvement in our understanding of the control of development and of viability of the early embryo. It is the poor viability of embryos, with consequent implantation failure, which is the major limiting factor to successful outcomes. While much of the research in this area has concentrated on strategies of ovulation induction, experimental models have shown that the major cause of reduced embryo viability is due to the actual process of fertilization in vitro and subsequent culture of the pre-embryo in synthetic culture medium. It is likely that this is due to the absence of critical nutrients or trophic factors of maternal origin and work with co-culture of embryos with somatic cells suggests improved viability can be achieved. Such co-culture is not an option for routine clinical use, however. It is essential therefore to understand by detailed study of the physiology of embryonic development their requirements for optimal development. The empirical approach of comparing different formulations of culture media is unlikely to be successful because of the vast range of parameters to be tested and the large number of pregnancies required to demonstrate a significant improvement in outcome. The strategy that is most likely to be successful in the future, therefore, is the use of appropriate experimental models, such as the developing rodent embryo, to understand the essential physiological changes in the embryo during its development, the control processes in place, and the effect of the embryo's environment on the processes. This will allow the rational design of culture media which can then be rigorously tested for improved outcome. An example of successful application of this approach is the discovery of embryo-derived platelet activating factor (PAF). The production of embryo-derived PAF was first described and validated in the rodent. In the same species it was shown to have an essential role in pregnancy and to act as an autocrine mediator of embryo viability. This fundamental observation in rodents was then confirmed in humans, and recent work has shown that supplementation of culture human embryo media with PAF results in a dramatic increase in their developmental and pregnancy potential. This example should be the first of many such improvements based on a more fundamental understanding of the embryo's developmental requirements.

REFERENCES

Acker G, Hecquet F, Etienne A, Braquet P & Mencia-Huerta JM (1988) Role of platelet activating factor (PAF) in the ovoimplantation in the rat: effect of the specific PAF-acether antagonist, BN 52021. *Prostaglandins* **35**: 233–241.

Amin J, Ananthan J & Voellmy R (1988) Key features of heat shock regulatory elements. *Molecular and Cellular Biology* **8**: 3761–3769.

Ammit AJ & O'Neill C (1991) Comparison of a bioassay and radioimmunoassay for embryo-derived PAF. *Human Reproduction* (in press).

Battye KM, Ammit AJ, Evans G et al (1990) Production of platelet activating factor *in vitro* by pre-implantation sheep embryos. *Proceedings of the Australian Society of Reproduction and Biology*, Perth.

Bavister BD & Minami N (1986) Use of cultured mouse oviducts to by-pass *in vitro* development block in cleavage stage hamster embryos. *Biology of Reproduction* **Supplement 34:** 191.

Bensaude O, Babinet C, Morange M & Jacob F (1983) Heat shock proteins, first major products of zygotic gene activity in mouse embryo. *Nature* **303:** 331–333.

Biggers JD, Gwatkin RBL & Brinster RL (1962) Development of mouse embryos in organ culture of fallopian tubes on a chemically defined medium. *Nature* **194:** 747–749.

Bolton VN, Oades PJ & Johnson MH (1984) The relationship between cleavage, DNA replication, and gene expression in the mouse 2-cell embryo. *Journal of Embryology and Experimental Morphology* **79:** 139–163.

Bolton VN, Hawes SM, Taylor CT & Parsons JH (1989) Development of spare human preimplantation embryos *in vitro*: an analysis of the correlations among gross morphology, cleavage rates, and development to the blastocyst. *Journal of In Vitro Fertilization and Embryo Transfer* **6:** 30–35.

Bongso A, Soon-Chye N, Santhananthan H et al (1989) Improved quality of human embryos when co-cultured with human ampullary cells. *Human Reproduction* **4:** 706–713.

Braude P, Bolton V & Moore S (1988) Human gene expression first occurs between the four- and eight cell stages of preimplantation development. *Nature* **332:** 459–461.

Collier M, O'Neill C, Ammit AJ & Saunders DM (1988) Biochemical and pharmacological characterisation of human embryo-derived platelet activating factor. *Human Reproduction* **3:** 993–998.

Collier M, O'Neill C, Ammit AJ & Saunders DM (1990) Measurement of human embryo-derived platelet-activating factor (PAF) using a quantitative bioassay of platelet aggregation. *Human Reproduction* **5:** 323–328.

Cummins JM, Breen TM, Harrison KL et al (1986) A formula for scoring human embryo growth rate in *in vitro* fertilization: its value in predicting pregnancy and in comparison with visual estimates of embryo quality. *Journal of In Vitro Fertilization and Embryo Transfer* **3:** 284–295.

De Robertis EM, Oliver G & Wright CVE (1990) Homeobox genes and the vertebrate body plan. *Scientific American* **July** 26–32.

Eyestone WH & First NL (1989) Co-culture of early cattle embryos to the blastocyst stage with oviducal tissue ovine conditioned medium. *Journal of Reproduction and Fertility* **85:** 715–720.

Flach G, Johnson MH, Braude PR, Taylor RAS & Bolton VN (1982) The transition from maternal to embryonic control in the 2-cell mouse embryo. *Journal of Embryology* **1:** 681–686.

Flaherty KM, DeLuca-Flaherty C & McKay DB (1990) Three-dimensional structure of the ATPase fragment of a 70 K heat shock cognate protein. *Nature* **346:** 623–628.

Gandolfi F & Moor RH (1987) Stimulation of early embryonic development in the sheep by co-culture with oviduct epithelial cells. *Journal of Reproduction and Fertility* **81:** 23–28.

Gardner DK & Leese AJ (1987) Assessment of embryo viability prior to transfer by non-invasive measurements of glucose uptake. *Journal of Experimental Zoology* **212:** 103–105.

Hardy K, Hooper MAK, Handyside AH et al (1989) Non-invasive measurement of glucose and pyruvate uptake by individual human oocytes and preimplantation embryos. *Human Reproduction* **4:** 188–191.

Holland PWH & Hogan BLM (1988) Expression of homeobox genes during mouse development: a review. *Genes and Development* **2:** 773–782.

Johnson MH, Handyside AH & Braude PR (1976) Control mechanisms in early mammalian development. In Johnson MH (ed.) *Mammalian Development*, pp 67–97. Amsterdam: Elsevier/North Holland Biomedical Press.

Lee T-C & Snyder F (1989) Overview of PAF biosynthesis and catabolism. In Barnes PJ, Page CP & Henson PM (eds) *Platelet Activating Factor and Human Disease*, pp 1–22. Oxford: Blackwell Scientific Publications.

Leese HJ (1987) Analysis of embryos by non-invasive methods. *Human Reproduction* **2:** 37–40.

Milligan SR & Finn CA (1990) Failure of platelet activating factor (PAF-acether) to induce decidualization in mice and failure of antagonists of PAF to inhibit implantation. *Journal of Reproduction and Fertility* **88:** 105–112.

Muggleton-Harris AL & Brown JJG (1988) Cytoplasmic factors influence mitochondrial reorganization and resumption of cleavage during culture of early mouse embryos. *Human Reproduction* **3**: 1020–1028.

Muggleton-Harris A, Whittingham DG & Wilson L (1982) Cytoplasmic control of pre-implantation development *in vitro* in the mouse. *Nature* **229**: 460–462.

Murakami M, Pain D & Blobel G (1988) 70-kD heat shock related protein is one of at least two distinct cytosolic factors stimulating protein import into mitochondria. *Journal of Cellular Biology* **107**: 2051–2057.

National Perinatal Statistics Unit (1989) *IVF and GIFT Pregnancies, Australia and New Zealand: 1988*, ISSN 1030–4711.

O'Neill C (1985a) Thrombocytopenia is an initial maternal response to fertilisation in mice. *Journal of Reproduction and Fertility* **73**: 567–577.

O'Neill C (1985b) Examination of the causes of early pregnancy associated thrombocytopenia in mice. *Journal of Reproduction and Fertility* **73**: 578–585.

O'Neill C (1987) Invited Review: Embryo derived platelet activating factor: a pre-implantation embryo mediator of maternal recognition of pregnancy. *Domestic Animal Endocrinology* **4**: 69–86.

O'Neill C, Gidley-Baird AA, Pike IL et al (1987) Use of a bioassay for embryo-derived platelet-activating factor as a means of assessing quality and pregnancy potential of human embryos. *Fertility and Sterility* **47**: 969–975.

O'Neill C, Ryan JP, Collier M et al (1989) Supplementation of IVF culture media with platelet activating factor (PAF) increased the pregnancy rate following embryo transfer. *Lancet* ii: 769–772.

O'Neill C, Wells X & Battye KM (1990a) Platelet activating factor: interactions with the arachidonic acid cascade and the establishment and maintenance of pregnancy. *Reproduction, Fertility and Development* **2**: 423–430.

O'Neill C, Collier M, Spinks NR et al (1990b) An autocrine role for PAF in early embryo-genesis. In Handley DA, Saunders R, Houlihan W & Tomesch J (eds) *Platelet Activating Factor in Endotoxin and Immune Diseases*, pp 207–220. New York: Marcel Dekker.

O'Neill C, Ammit AJ, Korth R et al (1990c) Inhibitors of platelet activating factor as well as PAF-receptor antagonist inhibit catabolism of PAF by washed rabbit platelets. *Lipids* (in press).

Plachot M, DeGrouchy J, Junca AM et al (1988) Chromosomal analysis of human oocytes and embryos in an *in vitro* fertilization programme. *Annals of the New York Academy of Sciences* **541**: 384–397.

Poueymirou WT, Conover JC & Schultz RM (1989) Regulation of mouse preimplantation development: differential effects of CZB medium and Whitten's medium on rates and patterns of protein synthesis in 2-cell embryos. *Biology of Reproduction* **41**: 317–322.

Roberts C & O'Neill C (1990) Examination of the effects of platelet activating factor (PAF) and PAF-receptor antagonists on fertilisation in vitro. *Proceedings of the Australian Society of Reproduction and Biology*, Perth.

Roberts TK, Adamson LM, Cheng Smart Y, Stanger JD & Murdoch RN (1987) An evaluation of peripheral blood platelet enumeration as a monitor of fertilization and early pregnancy. *Fertility and Sterility* **47**: 848–854.

Rosner MA, Vigano MA, Ozato K et al (1990) A POU-domain transcription factor in early stem cells and germ cells of the mammalian embryo. *Nature* **345**: 686–692.

Ryan JP, Spinks NR, O'Neill C, Ammit AJ & Wales RG (1989) Platelet activating factor (PAF) production by mouse embryos *in vitro* and its effects on embryonic metabolism. *Journal of Cellular Biochemistry* **40**: 387–395.

Ryan JP, O'Neill C & Wales RG (1990a) Oxidative metabolism of energy substrates by preimplantation mouse embryos in the presence of platelet activating factor. *Journal of Reproduction and Fertility* **89**: 301–307.

Ryan JP, Spinks NR, O'Neill C & Wales RG (1990b) Implantation potential and fetal viability of mouse embryos cultured in media supplemented with platelet activating factor. *Journal of Reproduction and Fertility* **89**: 309–315.

Sathananthan H, Bongso A, Ng SC et al (1990) Ultrastructure of preimplantation human embryos co-cultured with human ampullary cells. *Human Reproduction* **5**: 309–318.

Spinks NR & O'Neill C (1988) Antagonists of embryo-derived platelet activating factor prevent implantation of mouse embryos. *Journal of Reproduction and Fertility* **84**: 89–98.

Spinks NR, Ryan JP & O'Neill C (1990) Antagonists of embryo-derived platelet activating factor act by inhibiting the ability of the mouse embryo to implant. *Journal of Reproduction and Fertility* **88:** 241–248.

Tervit HR, Whittingham DG & Rowson LEA (1972) Successful culture *in vitro* of sheep and cattle ova. *Journal of Reproduction and Fertility* **30:** 493–497.

Vanderhyden BC & Armstrong DT (1988) Decreased embryonic survival of in-vitro fertilizated oocytes in rats is due to retardation of preimplantation development. *Journal of Reproduction and Fertility* **83:** 851–857.

Vanderhyden BC, Rouleau A, Walton EA & Armstrong DT (1986) Increased mortality during early embryonic development after in-vitro fertilization of rat oocytes. *Journal of Reproduction and Fertility* **77:** 401–409.

Walker SK, Seamark RF, Quinn P et al (1988) Culture of pronuclear embryos of sheep in a simple medium. *Proceedings of the 11th International Congress on Animal Reproduction and Artificial Insemination*, Dublin, **4:** 483–485.

Warner CM, Gollnick SO & Goldbard SB (1987) Linkage of the preimplantation embryo development (Ped) gene to the mouse major histocompatibility complex (MHC). *Biology of Reproduction* **36:** 606–610.

Warner CM, Brownell MS & Ewoldsen MA (1988) Why aren't embryos immunologically rejected by their mothers. *Biology of Reproduction* **38:** 17–29.

Wells X & O'Neill C (1990) The biosynthesis of platelet activating factor (PAF) by the mouse two-cell embryo. *Proceedings of the Australian Society of Reproduction and Biology*, Perth.

Whittingham DG (1968) Development of zygotes in cultured mouse oviducts. I. The effects of varying oviducal conditions. *Journal of Experimental Zoology* **169:** 891–898.

Wiemer KE, Cohen J, Amborski GF et al (1989a) In-vitro development and implantation of human embryos following culture on fetal bovine uterine fibroblast cells. *Human Reproduction* **4:** 595–600.

Wiemer KE, Cohen J, Wiker SR et al (1989b) Co-culture of human zygotes on fetal bovine uterine fibroblasts: embryonic morphology and implantation. *Fertility and Sterility* **52:** 503–508.

11

Frequency of implantation and early pregnancy loss in natural cycles

T. CHARD

It is generally accepted that couples having regular intercourse without contraception have a 25–30% chance of starting a recognizable pregnancy in a single menstrual cycle. In those couples who do not become pregnant in any one cycle, it is presumed that there has been either a failure of fertilization, or that fertilization has taken place but that the embryo is aborted before the first missed period; in other words, before there is obvious evidence for the pregnancy.

One of the earlier and more significant papers to draw attention to the fact that the potential number of conceptions greatly exceeds the number of clinically apparent pregnancies was that by Roberts and Lowe (1975). They made various assumptions and calculations and concluded that the number of actual pregnancies was only one-quarter that which would have been anticipated from the rate of conception. Since then, the problem of the missing pregnancies has been addressed by a number of authors. In particular it has stimulated work on the possibility that unexplained early pregnancy loss might be a feature of a number of congenital abnormalities and also might explain infertility in some subjects. Furthermore, knowing the rate of spontaneous early loss is highly relevant to judging the potential success of in vitro fertilization (IVF) procedures. For example, if the frequency of implantation following normal fertilization is only 30%, it is unreasonable to expect that IVF would achieve much higher rates.

WHAT IS THE EXPECTED NUMBER OF CONCEPTIONS?

For the answer to this question it is still difficult to better the original calculations of Roberts and Lowe (1975). They estimated that 78% of women abort their conceptus: the calculations leading to this conclusion are summarized in Table 1.

Studies of cumulative conception rates suggest that clinically apparent pregnancies might be expected in 12–20% of cycles (Cooke et al, 1981). Of these, some 12–16% will end in spontaneous abortion. However, the figures for spontaneous abortion are largely derived from hospital based studies, which might well miss some of the earliest losses.

Baillière's Clinical Obstetrics and Gynaecology—
Vol. 5, No. 1, March 1991
ISBN 0–7020–1533–4

Table 1. Estimated fetal loss for married women aged 20–29 in England and Wales, 1971.

	Number (millions)
Married women (aged 20–29)	2.4
Annual acts of coitus (mean of twice a week)	253.4
Annual acts of unprotected coitus (one in four unprotected)	63.4
Unprotected acts occurring within 2 days around ovulation	4.5
One in two of these results in fertilization	2.3
Actual number of infants born to these women	0.5
Estimated loss $(2.3 - 0.5)$	1.8
Percentage loss $((1.8 \div 2.3) \times 100)$	78%

Modified from Roberts and Lowe (1975).

WHAT IS THE EVIDENCE FOR EARLY PREGNANCY LOSS?

Theoretical calculations of the rate of very early pregnancy loss do not, of course, guarantee that such losses actually occur. There have therefore been many attempts to demonstrate objectively the existence of early pregnancy failure.

There are two lines of evidence which support the concept of unrecognized early pregnancy loss as a real phenomenon. The first is direct observation of such pregnancies. The second is the transient appearance in the woman of specific fetoplacental products during the luteal phase of an apparently normal menstrual cycle.

Direct evidence for early pregnancy loss

The earliest and still some of the best evidence on the frequency of early pregnancy loss came from the classic studies of Hertig and Rock (1959). They examined hysterectomy specimens collected from women in the course of potentially fertile cycles. Only 34% of the 107 specimens examined contained 'ova' (oocytes, preimplantation cleavage stages or implantation sites). Later, Hertig (1975) estimated that some 42% of women from 'ideal' fertile couples are pregnant in any one menstrual cycle at the time of the first missed menses. He further estimated that the greatest loss occurs in the preimplantation phase and that the next greatest loss occurs during the week following implantation.

More recent direct evidence comes from studies in women who were inseminated at the time of ovulation and from whom the 'ova' were retrieved 5 days later (Buster et al, 1985; Formigli et al, 1987). In only 41% of cycles studied were oocytes or preimplantation cleavage stages found. Even allowing for technical losses, this suggests that at least 50% of fertile cycles do not yield a conceptus. Similarly, Bolton and her colleagues (1988) found that fewer than 20% of oocytes fertilized in vitro formed a normal blastocyst; the majority failed at the 4- to 8-cell stage.

Biochemical evidence for early pregnancy loss

The best known of the biochemical studies have been based on the use of very sensitive assays for human chorionic gonadotrophin (hCG). Chorionic gonadotrophin is produced by the syncytiotrophoblast. It can be detected in culture medium from embryos at 7–8 days post fertilization (Fishel et al, 1984; Lopata and Hay, 1989) but not at 4 days (Shutt and Lopata, 1981) though messenger RNA for the beta-subunit of hCG has been shown in the 8-cell embryo (Bonduelle et al, 1988). The amount of hCG released increases greatly after hatching from the zona pellucida. Saxena (1989) has claimed that hCG is secreted into the mother prior to implantation of the blastocyst. Though it is difficult to entirely exclude this, most authors agree that hCG first appears in the maternal circulation shortly after the time of implantation. The appearance will be the result of the combination of hCG synthesis by the trophoblast, shedding of the zona pellucida and establishment of direct contact between the trophoblast and the maternal circulation. The timing has been studied in considerable detail by Lenton and colleagues (see Lenton and Woodward, 1988), who conclude that the time of first appearance is in the range of 7.5–9.5 days after the luteinizing hormone (LH) surge, following which the levels rise exponentially for several days (doubling time estimated at between 1.4 and 2.2 days). Hay (1985) showed that free β-subunit was detectable as early as 6.5 days after oocyte retrieval in IVF pregnancies. These figures suggest that the appearance of hCG in the mother is virtually

Table 2. Studies on the appearance of hCG in the luteal phase in women wearing an intrauterine contraceptive device.

Authors	Number of subjects	
Beling et al (1976)	131	Positive hCG in 32 of 73 samples from the second half of the cycle
Landesman et al (1976)*	200	12–19% had detectable serum hCG during luteal phase
Klein and Mishell (1977)	24	No hCG detected in luteal phase
Sharpe et al (1977)	201	No hCG detected at any stage of the cycle
Seppälä et al (1978)	34 women using oral contraceptives (OC) and 94 cycles from 69 women with an IUD	No positive hCG (or SP1) results in women on OCs. hCG detected in one cycle and SP1 in six cycles of women with an IUD
Orloff et al (1979)	9	No hCG detected in luteal phase
Segal et al (1985)	30 women with IUDs; 30 women with tubal ligation; 25 normal women	No detectable hCG in luteal phase in IUD users or women with tubal ligation
Tamsen and Eneroth (1986)	42 (73 cycles)	SP1 detectable in five cycles and hCG in two cycles

* Using a receptor assay.
SP1, Schwangerschafts protein 1.

coincident with the implantation process which occurs at an estimated 6–8 days from ovulation.

Much of the argument on the frequency of early pregnancy loss as judged by hCG determination has centred around the characteristics of the assays employed. Earlier work used the traditional assay with radiolabelled β-subunit and an antibody to the β-subunit of hCG (Vaitukaitis et al, 1972). Although these were a great improvement over earlier assays to the intact hormone (which could not readily distinguish between hCG and LH), they have now been replaced by the still more sensitive and specific immunometric assays (see Wilcox et al, 1985; Norman et al, 1990) which employ labelled antibodies, usually monoclonal. Some of the positive findings in earlier studies have been attributed to the relative non-specificity of the assay rather than to any real biological phenomenon (Baker et al, 1987; Whittaker, 1988; Walker et al, 1988).

Other factors which differ between studies are the fluid studied (blood or urine) and the definition of what constitutes a positive result. Quantitative

Table 3. Studies on the appearance of hCG in the luteal phase in women with apparently fertile cycles.

Authors	Number of subjects	Findings
Chartier et al (1979)	321 cycles in 2147 infertile women	71 cycles had detectable serum hCG and confirmed pregnancy. 72 cycles had detectable serum hCG but ended in normal menstruation; 49 of these had not received exogenous hCG
Miller et al (1980)	623 cycles in 197 normal women	Clinical pregnancy in 102 women (87 > 20 weeks). 50 women showed transient rise in hCG with no clinical evidence of pregnancy (33% of pregnancies)
Edmonds et al (1982)	50 cycles from 18 sterilized women; 198 cycles in 82 normal women	All urine samples from sterilized women had no hCG. Clinical pregnancy in 51 cycles, hCG detected in 118 cycles (59.6%)
Whittaker et al (1983)	226 ovulatory cycles in 91 normal women	Clinical pregnancy in 85 cycles (74 live births; 11 abortions). Seven cycles had detectable serum hCG but ended in normal menstruation (8% of pregnancies)
Sharpe et al (1986)	27 subfertile women	Clinical pregnancy in 11 women, nine of whom had a transient hCG rise in a previous cycle. Three of 16 women with no pregnancy also showed a transient hCG rise
Wilcox et al (1988)	707 cycles from 221 normal women	Clinical pregnancy in 155 women. In 43 cycles there was a transient increase in hCG with no clinical pregnancy
Sweeney et al (1988)	306 cycles from 88 normal women	Pregnancy diagnosed in 32 cases, of which 6 (18%) resulted in early fetal loss

cut-off levels which have been employed range from 0.5 to 30 units/litre. Some authors require that only a single specimen give a positive result; others demand that the result be positive on more than one occasion.

Clinical definitions can also present a problem in the analysis of studies on early pregnancy loss. For example, in studies based on potentially fertile cycles, some authors (Whittaker et al, 1983) provide specific evidence for ovulation by progesterone measurement, while others do not provide such evidence.

The earliest studies addressed women using an intrauterine contraceptive device (IUD) and suggested that hCG could often be detected during an apparently normal luteal phase (Table 2). However, later reports suggested that these positive results could be attributed to the presence of LH.

Subsequently, many workers have evaluated the frequency of unsuspected pregnancy loss by measuring urine hCG on one or more occasions in the luteal phase of normal (Table 3) or IVF cycles (Table 4). Estimates of the frequency of this phenomenon range from 8% (Whittaker et al, 1983) to 52% (Edmonds et al, 1982). In one of the most recent studies using 'state of the art' assays of exceptional sensitivity and specificity, Wilcox et al (1988) demonstrated that some 22% of conceptions which could be detected by elevated hCG levels in the late luteal phase did not survive as a clinically recognizable pregnancy.

Several workers have looked at the rate of 'biochemical pregnancy' or 'menstrual abortion' following in vitro fertilization (Table 4). A meta-analysis of some of these studies by Whittaker (1988) indicated that, of 566 pregnancies, 94 (17%) were preclinical abortions, 93 (16%) were clinical

Table 4. Studies on the frequency of pregnancy resulting from IVF.

Authors	Number of observations	Findings
Jones et al (1983)	190 cycles	36 pregnancies of which eight were 'pre-clinical' abortions and four were 'clinical' abortions
Hay (1985)	84 cycles	Clinical pregnancy in 21 women. 16 women showed a transient rise in serum hCG with no clinical evidence of pregnancy (43% of pregnancies)
Confino et al (1986)	303 pregnancies	Pregnancies in which more than one embryo was transferred showed cyclic variation in hCG levels, attributed to early embryo death
Deutinger et al (1986)	37 pregnancies	Clinical pregnancy in 30 women (21 normal, 9 abortions). Seven women showed increase in hCG with no clinical evidence of pregnancy) (19% of pregnancies)
Barlow et al (1988)	108 pregnancies	29 'chemical' pregnancies (27%), five ectopic pregnancies (5%), 15 abortions (14%) and 59 ongoing pregnancies (55%)
Hutchinson-Williams et al (1989)	22 cycles	Two biochemical pregnancies, two abortions, five term pregnancies

abortions and 19 (3%) were ectopics. At first sight the rate of pregnancy loss in IVF cycles appears to be similar to that in spontaneous cycles. However, Weinberg and Wilcox have suggested that, after correcting for the sensitivity of assays and the number of embryos replaced, the rate of loss is much higher following IVF than that following natural conception (Weinberg and Wilcox, 1988).

It should be emphasized that significant hCG secretion into the mother commences only *after* implantation. It is quite possible, indeed very likely, that substantial losses, which would not be detected by measurement of hCG, could occur before that time. A number of workers have suggested that preimplantation loss might be signalled by the transient appearance of 'early pregnancy factor' (see Chard and Grudzinskas, 1988). Early pregnancy factor appears in the mother shortly after fertilization. In the mouse, there is good evidence for such a factor. However, the human embryo is the same size as the mouse embryo but the size of the maternal compartment is vastly greater. It is not surprising, therefore, that the evidence for such a factor in humans is unconvincing.

WHAT MIGHT LEAD TO FAILURE OF EARLY PREGNANCY?

This topic has been well reviewed by Braude and colleagues (1991). There is no doubt that a great deal of knowledge about early human development has been yielded by the clinical practice of assisted reproduction. This has provided information on human oocytes and preimplantation embryos that is unlikely to have become available from experimental studies alone.

Braude has classified possible causes of early loss under the headings of (1) failure of gene activation, (2) chromosomal abnormalities, and (3) errors of cytokinesis and karyokinesis.

Failure of gene activation

There is a substantial increase of mRNA transcriptional activity at the 4- to 8-cell stage (Tesarik et al, 1988). This can be blocked by transcription inhibitors (Braude et al, 1988). This is also the stage at which there is a rapidly increasing risk of pregnancy loss, and Braude has suggested that the failure of development might be the result of failure of genomic expression. However, cleavage arrest does not seem to be associated with a failure of protein synthesis.

Chromosomal abnormalities

An abnormal karyotype is found in some 60–84% of spontaneously aborted fetuses (Boue et al, 1975; Plachot, 1989). Most of the abnormalities are trisomies or polyploidies; the monosomies, which should be equal in number to the trisomies, are presumed to be lost at an earlier stage. Around 20–30% of human embryos fertilized and cultured in vitro are aneuploid (Angell et al, 1983; Plachot et al, 1988). However, it is possible that at least some of these abnormalities are the result of the experimental procedures themselves. Deleterious effects include temperature: the spindle structure of the second meiotic division of the oocyte is very sensitive to small reductions in temperature. Freshly recovered human oocytes show spindle abnormalities after exposure to room temperature for as little as 10 min (Pickering et al, 1988).

Errors of cytokinesis and karyokinesis

The formation of a blastocyst does not guarantee normal development: it is possible for a blastocyst-like structure to form but for the inner cell mass to be reduced or absent. The surface trophoblast cells are still capable of implanting and secreting specific proteins. This might be the basis of the so-called anembryonic pregnancy, although it now seems more likely that this is the result of unperceived loss of the fetus rather than failure of embryo formation (Stabile et al, 1989).

CAN LOW hCG LEVELS PREDICT ABORTION?

It is well accepted that low levels of hCG are associated with the process of spontaneous abortion (Grudzinskas and Chard, 1990), but do low levels precede the clinical signs of the abortion process and can they, therefore, be used to predict the outcome of an apparently normal pregnancy? Both Chartier et al (1979) and Batzer and colleagues (1981) suggested that both single and serial estimates of hCG can be prognostic of pregnancy outcome in the first 30 days of gestation. Okamoto and colleagues (1987) have shown that a single measurement of plasma hCG 14 days after IVF is useful in predicting ectopic pregnancy. However, other workers have been less impressed with the value of this test prior to 30 days gestation (Braunstein et al, 1978).

IS EARLY PREGNANCY LOSS A SIGNIFICANT CAUSE OF 'INFERTILITY'?

It is often suggested that repeated, unrecognized early pregnancy loss might be responsible for a significant number of cases of apparent infertility. However, Sharp and colleagues (1986) showed that the frequency of a transient hCG increase in the luteal phase was greater in subjects who subsequently had a clinically recognizable pregnancy than in those who did not. Barlow and colleagues (1988) reported similar findings in IVF cases. Furthermore, Wilcox et al (1988) showed that 95% of 40 women with unrecognized early pregnancy loss (judged by the transient appearance of hCG) had normal pregnancies within 2 years.

CONCLUSIONS

It is generally agreed that large numbers of conceptuses fail to develop into a clinically recognizable pregnancy. Estimates of the rate of failure at various stages are shown in Figure 1. At least 50% of early failures (before 12 weeks) are due to chromosomal abnormalities and the proportion may be still higher with preimplantation loss. There is no evidence that repeated early pregnancy loss is a cause of infertility.

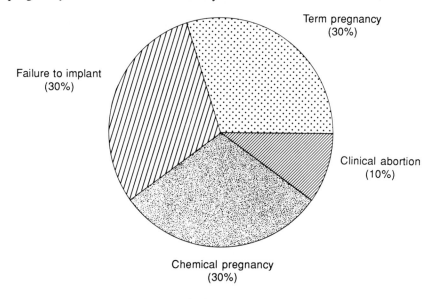

Figure 1. The fate of an early pregnancy.

REFERENCES

Angell RR, Aitken RJ, Van Look PFA, Lumsden MA & Templeton AA (1983) Chromosome abnormalities in human embryos after in vitro fertilization. *Nature* **303:** 336–338.
Barlow P, Lejeune B, Puissant F et al (1988) Early pregnancy loss and obstetrical risk after in-vitro fertilization and embryo replacement. *Human Reproduction* **3:** 671–675.
Batzer FR, Schlaff S, Goldfarb AF & Corson SL (1981) Early embryonic mortality in women. *Fertility and Sterility* **38:** 447–453.
Beling CG, Cederqvist LL & Fuchs F (1976) Demonstration of gonadotropin during the second half of the cycle in women using intrauterine contraception. *American Journal of Obstetrics and Gynecology* **125:** 855–858.
Bolton VN, Hawes SM, Taylor CT & Parsons JH (1988) Development of spare human preimplantation embryos in vitro: an analysis of the correlations among gross morphology, cleavage rates and development to the blastocyst. *Journal of In Vitro Fertilisation and Embryonic Transfer* **6:** 30–35.
Bonduelle RL, Dodd R, Liebaers I et al (1988) Chorionic gonadotrophin-β mRNA, a trophoblast marker, is expressed in human 8-cell embryos derived from tripronucleate zygotes. *Human Reproduction* **3:** 909–914.

Boue J, Boue A & Lazar P (1975) Retrospective and prospective epidemiological studies of 1500 karyotyped spontaneous human abortions. *Teratology* **12:** 11–26.

Braude PR, Bolton VN & Moor S (1988) Human gene expression first occurs between the four- and eight-cell stages of preimplantation development. *Nature* **332:** 459–461.

Braude P, Johnson M, Pickering S & Vincent C (1990) Mechanisms of early embryonic loss in vivo and in vitro. In Chapman MG, Grudzinskas JG & Chard T (eds) *The Embryo: Normal and Abnormal Development and Growth*. Berlin, Heidelberg, New York, Tokyo: Springer-Verlag (in press).

Braunstein GD, Karow WG, Rasor J & Wade ME (1978) First-trimester chorionic gonado-tropin measurements as an aid in the diagnosis of early pregnancy disorders. *American Journal of Obstetrics and Gynecology* **131:** 25–32.

Buster JE, Bustillo M & Rodi IA (1985) Biologic and morphologic description of donated human ova recovered by non-surgical uterine lavage. *American Journal of Obstetrics and Gynecology* **153:** 211–217.

Chard T & Grudzinskas JG (1987) Early pregnancy factor. *Biological Research in Pregnancy* **8:** 53–56.

Chartier M, Roger M, Barrat J & Michelon B (1979) Measurement of plasma human chorionic gonadotropin (hCG) and β-hCG activities in the late luteal phase: evidence of the occurrence of spontaneous menstrual abortions in infertile women. *Fertility and Sterility* **31:** 134–137.

Confino E, Demir RH, Friberg J & Gleicher N (1986) Does cyclic human chorionic gonado-tropin secretion indicate embryo loss in vitro fertilization? *Fertility and Sterility* **46:** 897–902.

Cooke ID, Sulaiman RA, Lenton EA & Parsons RJ (1981) Fertility and infertility statistics: their importance and application. *Clinical Obstetrics and Gynaecology* **8:** 531–548.

Deutinger J, Neumark J, Reinthaller A et al (1986) Pregnancy-specific parameters in early pregnancies after in vitro fertilization. *Fertility and Sterility* **46:** 77–80.

Edmonds DK, Lindsay KS, Miller JF, Williamson E & Woods PJ (1982) Early embryonic mortality in women. *Fertility and Sterility* **38:** 447–453.

Fishel SB, Edwards RG & Evans CJ (1984) Human chorionic gonadotropin secreted by pre-implantation embryos cultured in vitro. *Science* **223:** 816–818.

Formigli L, Formigli G & Roccia C (1987) Donation of fertilized uterine ova to infertile women. *Fertility and Sterility* **47:** 162–165.

Gordon Baker HW, Kovacs GT & Burger HG (1987) Failure of daily measurements of hCG in urine to demonstrate a high rate of early embryonic mortality. *Clinical Reproduction and Fertility* **5:** 15–25.

Grudzinskas JG & Chard T (1990) Endocrinology and metabolism in early pregnancy. In Chapman MG, Grudzinskas JG & Chard T (eds) *The Embryo: Normal and Abnormal Development and Growth*. Berlin, Heidelberg, New York, Tokyo: Springer-Verlag (in press).

Hay DL (1985) Discordant and variable production of human chorionic gonadotropin and its free α- and β-subunits in early pregnancy. *Journal of Clinical Endocrinology and Metabolism* **61:** 1195–1200.

Hertig AT, Rock J & Adams EC (1956) A description of 34 human ova within the first 17 days of development. *American Journal of Anatomy* **98:** 435–493.

Hertig AT (1975) Implantation of the human ovum. In Behrman SJ & Kistner RW (eds) *Progress in Infertility*, pp 411–421. Boston: Little Brown and Company.

Hutchinson-Williams KA, Lunenfeld B, Diamond MP, Lavy G, Boyers SP & DeCherney AH (1989) Human chorionic gonadotrophin, estradiol, and progesterone profiles in con-ception and nonconception cycles in an in vitro fertilization program. *Fertility and Sterility* **52:** 441–445.

Jones HW, Acosta AA, Andrews MC et al (1983) What is pregnancy? A question for programs of in vitro fertilization. *Fertility and Sterility* **40:** 728–733.

Klein TA & Mishell DR (1977) Absence of circulating chorionic gonadotropin in wearers of intrauterine contraceptive devices. *American Journal of Obstetrics and Gynecology* **129:** 626–628.

Landesman R, Coutinho EM & Saxena BJ (1976) Detection of human chorionic gonadotropin in blood or regularly bleeding women using copper intrauterine contraceptive devices. *Fertility and Sterility* **27:** 1062–1066.

Lenton EA & Woodward AJ (1988) The endocrinology of conception cycles and implantation in women. In Templeton AA & Weir BJ (eds) *The Early Days of Pregnancy*, pp 1–15. Proceedings of Symposium, Valedictory Meeting for Professor Arnold Klopper, Aberdeen, 1987.

Lopata A & Hay DL (1989) The potential of early human embryos to form blastocysts, hatch from their zona and secrete hCG in culture. *Human Reproduction* 4: 87–94.

Miller JF, Williamson E, Glue J, Gordon YB, Grudzinskas JG & Sykes A (1980) Fetal loss after implantation. *Lancet* ii: 554–556.

Norman RJ, Buck RH & De Medeiros SF (1990) Measurement of human chorionic gonadotropin (hCG): indications and techniques for the clinical laboratory. *Annals of Clinical Biochemistry* 27: 183–194.

Okamoto SH, Healy DL, Morrow LM, Rogers PAW, Trounson AO & Wood EC (1987) Predictive value of plasma human chorionic gonadotrophin β subunit in diagnosing ectopic pregnancy after in vitro fertilisation and embryo transfer. *British Medical Journal* 294: 667–670.

Orloff VS, Yamamoto S, Greenwood FC & Bryant-Greenwood GD (1979) Human chorionic gonadotropin β-subunit-like immunoreactive material in the plasma of women wearing an intrauterine progesterone contraceptive system. *American Journal of Obstetrics and Gynecology* 134: 632–637.

Pickering SJ, Johnson MH & Braude PR (1988) Cytoskeletal organisation in fresh, aged and spontaneously activated human oocytes. *Human Reproduction* 3: 978–979.

Plachot M (1989) Chromosome analysis of spontaneous abortions after IVF. A European survey. *Human Reproduction* 4: 425–429.

Plachot M, Veiga A, Montagut J et al (1988) Are clinical and IVF parameters correlated with chromosomal disorders in early life: a multicentric study. *Human Reproduction* 3: 627–635.

Roberts CJ & Lowe CR (1975) Where have all the conceptions gone? *Lancet* i: 495–499.

Saxena BB (1989) Measurement and clinical significance of preimplantation blastocyst and gonadotrophins. *Journal of Reproduction and Fertility* 37: 115–119.

Segal SJ, Alvarez-Sanchez F, Adejuwon CA, Branche de Mejia V, Leon P & Faundes A (1985) Absence of chorionic gonadotropin in women who use intrauterine devices. *Fertility and Sterility* 44: 214–218.

Seppälä M, Rutanen EM, Jalaniko H, Lehtovirta P, Stenman UH & Engvall E (1978) Pregnancy specific β₁-glycoprotein and chorionic gonadotropin-like immunoreactivity during the latter half of the cycle in women using intrauterine contraception. *Journal of Clinical Endocrinology and Metabolism* 47: 1216–1219.

Sharp NC, Anthony F, Miller JF & Masson GM (1986) Early conceptual loss in subfertile patients. *British Journal of Obstetrics and Gynaecology* 93: 1072–1077.

Sharpe RM, Wrixon W, Hobson BM, Corker CS, McLean HA & Short RV (1977) Absence of hCG-like activity in the blood of women fitted with intra-uterine contraceptive devices. *Journal of Clinical Endocrinology and Metabolism* 45: 496–499.

Shutt D & Lopata A (1981) The secretion of hormones during the culture of human pre-implantation embryos with corona cells. *Fertility and Sterility* 35: 413–416.

Stabile I, Olajide F, Chard T & Grudzinskas JG (1989) Maternal serum alpha-fetoprotein levels in anembryonic pregnancy. *Human Reproduction* 4: 204–205.

Sweeney AM, Meyer MR, Aarons JH et al (1988) Evaluation of methods for the prospective identification of early fetal losses in environmental epidemiology studies. *American Journal of Epidemiology* 127: 843–849.

Tamsen L & Eneroth P (1986) Serum levels of pregnancy-specific β₋₁-glycoprotein (SP₁) and human chorionic gonadotropin (β-hCG) in women using an intrauterine device. *Contraception* 33: 497–501.

Tesarik J, Kopeny V, Plachot M & Mandelbaum J (1988) Early morphological signs of embryonic genome expression in human preimplantation development as revealed by quantitative electron microscopy. *Developmental Biology* 128: 15–20.

Vaitukaitis JL, Braunstein GD & Ross GT (1972) A radioimmunoassay which specifically measures human chorionic gonadotropin in the presence of luteinizing hormone. *American Journal of Obstetrics and Gynecology* 113: 751–758.

Walker EM, Lewis M, Cooper W et al (1988) Occult biochemical pregnancy: fact or fiction? *British Journal of Obstetrics and Gynaecology* 95: 659–663.

Weinberg CR & Wilcox AJ (1988) Incidence rate of implantation in 'non-pregnant' patients. *Fertility and Sterility* **50:** 993.

Whittaker P (1988) Recognition of early pregnancy: human chorionic gonadotrophin. In Chapman M, Grudzinskas JG & Chard T (eds) *Implantation: Biological and Clinical Aspects*, pp 33–40. London, Berlin, Heidelberg, New York, Paris, Tokyo: Springer-Verlag.

Whittaker PG, Taylor A & Lind T (1983) Unsuspected pregnancy loss in healthy women. *Lancet* **i:** 1126–1127.

Wilcox AJ, Weinberg CR, Wehman RE, Armstrong EG, Canfield RE & Nisula BC (1985) Measuring early pregnancy loss: laboratory and field methods. *Fertility and Sterility* **44:** 366–374.

Wilcox AJ, Weinberg CR, O'Connor JF et al (1988) Incidence of early loss of pregnancy. *New England Journal of Medicine* **319:** 189–194.

12

Morphological and histochemical factors related to implantation

ELIZABETH JOHANNISSON

The rapid development of methods related to medically assisted procreation has opened new avenues for the treatment of infertility, and techniques related to human in vitro fertilization (IVF) have steadily improved since the first birth of an extracorporally fertilized baby in 1978. However, the current success rate rarely exceeds 25% per cycle of treatment (Ethics Committee of the American Fertility Society, 1990). Nevertheless, apparently-healthy embryos are achieved in vitro in about 75% of the cycles in some IVF programmes (Jones, 1984). This discrepancy of success rate between the number of apparently-healthy embryos transferred to the uterine cavity and attainment of pregnancy is an intriguing issue.

It has been repeatedly suggested that the low implantation rate in the IVF programmes could be related to disturbances of some endometrial factors which are usually important for implantation. The molecular events that accompany embryo attachment and implantation after the blastocyst enters the uterine cavity and hatches through its zona pellucida are unfortunately still incompletely understood. The lack of knowledge in this field may be partly due to the fact that the process of implantation in the human species is likely to be unique and that results from animal studies cannot be unconditionally extrapolated to human beings. Therefore, there is at this time no experimental animal model which could provide adequate information about the implantation process in humans.

Furthermore, for ethical and legal reasons the implantation of a human blastocyst in the human endometrium cannot be studied in vivo, and in many countries studies on the implantation process of a human blastocyst even in vitro are considered unethical. Studies on the factors important for implantation in human beings therefore have to be carried out in the full regard to current legal and ethical principles. However, in spite of all these limitations, it is widely recognized that IVF has become an accepted therapy for intractable infertility and that there is an urgent need to improve the techniques related to medically assisted procreation. Research in this area is therefore of paramount importance.

The complexity of the problem has called for a multidisciplinary approach involving not only gynaecologists but experts from a number of different research areas, e.g. biology, biochemistry, morphology, etc. Since the properties of the human blastocyst during the implantation process can not be studied for ethical and legal reasons, the uterine tissue in which the implantation normally takes place (the endometrium) has been the material of choice for most studies. Endometrial tissue usually obtained by biopsy or curettage has been processed for microscopic or electron microscopic examination, homogenized and analysed by biochemical methods or used for in vitro studies to investigate the composition of the secretory products of the human endometrium. Some material has also been obtained from women undergoing interruption of an early pregnancy. However, most investigators have focused their interest on the period empirically considered as the optimal time for a successful implantation (the 'implantation window'). To carry out such studies, endometrial biopsy has to be carefully timed in relation to ovulation, as reflected by the luteinizing hormone (LH) surge. Recent studies on the histological dating of the human endometrium in fertile women with a normal hormonal profile of circulating ovarian steroids have shown important individual variations in the length of the preovulatory and postovulatory phases (Johannisson et al, 1982, 1987; Dockery et al, 1988a, 1988b; Li et al, 1988). It would therefore be hazardous to assume that the preovulatory and postovulatory phases are invariably divided into periods of 14 days each; the period for the beginning of the implantation window calculated to occur on the 20th–21st day from the first day of the last menstrual period may correspond to any time between $LH-3$ to $LH+11$.

In view of the great variation in the implantation process among different species, the present review has mainly been concerned with the findings in humans. The results from animal studies have only been included when considered relevant to observations in the human implantation process. Furthermore, studies involving endometrial samples obtained with the onset of the menstrual bleeding as the only point of reference for a menstrual cycle have been treated with some reservation.

MORPHOLOGY OF THE ENDOMETRIUM DURING THE NORMAL MENSTRUAL CYCLE

During the normal physiological menstrual cycle the human endometrium undergoes significant morphological changes induced by the ovarian sex hormones produced (Noyes et al, 1950). In principle, ovulation divides the menstrual cycle into a preovulatory and a postovulatory phase. During the preovulatory phase the endometrium is mainly influenced by the oestrogens produced by the ovaries. Oestrogens stimulate the proliferative activity of the endometrium. The endometrium, which is composed of the epithelium lining the uterine cavity, the glandular epithelium and the stroma, then starts to grow. The lining epithelium and the glandular epithelium develop their endoplasmic reticulum and Golgi apparatus and there is also an increase of mitochondria (Cornillie et al, 1985). During the postovulatory phase the production of progesterone following ovulation introduces remarkable changes in the morphology of the endometrium. These changes occur with great precision, in particular during the first 6 days after ovulation

(Johannisson et al, 1987; Dockery et al, 1988a, 1988b; Li et al, 1988; Dockery and Rogers, 1989). Between days LH−1/0) and LH+1/+2 basal vacuoles start to appear in the glandular epithelium and their number gradually increases up to day LH+4. The glandular mitoses gradually decrease and after day LH+6 no more glandular mitoses can be found. The basal vacuoles have disappeared by day LH+6. Recent studies by Dockery et al (1990) have also revealed a dramatic increase in the packing density of the stroma between day LH+2 and LH+6. By day LH+6 the first half of the postovulatory phase, characterized by very precise changes in the endometrial glands, is over. This period, however, coincides with the passage of the oocyte through the fallopian tube. The arrival of a fertilized oocyte in the uterine cavity is believed to take place 4–5 days after ovulation (Findlay, 1984). At that time, the fertilized oocyte (the zygote) has hatched from the zona pellucida and is at the blastocyst stage, ready for the implantation process.

Between day LH+6 and LH+8 a substantial decrease ($P < 0.01$) has been found in the packing density of the endometrial stroma (Dockery et al, 1990). At this time, which is likely to correspond to the beginning of the implantation window, the stromal oedema is thought to be maximal. The last half of the postovulatory phase is characterized by extensive secretory activity of the glandular epithelium, reflected by an increase in the size of the glands and the presence of secretory products in the glandular lumina. The glandular diameter, as well as the volume density of the glandular lumen, shows a linear increase from day LH−1/0 to day LH+11/+12. Furthermore, major changes take place in the stroma 8–10 days after ovulation; for example, the development of predecidua around the spiral arteries as well as in the upper layer of the endometrium next to the epithelium lining the uterine cavity. Light microscopically, the predecidual cells are characterized by a vesicular nucleus and abundant clear cytoplasm. Electron microscopically, predecidual cells display a rounding of the nucleus and an increase and dilatation of the rough endoplasmic reticulum (Verma, 1983; Cornillie et al, 1985). If no implantation occurs, the endometrium undergoes regressive changes, starting at approximately days LH+11/+12 (Johannisson, 1990). The volume density of the glands diminishes and neutrophils start to invade the stroma.

MORPHOLOGY AND MOLECULAR EVENTS OF THE IMPLANTATION PROCESS

Implantation of the human blastocyst involves penetration of the endometrial surface epithelium by invading trophoblast. The penetration is preceded by apposition and then by adhesion (attachment) of the trophoblast to the endometrium.

Apposition phase

During apposition no visible functional connections are established between the blastocyst and the endometrium. The blastocyst is, however, exposed to the uterine milieu and the secretory products present in the uterine cavity may or may not have an embryo-toxic effect, depending on the short phase of uterine receptivity for embryonic implantation ('the implantation window'). The periods of receptivity and non-receptivity are likely to be hormone regulated in rodents (Psychoyos, 1963, 1973; Psychoyos and Martel, 1985), as well as in humans (Rosenwaks, 1987). Cholic acids have recently been found in high concentration in human uterine fluid obtained between the 22nd and 25th days of the menstrual cycle (Psychoyos et al, 1989). It was suggested that this substance could be responsible for the embryo-toxicity of the uterine environment in the non-receptive period of the postovulatory phase. The composition of the uterine milieu before and after the period of receptivity for embryonic implantation may therefore be one of the factors important for the apposition phase.

Adhesion phase

During the adhesion phase, functional connections are established between the blastocyst and the lining epithelium of the endometrium. The molecular events that accompany this adhesion are, however, still widely speculative. Taking into account that the human blastocyst usually implants in the upper part of the posterior wall of the uterine cavity (Boyd and Hamilton, 1970), the morphological structure of the lining epithelium in this area may be one of the factors important for the implantation process. Light microscopic (Hamperl, 1950) and transmission electron microscopic studies (Borell et al, 1959) have revealed cyclic changes in the lining epithelium of the endometrium during the normal menstrual cycle. Furthermore, scanning electron microscopic studies have confirmed the previous findings of cyclic changes occurring in the ciliated as well as in the non-ciliated cells in the lining epithelium (Johannisson and Nilsson, 1972; Ludwig and Metzger, 1976). Whereas the cilia were well developed in the preovulatory phase (Figure 1) clods were formed from the cilia and the microvilli of the cell surfaces during the postovulatory phase (Figure 2).

The ciliated cells were found to be unevenly distributed in the epithelium lining the endometrium. A scanty number of ciliated cells were observed in the tubal corners, whereas the ciliated cells were scattered all over the epithelial surface of the fundus area, with a concentration around the gland openings. The number of ciliated cells was increased towards the endocervix. The distribution of the ciliated cells seems to support the theory that the cilia are involved in the transport of endometrial secretory products.

It is noteworthy that secretory activity, e.g. the production of acid mucous glycoproteins, has been demonstrated in the lining epithelium of the human endometrium (Hester et al, 1968). This secretory activity may play an important role during the process of implantation. Cellular adhesion, or lack of it, is a property influenced by the electronegative cell-surface charges that are part of the glycoprotein cell-surface coat, the glycocalyx. In general, membrane glycoproteins are rich in the amino acids threonine and serine, the hydroxyl groups of which carry oligosaccharide side-chains similar to those of the mucous glycoproteins. Electron microscopical studies in

animals have revealed a quantitative decrease in thickness and electronegativity of the endometrial glycocalyx before the time of implantation
(Hewitt et al, 1979). By using a quantitative histochemical method specific
for carbohydrates on accurately timed endometrial biopsies, a similar
decrease in electronegativity of the glycocalyx was observed by Janssen et al
(1985) in normally menstruating women on the third day after the luteinizing
hormone peak. This was accompanied by a significant increase ($P = 0.005$)
in endometrial surface glycocalyx. In chemical terms, this represents
replacement of highly acid sulphated surface glycoprotein with moderately
acid sialyated glycoprotein. This decrease in electronegativity could be
important in reducing any impedance to implantation that a highly acid
endometrial glycocalyx might confer. One can therefore not exclude the
possibility that a decrease in electronegativity of the endometrial luminal

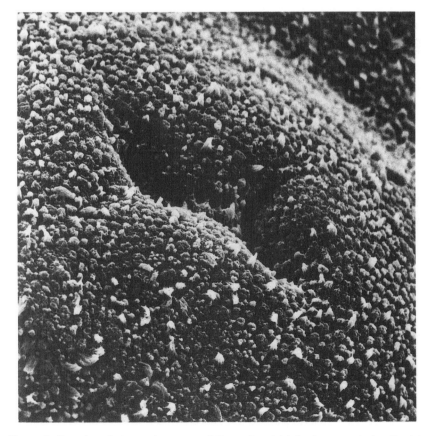

Figure 1. Scanning electron microscope of the endometrial fundus area during the late
proliferative phase. Note the gland opening with well-developed ciliated cells scattered all over
the region ($\times 1100$, reproduced at 80% of original).

surface glycocalyx is a necessary prelude to the adhesion between trophoblast and endometrium. The acquisition by the human endometrium of acid
mucous glycoproteins with the staining characteristics of sialyated substances in the early postovulatory phase is most likely to be part of the
influence of progesterone on the endometrium. By using a monoclonal
antibody technique, Thor et al (1987) demonstrated cyclic changes in the
composition of the glycocalyx of the lining epithelium during the normal
menstrual cycle. A hormone profile with levels of oestradiol and progesterone compatible with a normal menstrual cycle (Johannisson et al, 1982,
1987) may therefore be a prerequisite for a successful implantation.

Hester et al (1968) studied women on cyclic oestrogen and progesterone
therapy by using histochemical methods specific for acid mucous glycoproteins on endometrial biopsies. Highly acid sulphated mucous glycoproteins were observed at the cell surface under the influence of oestrogens,

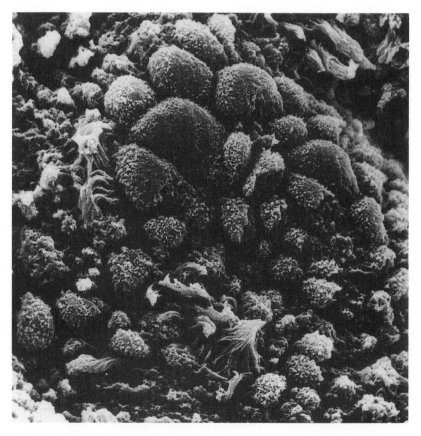

Figure 2. Surface structure of the endometrium at day LH+6/+7. Some epithelial cells are filled
with secretory products and bulging out from the surface. The ciliae are forming clods (×3700,
reproduced at 80% of original).

whereas the exposure to progestogens was accompanied by sialyated and less acid glycoproteins.

The results of more recent studies using the monoclonal antibody technique demonstrated two classes of polypeptide-associated keratan sulphate in the epithelial secretion of the human endometrium (Hoadley et al, 1990). One type of monoclonal antibody was bound to a hormonally regulated sialyated epitope associated with keratan sulphate sensitive to keratanase, endo-β-galactosidase and N-glycanase. The second type of monoclonal antibody was bound to a more highly sulphated type of keratan sulphate resistant to all three enzymes. These are again factors which may contribute to the environment of the implanting embryo.

Recently, an in vitro model for studying the adhesion of human blastocysts to uterine epithelial monolayer cultures, derived from curettage material in the midluteal phase of unstimulated menstrual cycles, has been developed (Lindenberg et al, 1985, 1986). The development, hatching and adhesion of the human blastocysts to the endometrial surface in vitro was delayed by one day compared with the implantation in vivo. However, the orientation and polarization of the implanting blastocyst in vitro during the adhesion phase were reported to be similar to that found in later implantation in vivo (Hertig et al, 1956; Larsen and Knoth, 1971; Knoth and Larsen, 1972). Transmission electron microscopic examinations of the material revealed the difference between species with regard to trophoblast outgrowth and the endometrial cell response. In the human material the trophoblast penetrated the intercellular spaces of the endometrial lining epithelium by forming long ectoplasmic protrusions. The human endometrial cells responded by a remarkable membrane activity adjacent to the trophoblast. In the trophoblast–endometrium contact zone, the rough endoplasmic reticulum of the endometrial cells was distended and numerous plasmolemmal vesicles were found at the surface of the endometrial cells next to the trophoblast. The in vitro model developed by Lindenberg et al (1985, 1989) might open new perspectives for studying factors of importance for the adhesion phase of the implantation process. As to other factors of importance for implantation, e.g. the decidualization of the stroma and components potentially involved in the nidatory mechanism, other techniques have been used.

Penetration phase

Although much attention has been paid to the histological and molecular events of the lining epithelium of the human endometrium in respect of the attachment of the blastocyst to the endometrium, products synthesized by the glands and/or the stroma of the underlying tissue may play a role in the penetration phase of the implantation process.

In mammals three types of penetration are recognized: intrusive, displacement and fusion penetration.

Intrusive penetration is characteristic of highly invasive embryos; the trophoblast penetrates between the epithelial lining cells, proliferates towards the basal lamina and invades the underlying stroma. In *displacement* penetration, the trophoblast phagocytoses epithelial cells and progresses to the basal lamina. In this case it is likely that the epithelial cells die by autolysis induced by embryonic signals (Schlafke and Enders, 1975; Lindenberg et al, 1989). Finally, in *fusion* penetration, the trophoblast fuses with the apical membrane of the lining epithelial cells. By cytoplasmic confluence the epithelial cells convert into a syncytium, which proliferates and penetrates the basal lamina.

In human being the penetration is intrusive and is likely to take place 8 days after ovulation (Hertig et al, 1956). The blastocyst is then completely embedded in the uterine stroma.

ENDOMETRIAL PRODUCTS POTENTIALLY RELATED TO IMPLANTATION

Based on the results from animal studies in rabbits (Krishman and Daniel, 1967; Beier, 1968) and in rats (Tzartos and Surani, 1979), it has been postulated that various substances synthesized by the human endometrium at specific moments after ovulation will affect the process of implantation. The results of such studies carried out in human material mainly refer to biochemical identification of various products in homogenates of human endometrial tissue obtained in the preovulatory or postovulatory phase. Unfortunately, the material investigated has rarely been timed in relation to the LH-peak. In view of the fact that the intrauterine implantation may take place only during a limited period of time ('the implantation window'), such studies of endometrial material obtained without LH timing do not give much information on the uterine environment; it could be indifferent, favourable or hostile to the embryo. In some of the studies, endometrial material from the proliferative phase has been compared with that of the postovulatory phase. The results of such studies may reveal the effect of progesterone on the endometrial products but they rarely allow any conclusion regarding factors important for implantation. In other studies endometrium from non-pregnant women has been compared with that obtained in early pregnancy or after full term. Such studies only provide information about the synthesis of endometrial products *after* a successful implantation has occurred.

Proteins produced by the endometrium during the postovulatory phase

Most of the biochemical investigations of the endometrium have involved studies on protein production. Several investigators have tried to identify certain proteins as markers specific for implantation but such studies are still at the experimental level.

Endometrial protein 14 or pregnancy-associated endometrial α_1-globulin (α_1-PEG) has been identified as a major secretory protein during the first trimester of pregnancy by radiolabelled amino acid incorporation in vitro (Bell et al, 1985). There is now strong evidence that the low-molecular mass of insulin-like growth factor-binding protein (IGF-BP) and placental protein 12 (PP12) are identical proteins (Julkunen et al, 1988). During the first trimester of the pregnancy this protein correlates with the extent of decidualization of the endometrium and by using monoclonal antibody technique it has also been localized to 'classically' defined decidual cells (Waites et al, 1989). The α_1-PEG is not, however, a pregnancy-specific protein. During the normal menstrual cycle this protein is a minor product, but an increase in synthesis and secretion has been reported during the latter stage of the luteal phase (Bell et al, 1986). Other investigators have demonstrated the presence of PP12 in human serum, amniotic fluid, the decidua and in the glandular epithelium from day 4 after ovulation (Wahlström and Seppälä, 1984; Rutanen et al, 1984). Furthermore, by using monoclonal antibodies the α_1-PEG was also found to be localized to stromal fibroblasts around the spiral arteries and to the upper layer of the endometrial mucosa next to the lining epithelium (Waites et al, 1988). The localization of the protein would then be consistent with the predecidualization taking place in the endometrium from day LH+9 in the normal physiological cycle. The balance of evidence indicates that the importance of the protein PP12 (or IGF-BP) for the preimplantation and the implantation period is still not fully understood.

A second protein, PP14, has been demonstrated in the post-ovulatory endometrium (Julkunen et al, 1986). PP14 is immunologically similar to α_2-PEG and to progestagen-dependent endometrial protein (Seppälä et al, 1988). As a matter of fact, the protein PP14 is immunologically indistinguishable from the progestagen-dependent endometrial protein (Julkunen et al, 1986). PP14 was found to be localized to the glandular surface epithelium of the endometrium from the fourth postovulatory day and onwards. However, the intensity of the staining varied from one gland to another in the late secretory phase also (Seppälä et al, 1988). Recently PP14 was demonstrated histochemically using the RNAs encoding a uterine β-lactoglobulin homologue (βLG/PP14) (Julkunen et al, 1990).

The progestagen specificity of PP14 in the postovulatory phase has been used to distinguish ovulatory from anovulatory cycles using serum samples of non-pregnant women (Seppälä et al, 1988). PP14 was reported to be present in the endometrium of infertile women on stimulated cycles for IVF (Manners, 1990). In this latter case, it was noteworthy that an atypical pattern of protein secretion occurred in spite of a histological dating classified as 'normal'. The concentration of the endometrial protein PP14 has also been described to be increased following the suppression of prolactin secretion (Seppälä et al, 1989). The treatment resulted in increased oestradiol levels in the mid- and late preovulatory phase. It was therefore suggested that low prolactin and high oestradiol levels during the preovulatory phase led to an influence on the subsequent secretory capacity of the endometrium (Seppälä et al, 1989).

Bell et al (1986) have also described other proteins synthesized by the human endometrium and associated with the menstrual cycle, e.g. EP13 which is the major product of the proliferative phase and EP9 and EP11 whose secretions are inhibited by progesterone.

Strong immunoreactivity has recently been demonstrated in the glandular compartment of the endometrial decidua during early pregnancy with poly-clonal S-100 protein antisera and monoclonal S-100 α-subunit antiserum (Nakamura et al, 1989). Although the function of S-100 protein is not known, a relationship was postulated between humoral factors related to implantation and the expression of the S-100 protein gene.

Pregnancy associated plasma protein (PAPP-A) is a macromolecular glycoprotein produced during human pregnancy and widely considered to be of trophoblastic origin. However, in non-pregnant women the concentration of PAPP-A has been reported to be increased in the uterine luminal fluid (Bischof et al, 1984) as well as in the endometrial tissue (Bischof et al, 1982), during the postovulatory phase. In vitro studies of monolayer cultures of non-decidualized human endometrial cells have also revealed increased production of PAPP-A following stimulation by progesterone (Bischof and Tseng, 1986). The synthesis of PAPP-A is likely to be dependent on progesterone stimulation but so far it is not yet clear if this endometrial product is a prerequisite for implantation. However, more recent histochemical studies have revealed that PAPP-A is localized to the cytoplasm of the cytotrophoblast of the early blastocyst, to the superficial epithelium of the endometrium adjacent to the implantation site, and to the decidual cells around the implantation site (Sabet et al, 1989).

In most studies dealing with the identification of proteins and growth factors specific for implantation, the development of the predecidua associated to the progesterone production in the late postovulatory phase of the menstrual cycle has been considered as an important factor for the nidatory mechanism of the implantation process. Among the factors which are likely to be involved in the development of the decidualization of the human endometrium, insulin-like growth factors (IGFs) or somatomedins have been claimed to play a significant role (Koistinen et al, 1986). IGFs are polypeptide hormones which specifically bind to cell membrane receptors. However, the IGFs also bind with high affinity to binding proteins (IGFBPs) in plasma and other body fluids. Human follicular fluid contains the insulin-like growth factor-binding protein (IGFBP 1) synthesized by ovarian granulosa cells. The production has been shown to be regulated via protein kinase-C- and adenylate cyclase-dependent pathways (Jalkanen et al, 1989). The synthesis of the IGFBP has also recently been reported to be associated with stromal fibroblast populations of the human endometrium (Bell, 1989). Furthermore, it has been postulated that this protein could be involved in specifying the proliferation of those fibroblasts which later differentiate into decidual cells in the human endometrium (Bell, 1989).

By using immunohistochemical techniques, IGFBP was recently demonstrated to be localized to decidual cells, at least in tissue of pregnancy endometrium (Bell, 1989). By accepting the concept that the formation of the predecidua in the human endometrium during the late postovulatory phase is essential for the nidation, IGFBP synthesis might be one of the factors modulating this part of the implantation process. However, the process of decidualization of the endometrium is biochemically complex. Apart from progesterone, which is implicated in the production of most proteins derived from the endometrial tissue during the postovulatory phase, additional factors may be involved for the induction of IGFBP synthesis in human endometrium.

Extracellular matrix in the endometrium during the postovulatory phase

Several studies have revealed that the decidual cells in early pregnancy are surrounded by large amounts of laminin (Charpin et al, 1985; Wewer et al, 1985). During the normal menstrual cycle very little laminin is seen in the preovulatory phase, whereas this protein begins to appear in larger amounts during the postovulatory phase. It has therefore been suggested that progesterone could be a stimulus for laminin synthesis (Faber et al, 1986; Irwin et al, 1989). In vitro systems have been developed from endometrial tissue using separation techniques for epithelial and stromal cells (Osteen et al, 1989; Schatz et al, 1990). By such techniques endometrial stromal cells were grown in vitro and stimulated by oestradiol and/or progesterone in more or less physiological doses and an in vitro model system for decidualization of the human endometrium has been developed (Irwin et al, 1989). Such studies have demonstrated that treatment with physiological doses of oestradiol and progesterone can induce an increase in fibronectin and laminin forming the pericellular matrix (Irwin et al, 1989). The pattern of pericellular distribution of laminin around the individual decidual cells cultured in vitro was identical to that observed in vivo (Loke et al, 1989).

In view of the hypothesis that the predecidual reaction of the human endometrium during the postovulatory phase may provide the initial anchorage of the blastocyst and facilitates the trophoblast migration, further studies have been carried out on the interaction in vitro between human trophoblast and laminin. In controlled in vitro studies it was observed that the number of trophoblast cells attached to areas coated with laminin was significantly higher than that attached to areas coated with collagen type IV ($P<0.01$) and coated with bovine serum albumin (BSA, $P<0.001$) (Loke et al, 1989). Therefore, there is reason to believe that the development of the decidua including the laminin production in the human endometrium during the postovulatory phase is important for the nidation of the blastocyst.

Hormones produced by the endometrium

The decidualization of the human endometrium during the postovulatory phase is not only associated with characteristic morphological patterns and a significant increase in the extracellular matrix containing laminin and fibronectin (Wewer et al, 1985): it is also accompanied by prolactin secretion, the production of which has been shown to correlate with the degree of the histological decidualization (Maslar and Riddick, 1979). It has also been shown that progesterone can induce and maintain decidualization and prolactin synthesis in organ cultures of the human endometrium (Maslar et al, 1986). More recent in vitro studies by Irwin et al (1989) have shown that the prolactin production by the stromal cells can be stimulated by progesterone in vitro in a dose-dependent manner. Further in vitro studies have also confirmed that non-gestational endometrial prolactin is of stromal origin and that the stromal prolactin production cannot only be induced, but also maintained, by progesterone (Randolph et al, 1990). The importance of this finding in respect of implantation is not fully known. However, it has been suggested that late appearance or absence of prolactin can have an impeding effect on the nidatory mechanism of implantation (McRae et al, 1986).

The decidual tissue has also been reported to be able to synthesize prorenin and renin, and it has been suggested that pregnancy enhances renin production by decidua formation (Shaw et al, 1989). Again, the importance of renin (if any) for the penetration and anchorage of the trophoblast is incompletely understood.

The endometrium has been reported to secrete prostaglandins ($PGF_{2\alpha}$ and PGE_2) (Abel et al, 1980; Kasamo et al, 1986). In vitro studies using $PGF_{2\alpha}$ have revealed that progesterone interferes with the prostaglandin synthesis (Brumsted et al, 1989). An increase in $PGF_{2\alpha}$ output was found in the late luteal phase of the menstrual cycle, but this finding may result not only from increased synthesis but also from a decrease in the catabolism (Brumsted et al, 1989). Very few $PGF_{2\alpha}$ binding sites have been found in the human endometrium. On the other hand PGE_2 binding sites have been demonstrated in the stromal cells, the glandular epithelium, elongated and circular smooth muscles, and arterioles (Chegini et al, 1986). The number of PGE_2 binding sites on the endometrial cells of the preovulatory phase was higher than in the postovulatory phase. The significance of this finding for the implantation process is not clear. However, it is noteworthy that prostaglandin endoperoxide synthase has been localized in the decidualized endometrial stromal cells in early pregnancy (Price et al, 1989).

Relaxin may also play a role in the implantation process via the aromatase activity stimulated by progesterone in human endometrial stromal cells (Tseng et al, 1987). Relaxin seems to exert a synergistic effect on the aromatase activity of the stromal cells in the presence of this steroid.

Little is known about the presence of gonadotrophin receptors in non-pregnant human endometrium. Recent studies using immunostaining techniques have displayed a higher concentration of hCG/LH receptors in the postovulatory phase when compared with the preovulatory phase (Reshef et al, 1990). In the preovulatory phase the receptors were mainly found in the luminal and glandular epithelium, whereas receptors were also found in the decidua cells during the postovulatory phase.

Immunoprotective factors

Immunoproteins have been studied in the endometrium in order to elucidate the immunoprotecting role of the uterus. From an immunological point of view it is difficult to explain that the genetically alien embryo, once implanted, is not rejected by the immunocompetent mother. Certain immunoglobulins (IgG and IgA) have been identified in endometrial homogenates (Tauber et al, 1985) and immunosuppressive factors have been reported in the endometrial decidua in pregnant women (Daya et al, 1985, 1987; Tatsumi et al, 1987). These factors have been shown to inhibit mixed lymphocyte reaction

(Tatsumi et al, 1987; Wang et al, 1988). The immunosuppressive factors are likely to be progesterone dependent but the immunoprotective mechanism in the implantation process is still incompletely understood and requires further investigation.

ENDOMETRIAL VASCULARIZATION AND THE NIDATORY MECHANISM

During the normal menstrual cycle the human endometrium undergoes extensive changes in vascularization, including the spiral arteries, the arterioles, the capillaries, the venous lakes and the veins. These changes are usually found in the functional layer of the endometrium, which is likely to be highly sensitive to the ovarian hormone stimulation. The preovulatory phase is characterized by rapid growth of the whole vascular system. The most distal part of the spiral arteries becomes connected to the subepithelial capillary plexus via arterioles, but they also develop small branches at irregular intervals in the functional layer (Fanger and Barker, 1961; Ramsey, 1977).

The subepithelial capillary plexus itself undergoes dynamic changes during the normal menstrual cycle. During the preovulatory phase the capillaries are thin walled and have a narrow lumen. However, the lumen progressively increases in diameter (Sheppard and Bonnar, 1980). Later, in the secretory phase, a complex meshwork of capillaries is present in the upper functional layer of the endometrium. There is a close connection between the thin capillaries and the arterioles, as well as with the venules, which often are dilated and form venous lakes. These lakes are probably dilated venules, the function of which has been claimed to be the regulation of the blood volume and the rate of blood flow in the upper part of the functional layer of the endometrium (Ramsey, 1977). The dilatation observed in the subepithelial capillaries reaches its maximum around LH+7 to LH+10, at the time when the nidation of the blastocyst is likely to take place (M. Peek and E. Johannisson, unpublished data). This observation supports the data reported from animal experiments that the vascular dynamics and the functional properties of the endothelial cells may be factors important for the nidatory mechanism of the implantation process.

Psychoyos (1971) demonstrated that an increase of the capillary permeability was the earliest detectable response of the endometrium to the blastocyst adhesion in rodents. Later, Abrahamsohn et al (1983) reported an increased capillary permeability in the rat endometrium at the beginning of the implantation process. It is likely that such an increase in capillary permeability will permit complexes composed of serum proteins to cross the blood vessel walls. It is also likely that the increased permeability of the capillaries facilitate the formation of the stromal oedema observed not only in rodents but also in the human endometrium at the time of implantation. The stromal oedema reaches its maximum around LH+10/+11 in the normal menstrual cycle of the human endometrium (Johannisson et al, 1987). It has been claimed that, in general, the vascular density is decreased because of the stromal oedema, thereby permitting volume expansion of the decidual cells and offering a loose interstitium within which vascular sprouts may elongate (Christoffersson and Nilsson, 1988).

In rodents a 'vascular shut-down' has been reported to occur in the primary decidual zone prior to implantation (Christoffersson and Nilsson, 1988). This may be due to a swelling of the capillary and venular endothelium and a volume expansion of the decidua surrounding the vessels (Enders and Schlafke, 1967; Rogers et al, 1983; Parr et al, 1986). Patent and collapsed capillaries then give rise to an avascular area in the primary decidual zone. The importance of this vascular shut-down for the implantation process is not fully known. It has been suggested that this phenomenon might 'weaken' the epithelium and the underlying mucosa and thereby facilitate the invasion of the blastocyst in rats (Rogers et al, 1982). It has also been suggested that this avascular zone might form an immunological barrier (Parr and Parr, 1986). However the same authors report on the presence of labelled bovine IgG in the primary decidual zone and in the rat embryo on day 7 of pregnancy. Acting as an immunological barrier may therefore not be the primary function of the avascular zone in rats.

Any vascular shut-down related to the implantation process has not, as yet, been reported in the human endometrium. This may be explained by the differences among species with regard to implantation. The penetration phase of the implantation process in rats and mice is a *displacement* penetration. In this case the trophoblast phagocytoses dead epithelial cells and progresses to the basal lamina. The embryo is only weakly invasive. In humans, penetration is *intrusive*. The trophoblast penetrates between adjacent epithelial cells, invades the underlying stroma and incorporates into the walls of the endometrial vessels. This invasion of the arteries, capillaries and veins is thought to lead to extensive fibrinoid necrosis and ultimate conversion of the vascular structures into sinusoidal vessels, changes which are considered to be important for the establishment of the required low resistance blood supply to the developing placenta (Robertson, 1987).

CONCLUSIONS

Implantation of a blastocyst in the human endometrium represents a highly complex system of hormonally regulated events. The discrepancy in the success rate between transfer of an apparently healthy embryo and attainment of pregnancy is an intriguing issue in most IVF programmes. Research in the field of human implantation is difficult and restricted by legal and ethical regulations. Nevertheless, the development of precise and accurate technology, and multidisciplinary efforts involving gynaecologists, biologists, biochemists, morphologists and experts in various research areas, are essential and of paramount importance for a better understanding of the factors involved in human implantation. Such multidisciplinary efforts may also contribute to specifying the gaps of knowledge now existing in this field and to defining more goal-oriented areas of research in the future.

REFERENCES

Abel MH, Smith SK & Baird DT (1980) Suppression of concentration of endometrial prostaglandin in early intra-uterine and ectopic pregnancy in women. *Journal of Endocrinology* **85:** 379–381.

Abrahamsohn P, Lundkvist O & Nilsson O (1983) Ultrastructure of the endometrial blood vessels during implantation of the rat blastocyst. *Cell Tissue Research* **229:** 269–280.

Beier H (1968) A hormone sensitive endometrial protein in blastocyst development. *Biochimica et Biophysica Acta* **160:** 289–291.

Bell SC (1989) Decidualization and insulin-like growth factor (IGF) binding protein: implications for its role in stromal cell differentiation and the decidual cell in haemochorial placentation. *Human Reproduction* **4:** 125–130.

Bell SC, Hales MW, Patel S et al (1985) Protein synthesis and secretion by the human endometrium and decidua during early pregnancy. *British Journal of Obstetrics and Gynaecology* **92:** 793–803.

Bell SC, Patel SR, Kirman PH & Drife JO (1986) Protein synthesis and secretion by human endometrium during the menstrual cycle and the effect of progesterone in vitro. *Journal of Reproduction and Fertility* **77:** 221–231.

Bischof P & Tseng L (1986) In vitro release of pregnancy-associated plasma protein-A (PAPP-A) by human endometrial cells. *American Journal of Reproductive Immunology and Microbiology* **10:** 139–142.

Bischof P, DuBerg S, Schindler AM et al (1982) Endometrial and plasma concentrations of pregnancy-associated plasma protein-A (PAPP-A). *British Journal of Obstetrics and Gynaecology* **89:** 701–703.

Bischof P, Schindler AM, Urner F, Mensi N, Herrmann WL & Sizonenko PC (1984) Pregnancy-associated plasma protein-A (PAPP-A): concentration in uterine fluid and immunohistochemical localization in the endometrium. *British Journal of Obstetrics and Gynaecology* **9:** 863–869.

Borell U, Nilsson O & Westman A (1959) The cyclic changes occurring in the epithelium lining the endometrial glands. An electron-microscopic study in the human being. *Acta Obstetricia et Gynecologica Scandinavica* **38:** 364–377.

Boyd JD & Hamilton WJ (1970) *The Human Placenta.* Cambridge: Heffer & Sons.

Brumsted JR, Chapitis J, Deaton JR, Riddick DH & Gibson M (1989) Prostaglandin F$_{2\alpha}$ synthesis and metabolism by luteal phase endometrium in vitro. *Fertility and Sterility* **52:** 769–773.

Charpin C, Kopp F, Pourreau-Schneider N et al (1985) Laminin distribution in human decidua and immature placenta. *American Journal of Obstetrics and Gynecology* **151:** 822–826.

Chegini N, Rao CV, Wakim N & Sanfilippo J (1986) Prostaglandin binding to different cell types of human uterus: quantitative light microscope autoradiographic study. *Prostaglandins, Leukotrienes and Medicine* **22:** 129–138.

Christofferson RH & Nilsson O (1988) Morphology of the endometrial microvasculature during early placentation in the rat. *Cell and Tissue Research* (in press).

Cornillie FJ, Lauweryns JM & Brosens I (1985) Normal human endometrium. An ultrastructural survey. *Gynecologic and Obstetric Investigation* **20:** 113–129.

Daya S, Clark DA, Devlin C & Jarrell J (1985) Preliminary characterization of two types of suppressor cells in the human uterus. *Fertility and Sterility* **44:** 778–785.

Daya S, Rosenthal KL & Clark DA (1987) Immunosuppressor factor(s) produced by decidua-associated suppressor cells: A proposed mechanism for fetal allograft survival. *American Journal of Obstetrics and Gynecology* **156:** 344–350.

Dockery P & Rogers AW (1989) The effects of steroids on the fine structure of the endometrium. *Baillière's Clinical Obstetrics and Gynaecology* **3:** 248.

Dockery P, Li TC, Rogers AW, Cooke ID & Lenton EA (1988a) The ultrastructure of the glandular epithelium in the timed endometrial biopsy. *Human Reproduction* **3:** 826–834.

Dockery P, Li TC, Rogers AW, Cooke ID, Lenton EA & Warren MA (1988b) An examination of the variation in timed endometrial biopsies. *Human Reproduction* **3:** 715–720.

Dockery P, Warren MA, Li TC, Rogers AW, Cooke ID & Mundy J (1990) A morphometric study of the human endometrial stroma during the periimplantation period. *Human Reproduction* **5:** 112–116.

Enders AC & Schlafke S (1967) A morphological analysis of the early implantation stages in the rat. *American Journal of Anatomy* **120**: 185–226.

Ethics Committee of the American Fertility Society (1990) Ethical considerations of the new reproductive technology. *Fertility and Sterility* **53** (supplement 2): 378–388.

Faber M, Wewer UM, Berthelson JG, Liotta LA & Albrechtsen R (1986) Laminin production by human endometrial stromal cells relates to the cyclic and pathologic state of the endometrium. *American Journal of Pathology* **124**: 384–391.

Fanger H & Barker BE (1961) Capillaries and arteriales in normal endometrium. *Obstetrics and Gynecology* **17**: 543–550.

Findlay JK (1984) Implantation and early pregnancy. In Trounson A & Wood C (eds) *In Vitro Fertilization and Embryo Transfer*, pp 57–74. London: Churchill Livingstone.

Hamperl H (1950) Ueber die 'hellen' Flimmerepithelzellen der menschlichen Uteruschleimhaut. *Virchows Archiv; A: Pathological Anatomy and Histopathology* **319**: 265–281.

Hertig AT, Rock J & Adams EC (1956) A description of 34 human ova within the first 17 days of development. *American Journal of Anatomy* **98**: 435–441.

Hester LL, Kellett WW III, Spicer SS, Williamsson HO & Pratt-Thomas HR (1968) Effects of sequential oral contraceptive on endometrial enzyme and carbohydrate histochemistry. *American Journal of Obstetrics and Gynecology* **102**: 771–783.

Hewitt K, Bear AE & Grinnell F (1979) Disappearance of anionic sites from the surface of the rat endometrial epithelium at the time of blastocyst implantation. *Biology of Reproduction* **21**: 691–695.

Hoadley ME, Seif MW & Aplin JD (1990) Menstrual cycle dependent expression of keratan sulphate in human endometrium. *Biochemical Journal* **266**: 757–763.

Irwin JC, Kirk D, King RJ, Quigley MM & Gwatkin RB (1989) Hormonal regulation of human endometrial stromal cells in culture: an in vitro model for decidualization. *Fertility and Sterility* **52**: 761–768.

Jalkanen J, Suikkari A-M, Koistinen R et al (1989) Regulation of insulin-like growth factor-binding protein 1 production in human granulosa luteal cells. *Journal of Clinical Endocrinology and Metabolism* **69**: 1174–1179.

Jansen RPS, Turner M, Johannisson E, Landgren BM & Diczfalusy E (1985) Cyclic changes in human endometrial surface glycoproteins: a quantitative histochemical study. *Fertility and Sterility* **44**: 85–91.

Johannisson E (1990) Endometrial morphology during the normal cycle and under the influence of contraceptive steroids. In d'Arcangues C, Fraser I, Newton JR & Odlind V (eds) *WHO Symposium on Contraception and Endometrial Bleeding*, pp 53–80. Cambridge: Cambridge University Press.

Johannisson E & Nilsson L (1972) Scanning electron microscopic study of the human endometrium. *Fertility and Sterility* **23**: 613–625.

Johannisson E, Parker RA, Landgren BM & Diczfalusy E (1982) Morphometric analysis of the human endometrium in relation to peripheral hormone levels. *Fertility and Sterility* **38**: 564–571.

Johannisson E, Landgren BM, Rohr HP & Diczfalusy E (1987) Endometrial morphology and peripheral hormone levels in women with regular menstrual cycles. *Fertility and Sterility* **48**: 401–408.

Jones GS (1984) Update on in vitro fertilization. *Endocrine Reviews* **5**: 62–69.

Julkunen M, Raikar RS, Joshi SG et al (1986) Placental protein 14 and progestagen-dependent endometrial protein are immunologically indistinguishable. *Human Reproduction* **1**: 7–8.

Julkunen M, Koistinen R, Aalto-Setälä K et al (1988) Primary structure of human insulin-like growth factor-binding protein/placental protein 12 and tissue-specific expression of its mRNA. *FEBS Letters* **236**: 295–302.

Julkunen M, Koistinen R, Suikkari A-M et al (1990) Identification by hybridization histochemistry of human endometrial cells expressing mRNAs encoding a uterine β-lactoglobulin homologue and insulin-like growth factor-binding protein-1. *Molecular Endocrinology* **4**: 700–707.

Kasamo M, Ishikawa M, Yamashita K, Sengoku K & Shimizu T (1986) Possible role of prostaglandin F in blastocyst implantation. *Prostaglandins* **31**: 321–323.

Knoth M & Larsen JF (1972) Ultrastructure of the human implantation site. *Acta Obstetricia et Gynecologica Scandinavica* **51**: 385–393.

Koistinen R, Kalkkinen N, Huhtala ML et al (1986) Placental protein 12 is a decidual protein that binds somatomedin and has an identical N terminal amino acid sequence with somatomedin-binding protein from human amniotic fluid. *Endocrinology* **118**: 1375–1378.

Krishman RS & Daniel JC (1967) Blastokinin inducer and regulator of the blastocyst development in rabbit uterus. *Science* **158**: 490–492.

Larsen JF & Knoth M (1971) Ultrastructure of the anchoring villi and trophoblast shell in the second week of placentation. *Acta Obstetricia et Gynecologica Scandinavica* **50**: 117–128.

Li TC, Rogers AW, Dockery P, Lenton EA & Cooke ID (1988) A new method of histologic dating of human endometrium in the luteal phase. *Fertility and Sterility* **50**: 52–60.

Lindenberg S, Nielsen MH & Lenz S (1985) In vitro studies of human blastocyst implantation. *Annals of the New York Academy of Sciences* **442**: 368–374.

Lindenberg S, Hyttel P, Lenz S & Holmes PV (1986) Ultrastructure of early human implantation in vitro. *Human Reproduction* **1**: 533–538.

Lindenberg S, Hyttel P, Sjögren A & Greve T (1989) A comparative study of attachment of human, bovine and mouse blastocysts to uterine epithelial monolayer. *Human Reproduction* **4**: 446–456.

Loke YW, Gardner L, Burland K & King A (1989) Laminin in human trophoblast–decidua interaction. *Human Reproduction* **4**: 457–463.

Ludwig H & Metzger H (1976) The human female reproductive tract. In *A Scanning Electron Microscopic Atlas*, New York: Springer-Verlag.

Manners CV (1990) Endometrial assessment in a group of infertile women on stimulated cycles for IVF: immunohistochemical findings. *Human Reproduction* **5**: 128–132.

McRae MA, Newman GR, Walker SM & Jasani B (1986) Immunohistochemical identification of prolactin and 24K protein in secretory endometrium. *Fertility and Sterility* **45**: 643–648.

Maslar IA & Riddick DM (1979) Prolactin production by human endometrium during the normal menstrual cycle. *American Journal of Obstetrics and Gynecology* **135**: 731–734.

Maslar IA, Powers-Craddock P & Ansbacher R (1986) Decidual prolactin production by organ cultures of human endometrium: effects of continuous and intermittent progesterone treatment. *Biology of Reproduction* **34**: 741–750.

Nakamura Y, Moritsuka Y, Ohta Y et al (1989) S-100 protein in glands within decidua and cervical glands during early pregnancy. *Human Pathology* **20**: 1204–1209.

Noyes RW, Hertig AT & Rock J (1950) Dating the endometrial biopsy. *Fertility and Sterility* **1**: 3–25.

Osteen KG, Hill GA, Hargrove JT & Gorstein F (1989) Development of a method to isolate and culture highly purified populations of stromal and epithelial cells from human endometrial biopsy specimens. *Fertility and Sterility* **52**: 965–972.

Parr MB & Paar EL (1986) Permeability of the primary decidual zone in the rat uterus: studies using fluorescein-labeled proteins and dextrans. *Biology of Reproduction* **34**: 393–403.

Parr MB, Tung HN & Parr EL (1986) The ultrastructure of the rat primary decidual zone. *American Journal of Anatomy* **176**: 423–436.

Price TM, Kauma SW, Curry TE & Clark MR (1989) Immunohistochemical localization of prostaglandin endoperoxidase synthase in human fetal membranes and decidua. *Biology of Reproduction* **41**: 701–705.

Psychoyos A (1963) Precisions sur l'état de 'non-receptivé' de l'uterus. *Comptes Rendus Hebdomadaires des Séances de l'Academie des Sciences* **257**: 1153–1156.

Psychoyos A (1971) Methods for studying changes in capillary permeability in the rat endometrium. In Daniel JC (ed.) *Methods in Mammalian Embryology*, pp 334–338. San Francisco: WH Freeman.

Psychoyos A (1973) Hormonal control of ovoimplantation. *Vitamins and Hormones* **31**: 201–256.

Psychoyos A & Martel D (1985) Embryo-endometrial interactions at implantation. In Edwards RG, Purdy JM & Steptoe PC (eds) *Implantation of the Human Embryo*, pp 195–218. London: Academic Press.

Psychoyos A, Roche D & Gravanis A (1989) Is cholic acid responsible for embryo-toxicity of the postreceptive uterine environment? *Human Reproduction* **4**: 832–834.

Ramsey EM (1977) Vascular anatomy. In Wynn RM (ed.) *Biology of the Uterus*, pp 59–76. New York: Plenum Press.

Randolph JF Jr, Peegel H, Ansbacher R & Menon KM (1990) In vitro induction of prolactin production and aromatase activity by gonadal steroids exclusively in the stroma of separated proliferative human endometrium. *American Journal of Obstetrics and Gynecology* **162:** 1109–1114.

Reshef E, Lei ZM, Rao CV, Pridham DD, Chegini N & Luborsky JL (1990) The presence of gonadotropin receptors in non-pregnant human uterus, human placenta, fetal membranes and decidua. *Journal of Clinical Endocrinology and Metabolism* **70:** 421–430.

Robertson WG (1987) Pathology of the pregnant uterus. In Fox H (ed.) *Obstetrical and Gynecological Pathology*, pp 1149–1176. Edinburgh: Churchill Livingstone.

Rogers PAW, Murphy CR & Gannon BJ (1982) Absence of capillaries in the endometrium surrounding the implanting rat blastocyst. *Micron* **13:** 373–374.

Rogers PAW, Murphy CR, Rogers AW & Gannon BJ (1983) Capillary patency and permeability in the endometrium surrounding the implanting rat blastocyst. *International Journal of Microcirculation: Clinical and Experimental* **2:** 241–249.

Rosenwaks Z (1987) Donor eggs: their application in modern reproductive technologies. *Fertility and Sterility* **47:** 895–909.

Rutanen EM, Koistinen R, Wahlström T, Stenman U-H & Seppälä M (1984) Placental protein 12 (PP12) in the menstrual fluid. *British Journal of Obstetrics and Gynaecology* **91:** 1025–1030.

Sabet LM, Daya D, Stead R, Richmond H & Jimeneze CL (1989) Significance and value of immunohistochemical localization of pregnancy specific proteins in the feto-maternal tissue throughout pregnancy. *Modern Pathology* **2:** 227–232.

Schatz F, Gordon RE, Laufer N & Gurpide E (1990) Culture of human endometrial cells under polarizing conditions. *Differentiation* **42:** 184–190.

Schlafke S & Enders A (1975) Cellular basis of interaction between trophoblast and uterus at implantation. *Biology of Reproduction* **12:** 41–65.

Seppälä M, Julkunen M, Koskimies A et al (1988) Proteins of the human endometrium. In: In vitro fertilization and other assisted reproduction. *Annals of the New York Academy of Sciences* **541:** 432–444.

Seppälä M, Martikainen H, Rönnberg L et al (1989) Suppression of prolactin secretion during ovarian hyperstimulation is followed by elevated serum levels of endometrial protein PP14 in the late luteal phase. *Human Reproduction* **4:** 389–391.

Shaw KJ, Do YS, Kjos S et al (1989) Human decidua is a major source of venin. *Journal of Clinical Investigation* **83:** 2085–2092.

Sheppard BL & Bonnar J (1980) The development of vessels of the endometrium during the menstrual cycle. In Diczfalusy E, Fraser IS & Webb FTG (eds) *Endometrial Bleeding and Steroidal Contraception*, pp 65–77. Bath: Pitman Press.

Tatsumi K, Mori T, Mori E & Kauzaki H (1987) Immunoregulatory factor released from a cell line derived from human decidual tissue. *American Journal of Reproductive Immunology and Microbiology* **13:** 87–92.

Tauber PF, Wettig W, Nohlen M & Laneveld LJD (1985) Diffusible proteins of the mucosa of the human cervix, uterus and fallopian tubes: distribution and variation during the menstrual cycle. *American Journal of Obstetrics and Gynecology* **15:** 1115–1125.

Thor A, Viglione MJ, Muraro R, Ohuchi N, Schlum J & Gorstein F (1987) Monoclonal antibody B72.3 reactivity with human endometrium: a study of normal and malignant tissues. *International Journal of Gynecological Pathology* **6:** 235–247.

Tseng L, Mazella J & Chen GA (1987) Effect of relaxin on aromatase activity in human endometrial stromal cells. *Endocrinology* **120:** 2220–2226.

Tzartos SJ & Surani MAH (1979) Affinity of uterine luminal proteins for rat blastocysts. *Journal of Reproduction and Fertility* **56:** 579–586.

Verma V (1983) Ultrastructural changes in human endometrium at different phases of the menstrual cycle and their functional significance. *Gynecologic and Obstetric Investigation* **15:** 193–212.

Wahlström T & Seppälä M (1984) Placental protein 12 (PP12) is induced in the endometrium by progesterone. *Fertility and Sterility* **41:** 781–784.

Waites GT, James RFL & Bell SC (1988) Immunohistological localization of the human secretory protein pregnancy-associated endometrial α_1-globulin (α-PEG), an insulin-like growth factor binding protein, during the menstrual cycle. *Journal of Clinical Endocrinology and Metabolism* **67:** 1100–1104.

Waites GT, James RFL & Bell SC (1989) Human 'pregnancy-associated endometrial α_1-globulin', an insulin-like growth factor binding protein: immunohistological localization in the decidua and placenta during pregnancy employing monoclonal antibodies. *Journal of Endocrinology* **120**: 351–357.

Wang HS, Kanzaki H, Tokushige M, Sato S, Yoshida M & Mori T (1988) Effect of ovarian steroids on the secretion of immunosuppressive factor(s) from human endometrium. *American Journal of Obstetrics and Gynecology* **158**: 629–637.

Wewer UM, Faber M, Liotta LA & Albrechtsen R (1985) Immunochemical and ultrastructural assessment of the nature of the pericellular basement membrane of human decidual cells. *Laboratory Investigation* **53**: 624–633.

13

Implantation failure: clinical aspects

JOHN YOVICH
ADRIAN LOWER

Successful embryo implantation in the human involves a complex inter-action between the hatched blastocyst and the luteal phase endometrium. The physiological aspects of this interaction have been covered in other chapters. The clinical perspectives concerning the factors of importance for implantation are brought into sharp focus in four areas:

1. Controlling fertility.
2. Treating infertility.
3. Managing threatened pregnancy wastage.
4. Managing the problem of recurrent pregnancy wastage.

This chapter will deal with the clinical implications of enhancing implan-tation and treating disorders of implantation in the last three areas of infertility and pregnancy wastage. In particular, it will examine clinical strategies, including specific treatments, to enhance and maintain successful embryo implantation.

TREATING INFERTILITY

Current developments

The last decade has witnessed a rapid evolution in the application of new knowledge and techniques in reproductive medicine to treat infertility. Specialized clinics adopting a team approach have emerged around the world for the specific treatment of infertility and early pregnancy disorders. This follows on the model introduced by the pioneers of in vitro fertilization and embryo transfer (IVF-ET) (Edwards et al, 1980), and which requires a very close working relationship between clinic and laboratory, particularly where any form of gamete handling is used. Today's teams generally comprise clinicians, nurse co-ordinators, scientists, specialized laboratory technologists and counsellors who provide information, emotional support and psychological services. Such organizations are in addition to con-ventional medical facilities and are generally supervised by institutional ethics committees and a central supervising body, e.g. the Interim Licensing Authority in the United Kingdom, the Society for Assisted Reproductive

Baillière's Clinical Obstetrics and Gynaecology—
Vol. 5, No. 1, March 1991
ISBN 0–7020–1533–4

Technology in the United States of America, and the Reproductive Technology Accreditation Committee in Australia. In some countries there are statutory controls governing and limiting both service and research applications.

Aetiological factors

The aetiological factors underlying infertility are numerous and the predominant causes vary with geographical location, socioeconomic factors and the changing face of health problems within different areas in given periods of time. For example, tuberculous disease was the prominent underlying condition in one location (Bahadori, 1986), whilst ovulatory disorders appeared most common in another (Cox, 1975). The broad categories of infertility recognized in industrialized societies are ovulatory dysfunction (25–45%), spermatozoal disorders (mostly unexplained; 20–35%), tubal disease (15–30%), pelvic endometriosis (10–15% as the attributed cause; up to 45% as an identified factor), poor sperm–mucus interaction (5–15%), antispermatozoal antibodies (ASABs; 5–15%) and completely unexplained (5–15%). Following the comprehensive investigation of both partners the infertility problem will often be identified as having a multifactorial basis, although one underlying condition usually predominates. Some uncommon causes of infertility include genital tract anomalies, such as congenital absence of vital structures (e.g. müllerian agenesis, androgen insensitivity syndromes, congenital absence of vasa deferentia), as well as those caused by surgical procedures, diethylstilboestrol (DES) exposure in utero, and uterine synechiae causing Asherman's syndrome. Sexual dysfunctions and ejaculatory disorders are occasional causes of infertility due to failure of sperm deposition in the vagina.

Range of procedures

A wide range of techniques and procedures enables a much improved chance of achieving conception for infertile couples than was achievable in the early 1980s. These include tubal microsurgery, ovarian stimulation with close monitoring, a variety of techniques involving gamete handling or manipulation namely, donor insemination (DI), the intrauterine insemination of husband's washed spermatozoa (AIH or IUI), IVF-ET and related procedures such as gamete intrafallopian transfer (GIFT), pronuclear or zygote intrafallopian transfer (PROST or ZIFT), and tubal embryo stage transfer (TEST). Additional procedures which have been described but are not widely used include direct intraperitoneal insemination (DIPI), peritoneal ovum and sperm transfer (POST), and fallopian replacement of eggs with delayed insemination (FREDI). Ovum donation of supernumerary oocytes from GIFT programmes is widely practised but ovum donation with in vivo insemination and uterine lavage is not widely accepted for ethical reasons. Surrogacy arrangements may involve the surrogate woman allowing her own egg to be fertilized, which is the common form of commercial surrogacy practised in some American States. Alternatively, the surrogate woman may carry the embryo resulting from the fertilization of the gametes of an infertile couple (IVF surrogacy). The latter is usual in altruistic compassionate surrogacy arrangements within families.

INFLUENCING IMPLANTATION

In counselling and treating couples who present with infertility the clinician will be concerned with: (1) the available treatment options for the underlying diagnosis; (2) the relative chance of achieving pregnancy by any given treatment option; and (3) the chance of the resultant pregnancy ending in the birth of a healthy live infant. Extensive data is available covering these considerations but the prognosis for the individual case is uncertain because of the numerous variables involved in a treatment cycle, the wide range of results reported from clinics and the changes occurring in the technology, in addition to other factors within clinics, over time.

Treatment by IVF has provided an excellent model for studying the question of influencing the chance of implantation, as it maximizes the opportunity of measuring the various parameters, and there has been an enthusiastic response by infertile couples invited to participate in approved research studies. A number of developments in the procedure over the past 3 years have significantly improved the chance of pregnancy (Yovich et al, 1989d) and will be considered with respect to their respective impact on implantation. In general terms, the likelihood of successful implantation in IVF is dependent upon embryo factors, uterine receptivity and certain technical or mechanical considerations.

EMBRYO FACTORS

The quality of embryos generated from IVF is dependent upon the quality of the oocyte fertilized, the normality of fertilization and the laboratory conditions for in vitro culture.

Oocyte quality

In practice, oocyte quality is measured directly by morphological criteria and the ability to undergo fertilization. It is also measured indirectly by the morphological quality characteristics of the resultant embryos and their outcome following transfer. Reported oocyte grading systems are based on that originally proposed by Marrs and his colleagues (Marrs et al, 1984). Criteria considered include characteristics of the cumulus, the coronal layer, the presence of the first polar body and evidence of germinal vesicle breakdown (Figure 1).

Several influencing factors govern the quality of oocytes recovered from follicle aspirations. These are considered below.

Stimulation regimen. Until recently clomiphene citrate (CC) and human

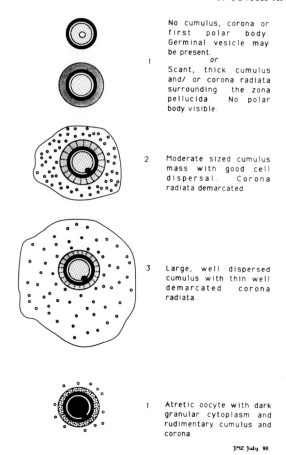

No cumulus, corona or first polar body. Germinal vesicle may be present.
1   or
Scant, thick cumulus and/ or corona radiata surrounding the zona pellucida. No polar body visible.

2   Moderate sized cumulus mass with good cell dispersal. Corona radiata demarcated.

3   Large, well dispersed cumulus with thin well demarcated corona radiata.

1   Atretic oocyte with dark granular cytoplasm and rudimentary cumulus and corona.

JMC July '90

Figure 1. Schematic diagram indicating oocyte grading system in use at PIVET. After Marrs et al, 1984.

menopausal gonadotrophins (hMGs) have been widely used both separately or in combination to develop ovarian follicles to an 'appropriate' stage for oocyte recovery. Based on the ultrasonic determination of the size of follicles and/or the pattern of the oestradiol-17β (E_2) rise during the follicular phase, a clinical decision is made to trigger the final stage of follicle and oocyte maturation using human chorionic gonadotrophin (hCG) rather than await the spontaneous luteinizing hormone (LH) surge. Some programmes do monitor LH and progesterone, with a view to collecting oocytes on the basis of a spontaneous surge or an hCG-augmented surge. However, most prefer the hCG trigger mainly, for logistic reasons (e.g. for more orderly and convenient scheduling of retrieval procedures).

Marked improvements in IVF results have recently ensued from the diminishing use of CC and the increasing use of gonadotrophin releasing hormone agonist analogues (GnRHa) such as buserelin (Suprefact, Hoechst Laboratories) and leuprolide acetate (Lucrin, Abbott Laboratories). These

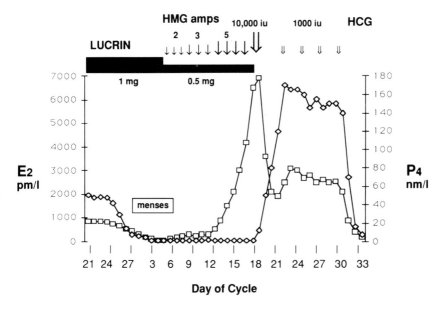

Figure 2. Preferred stimulation regimen for IVF and related procedures. hCG trigger is given on seventh day of E_2 rise. Courtesy of Blackwell Scientific Publications Ltd.

agents can be used in various regimens combined with hMG. Optimum results appear with a pituitary downregulation schedule. A successful regimen is shown in Figure 2 and involves commencing Lucrin 1 mg s.c. daily in the midluteal phase of the preceding cycle. Pituitary downregulation is usually achieved by day 3–5 of the ensuing cycle and is demonstrated by serum follicle stimulating hormone (FSH) and LH levels both <5 IU/litre and E_2 <200 pmol/litre. Thereafter 0.5 mg Lucrin daily will maintain suppression and hMG injections are given daily, with appropriate increases after 3 days of any given dosage, in order to increase E_2 by approximately 50% per day, and the hCG trigger is given on the 7th day of sustained E_2 rise. Spontaneous LH surges do not occur with this regimen. Ultrasound monitoring can provide additional useful information and may occasionally lead to delaying the LH trigger until a cohort of follicles have reached 1.6 cm or greater. However, follicle dimensions are not closely correlated with oocyte quality, as satisfactory fertilization, embryo development and pregnancy may be achieved across the range of 10–30 mm diameter follicles (Haines et al, 1989). One aims for E_2 levels around 6000 pmol/litre which equates with the recovery of 6–8 oocytes. It is unwise to stimulate higher E_2 levels as the generation of higher numbers of follicles increases the risk of the ovarian hyperstimulation syndrome (OHSS), which can be life threatening.

The use of GnRHa has been shown to have significant benefits in older patients (>35 years), those with underlying polycystic ovary (PCO) disease, those with raised androgens, those with raised basal LH or those with previous premature LH surges (Cummins et al, 1989). There are also advantages in using GnRHa in women who normally respond well to conventional regimens, but this is mainly by preventing a premature LH surge, thereby reducing the cancellation rate. Those who have previously demonstrated poor ovarian responsiveness to a downregulation regimen may often respond to the *flare technique* which involves commencing both the GnRHa and hMG together at the beginning of the cycle, when the analogue will initiate pituitary release of gonadotrophins as a normal effect prior to downregulation, and so supplement the exogenous drug. An *ultra-short flare regimen* (Macnamee et al, 1989) has also been described and may prove equally useful and have certain cost benefits. However, the persistently poor responder group remains difficult to treat effectively and cancellation rates due to an inadequate response is of the order of 5–8%. Current research indicates the *combined use of growth hormone* may improve the response or at least reduce the amount of hMG required to effect successful stimulation (Homburg et al, 1988, 1990). However, the expense of such treatment is currently prohibitive for consideration in clinical service.

In one study, comprising patients whose clinical characteristics combined with their previous IVF experience identified them as having a poor prognosis, the use of GnRHa treatment lifted their performance into line with that seen in 'good' prognosis groups (Cummins et al, 1989). In evaluating the advantage of one stimulation regimen over another, it is not always clear whether the difference relates to an improvement in the overall quality of oocytes recovered, or, if only a fixed proportion of oocytes within the ovary have the full potential for normal pregnancy, that simply more oocytes are recovered, leading to a greater chance that at least one oocyte will have the optimal characteristics. Furthermore, the drugs used in ovarian stimulation may influence luteal phase endometrial characteristics, thereby inhibiting the implantation of all embryos, regardless of their intrinsic potential for implantation.

Natural (unstimulated) cycles. Because there remain uncertainties regarding the effects of ovarian stimulation upon oocyte quality, some clinics have explored IVF in natural cycles. Indeed, the very first successful implantations which proceeded to livebirths were in IVF-ET treatment cycles involving the retrieval of an oocyte from the single, naturally developed follicle by monitoring the oestrogen output and spontaneous LH surge of natural cycles. It is salutary to recall that Louise Brown (born July 1978) was one of two livebirths after four such natural cycle pregnancies were achieved when embryos had been transferred to 32 women (i.e. pregnancy rate 12.5% per transfer in 1978–1979). However, the overall methodology was inefficient as 78 cycles were monitored in that series, leading to 68 attempts to collect the oocyte at laparoscopy, of which an oocyte was recovered from 45 women (i.e. pregnancy rate 5.9% per collection attempt). Other groups exploring IVF at the time experienced even less efficiency with natural cycle IVF; hence, it was not pursued very extensively, even by the original workers. However, given the methodological improvements in cycle monitoring, other technical developments for oocyte recovery (see below) and the possible benefits of oocyte preincubation (Garcia, 1989), natural cycle treatments are being explored once again. A recent study from Paris (Foulot et al, 1989) reported

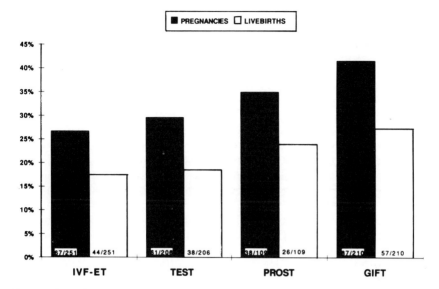

Figure 3. Data from PIVET for the 2-year period 1988–1989, showing pregnancy rates and livebirth rates (one or more infants) per transfer procedure for different IVF related techniques.

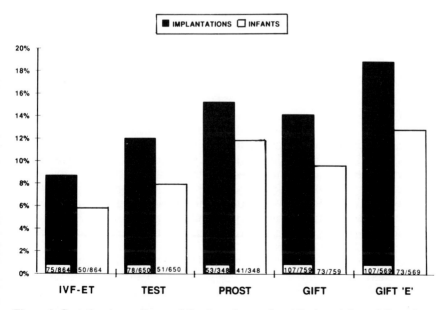

Figure 4. Gestational sacs diagnosed (implantation rate) and liveborn infants delivered per oocyte or embryo transferred for various IVF related procedures. GIFT 'E' refers to the rates obtained per estimated 'embryo' transferred if one assumes that 75% of oocytes will fertilize.

14 pregnancies advanced beyond 20 weeks from 80 unstimulated IVF cycles where the main infertility category was tubal disease and male factor cases were excluded (i.e. ongoing pregnancy rate 17.5% per cycle). Oocytes were recovered in 63 of 68 attempts (92.6%) and 53 oocytes fertilized (77.9%), with an apparently higher rate for those oocytes collected after an hCG trigger injection (37/41, 90.2% versus 16/22, 72.7%; not significant).

The best results reported from comprehensive annualized data in large series of stimulated cycles (e.g. Figures 3 and 4) indicate that around 10–15% of selected embryos have the capacity for implantation and complete development to a livebirth infant. The three embryos transferred are selected from a mean of 8–10 recovered oocytes. The supernumerary oocytes are known to have a reduced potential for fertilization (around 50%) (Yovich et al, 1989a), and probably for further development as well; hence, it appears that less than 10% of oocytes recovered from stimulated IVF cycles are of optimal quality. The data on unstimulated cycles should be considered in this context (i.e. a higher ongoing implantation rate per oocyte recovered) and, if the rates reveal a persisting difference, a possible adverse effect of stimulation on oocyte quality must be examined, along with the consideration that stimulation is 'capturing' a number of oocytes otherwise destined for the process of natural atresia.

Technical aspects of oocyte collection. Traditionally, oocyte recovery developed as a laparoscopic procedure but has increasingly become replaced by ultrasound-directed techniques, particularly the transvaginal approach. The optimization of oocyte recovery has been shown to depend upon three main aspects (Yovich et al, 1989c):

1. Timing the recovery following LH surge or hCG induction and inducing the surge at the appropriate stage of follicle maturation.
2. The instrumentation and techniques applied for aspiration of the oocytes from follicles.
3. Accessibility of the ovaries for aspiration.

With respect to timing, the LH surge or hCG trigger should occur on day 6 or 7 of the E_2 rise for CC/hMG cycles, and the optimal trigger is day 7 of the E_2 rise for cycles downregulated with GnRHa. Thereafter, follicles are aspirated 36 ± 2 h after initiation of the LH surge or hCG trigger. Oocytes aspirated earlier than 34 h may benefit by compensatory in vitro culture prior to insemination but embryo quality is poor and pregnancy rates are low if oocytes are recovered 4 or more hours earlier than optimal. Oocytes collected up to 4 h after the optimal time remain equally suitable but the risk of spontaneous oocyte release increases, although this appears to be $< 10\%$ up to 42 h in GnRHa cycles.

The first reports using ultrasound guidance for follicle aspirations were from Scandinavia (Lenz et al, 1981) and described a transcutaneous trans-vesical method. Subsequently, a transurethral method was explored briefly, and finally the transvaginal method has found popular acceptance (Wikland et al, 1989). The optimization of transvaginal ultrasound-directed aspiration is achieved by minimal anaesthesia (premedication is usually sufficient), an abdominal pressure band to stabilize the ovaries, sharp disposable double-lumen needles which enable combined aspiration and follicle flushing (PIVET–Cook needles from William Cook, Australia, are ideal), controlled aspiration pressures which take into account the needle diameter and its length, a high resolution ultrasound image (e.g. General Electric electronic phased array sector scanner with 5.0 MHz vaginal probe is popular), and avoidance of oocyte-toxic sterilizing fluids in the vagina (10 ml culture medium provides a suitable cleansing and coupling medium) (Yovich and Grudzinskas, 1990).

Chromosome abnormalities in gametes

Oocyte karyotypes. The major causes of preimplantation embryo loss, implantation failure and spontaneous early pregnancy wastage are known to be chromosomal abnormalities and abnormal embryonic development. A reasonably large multicentre (IVF) study examined the chromosomal status of unfertilized oocytes, errors at fertilization and the chromosomal complement of cleaved embryos (Plachot et al, 1988). With respect to oocytes the study revealed:

1. Of 316 mature unfertilized oocytes, 234 were of the normal 23,X haploid status (74.0%). The abnormal findings were mostly oocytes with aneuploidy (76) and a few with diploidy (6). The rate of abnormal chromosomes was not related to the underlying infertility category, the stimulation regimen nor the amount of hMG used in the stimulation regimen. There was, however, a significant increase in the rate of aneuploidy for women > 35 y (38%).

2. Of 1393 supernumerary oocytes examined at around 18 h postinsemination for pronuclear (PN) status, 92.4% showed a normal 2 PN complement, 6.4% showed multiple PN suggesting polyploidy, and 1.6% showed a single PN implying parthenogenetic activation. The fertilization abnormalities bore no relationship to maternal age or total dosage of gonadotrophins (in contrast to observations of pregnant mare's serum gonadotrophins in mice (Maudlin and Fraser, 1977)). Some minor differences in triploidy rates in relationship to stimulation schedules probably reflect total oocyte numbers collected, in that higher retrieval numbers are more likely to comprise some part-atretic or dysmature oocytes. With respect to the category of infertility, unexplained cases had a significantly higher rate of parthenogenetic zygotes (4.2%). Such causes might reflect oocyte abnormalities which are sensitive to activation of the oocyte under conventional IVF laboratory conditions. On the improvement side, there were fewer triple PN oocytes in male factor cases and this probably reflects a generally reduced fertilization (oocyte penetration) potential of such cases. This infers that multi-PN oocytes are due to polyspermic fertilization. There was also less triploidy when the preincubation of oocytes prior to insemination was short (2 h), rather than the usual longer (2–6 h) period.

Spermatozoal karyotypes. It is relevant in this discussion also to consider chromosomal abnormalities in spermatozoa. The technique of sperm karyotyping is more complex than that for other cells and relies on a technique involving sperm preparation in a manner similar to that used for IVF, followed by insemination of zona-denuded hamster oocytes (Rudak et al, 1978). After 12–12.5 h incubation, a Colcemid solution is added to the oocytes, which are then incubated for a further period prior to fixation, staining with quinacrine dihydrochloride and reading under fluorescence microscopy. If one considers the combined results from three groups, involving the examination of more than 6000 spermatozoa from 78 donors (Martin, 1988), the following conclusions can be drawn:

1. Total karyotypic abnormalities can be identified in around 10% of spermatozoa from men with normal semen parameters (range 8.5–13.9%).
2. Aneuploidies occur in around 2% and these can be subdivided into hyperhaploids (range from 0.5% in Japan to 2.4% in North America) and hypohaploids (range from 0.5% in Japan to 3.4% in North America). All chromosome groups appear to have the same frequency of non-dysjunction, with the exception of group G, in which there is a significant excess of hyperhaploidy ($\times 2.4$). These observations should be considered against the finding that human newborns display abnormalities, especially trisomies, of chromosomes 13, 18, 21 and X or Y far more often than any of the others and some, e.g. trisomy 1, are extremely rare.
3. Structural chromosome abnormalities occur in around 8% of spermatozoa (range from 3.3% in North America to 13.0% in Japan).
4. From studies in mice, it is apparent that chromosome constitution does not influence the ability of sperm to effect fertilization. The hamster studies on human sperm confirm that chromosomally abnormal sperm are not at a disadvantage in fertilizing zona-free hamster oocytes.
5. Sperm preparation techniques used for IVF, such as the overlay or swim-up method, do not show a difference in the frequency of sperm chromosomal abnormalities compared with sperm unselected for motility. Furthermore, other in vitro conditions, including cryopreservation, do not alter the sex ratio or the frequency of either numerical or structural abnormalities.
6. There was no relationship demonstrated between age of the male and the frequency of numerical chromosome abnormalities in sperm, although there may be some change in the ratio of the various complements (i.e. more hyperhaploids with advancing age). Furthermore, three independent studies find a negative association between non-dysjunction and paternal age. It is concluded that, unlike the situation with oocytes, there is no increased risk of trisomy with paternal age.
7. Structural spermatozoal chromosome abnormalities do show an increase with age, raising the question of a possible effect from mutagens. The technique of sperm karyotyping is therefore currently being widely explored with a view to developing a possible mutagen 'screening' system.

Laboratory conditions

Laboratory techniques have not changed significantly from the original model (Purdy, 1982), except where specialized sperm preparation, sperm enhancement and micromanipulation procedures are used to enhance the chance of fertilization. Some studies assessing co-culture of embryos with endometrial cells or endosalpingeal cells suggest a benefit, but this has not yet been clearly demonstrated. The methodology of IVF is very simple but does require rigid control over:

1. *Temperature*, particularly for oocyte handling, sperm–oocyte incubation and the PN check at 16–20 h postinsemination.
2. *pH*, which should be appropriately set and buffered for follicle flushing, sperm preparation, insemination and postfertilization media (involves high carbon dioxide gassing for bicarbonate buffered solutions).
3. *Osmolality*, which for all media should be held constant at the appropriate level in the range of 280–295, depending on the solutions used. Generally high humidification is required in incubators and during handling procedures which must, therefore, be carried out deftly and rapidly.

Probably the most important laboratory influence over the chromosomal integrity of oocytes occurs during the metaphase stages of meiosis and fertilization. During this period the meiotic spindles are most prone to depolymerization followed by disruption and disorganization as a consequence of relatively minor reductions in temperature. For example, a reduction to room temperature for as little as 10 min caused a high proportion of changes, including chromosome dispersal from the metaphase plate (Pickering et al, 1990). The effects have been known for some time but many IVF units do not rigidly control for reductions in temperature during the crucial oocyte recovery, gamete handling and early insemination stages, possibly in the mistaken belief that meiotic spindles will repolymerize and reorganize normally when the temperature is raised to 37°C. Indeed, this does occur in the mouse (Pickering and Johnson, 1987) but the damage to human oocytes is usually irreversible, the difference being due to the manner in which the pericentriolar material is located in the human. It appears likely, therefore, that poor temperature control during IVF procedures may affect the rate of aneuploidies in the resultant embryos.

Embryo quality

Following fertilization the resultant embryos are selected on morphological criteria prior to transfer. Other methods of assessment, including karyotypic analysis, biochemical microassays and genetic analysis by deoxyribonucleic acid (DNA) probes, have to date been conducted as research studies. However, the pace of development in both embryology (particularly with embryo biopsy) and molecular biology (especially the development of polymerase chain reaction (PCR) techniques) means that direct clinical applications are now feasible.

Morphological aspects

Embryos can usefully be graded according to four main criteria (Yovich, 1985; Cummins et al, 1986):

1. Clarity of blastomeres.
2. Regularity of blastomeres.
3. Degree of cytoplasmic fragmentation.
4. Time frame of cleavage stages.

At PIVET a point scoring system using these criteria is in current use (Yovich and Grudzinskas, 1990). High quality embryos can achieve a maximum of 4 points with ½ or 1 point deducted in accordance with the degree of deviation from the optimum for each parameter. The findings with respect to implantation rates (i.e. pregnancy sacs detected by ultrasound around the seventh week of pregnancy) are similar to those of other reports (Puissant et al, 1987; Grillo et al, 1991) and can be summarized as follows:

1. Grossly abnormal embryos with irregular, dark, granular and highly fragmented blastomeres do not have the capacity for successful implantation and should be discarded.
2. The implantation rate is significantly reduced when two or more blastomeres of a 4-cell embryo are irregular in size and shape when compared with the other two.
3. The implantation rate is significantly reduced if the degree of fragmentation is greater than 20% of total blastomere volumes.
4. If all blastomeres display dark, granular cytoplasm, indicating vacuolation, this indicates the likelihood of some toxic influence within the culture medium or infection and such embryos rarely implant.
5. Mild degrees of single criteria are insignificant but if total scores of embryos fall below 2/4, there will be significant reductions in implantation rates.

There remains a question of one embryo influencing the chance that another will implant, a concept which has been proposed and debated but so far remains unresolved (see discussion arising at second Bourn Hall meeting following an assessment of two mathematical models for embryo implantation (Walters, 1985)). There is some supportive data for the concept, particularly when one compares single embryo transfers (success clearly dependent upon grade of embryo) with the transfer of several embryos of mixed quality (when the individual embryo implantation rate may be higher than expected). From the later discussion on luteal support therapy, a suggested mechanism may be via an embryo–endometrial signal enhancing uterine receptivity.

Chromosome abnormalities in preimplantation embryos

In the aforementioned multicentre study by Plachot and her colleagues, 252 embryos were examined with the following findings:

1. Ninety-two per cent of the embryos were diploid, with 1.6% haploid, presumed to be parthenogenetically activated oocytes (all had an X chromosome), and 6.4% showed triploidy, presumed to be a consequence of polyspermy.
2. Of the diploid embryos which appeared morphologically normal,

21.4% displayed chromosome abnormalities as described for the PN oocytes.
3. There was a higher proportion of chromosome abnormalities (32.6%) in diploid embryos which were graded as morphologically abnormal.

From these and other karyotype studies on human gametes and embryos, some of which have been specifically generated for research (Angell et al, 1986; Veiga et al, 1987), a model on the natural selection process against chromosome abnormalities has been proposed and is summarized in Figure 5. Regardless of the severity of chromosomal defects, it is apparent that early cleavage stages usually proceed normally. However, once embryonic gene expression is manifested, the anomalies undoubtedly cause implantation failure or early pregnancy failure.

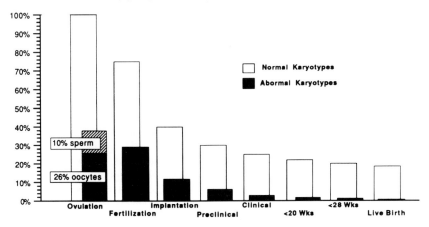

Figure 5. Bar chart displaying the inefficiency of normal human reproduction (19 infants per 100 ovulations) but a selective trend against generating infants with chromosomal abnormalities (e.g. 30–40% abnormal embryos but only 0.6% abnormal infants).

Other assessment of embryos

Over the past three years, research has focused on improvements in culturing blastomeres obtained from embryo biopsy as well as by advances in diagnostic methods. The stage has now been reached whereby genetic diagnoses can be made on a small number of cells, often a single cell, and this can obviate the need for propagating blastomere cell lines or having to cryopreserve biopsied embryos pending the outcome of such culture. Diagnostic methods have proceeded along three lines: biochemical microassays, chromosome analysis and probing DNA sequences.

Biochemical microassays. For example, a model has been developed with the potential for a four-enzyme study from a single assay of a single cell, i.e. HPRT (hypoxanthine phosphoribosyl transferase; a deficiency of which causes Lesch–Nyhan syndrome), ADA (adenosine deaminase; a deficiency of which causes severe combined immunodeficiency), PNP (purine nucleo-tide phosphorylase; a deficiency of which causes combined immunological and neurological disease) and APRT (adenine phosphoribosyl transferase; a deficiency of which causes another disorder of purine metabolism with nephrolithiasis and renal failure) (Monk, 1989).

Chromosome analysis. Obtaining unequivocal chromosome data from the few cells available in a human preimplantation embryo presented significant technical difficulties to the cytogeneticists undertaking the previously described studies on research embryos. Improved methods of fixation of human and mouse preimplantation embryos have been described to facilitate G banding and karyotypic analysis, enhancing the possibility of diagnosis on a single biopsied blastomere (Roberts and O'Neill, 1988), but this has not yet reached the stage of clinical feasibility. For sexing human embryos, Y-chromosome-specific DNA probes are now preferred. Success-ful probes have been described using in situ hybridization methods on entire 2–8-cell embryos (West et al, 1988), and recently PCR amplification (see below) has been applied to the single biopsied blastomere from 30 human embryos at the 6–10-cell stage (Handyside et al, 1989). The results of the latter technique matched the former (applied to the whole embryos) accurately. This development has now been applied successfully in clinical practice with two women, both carriers of X-linked disorders, implanting twin female pregnancies after preimplantation biopsy of a single cell at the 6–8-cell stage, and sexing by DNA amplification of a Y-chromosome-specific repeat sequence (Handyside et al, 1990). Subsequent chorionic villus sampling (CVS) and delivered outcomes have confirmed that the diagnoses have been accurate.

Probing DNA sequences. A rapidly increasing number of genetic diseases have had their specific gene sequence encoded, the most recent exciting report being the identification of the cystic fibrosis gene (Rommens et al, 1989), including the cloning and characterization of its cDNA (Riordan et al, 1989) and its complete genetic analysis (Kerem et al, 1989). Applying DNA probes for preimplantation embryo diagnosis using restriction fragment length polymorphisms required a large number of cells, initially many thousands. Subsequent DNA amplification methods reduced the numbers required to around a hundred but the development of the polymerase chain reaction (PCR), which can amplify DNA sequences by 10^7–10^{10}, enables the detection of a single copy gene from a single cell by amplification of the specific base sequence of that gene (Saiki et al, 1985, 1988). The feasibility of diagnosing cystic fibrosis and muscular dystrophy from a single biopsied cell has been demonstrated by applying the PCR technique to the DNA from a single human oocyte and detecting markers closely linked to those genes within a few hours of cell isolation (Coutelle et al, 1989). Now that the actual gene for cystic fibrosis has been cloned, greater diagnostic specificity is achievable. Similarly the feasibility of diagnosing β-thalassaemia has been demonstrated in single blastomeres from mouse preimplantation embryos using this approach (Holding and Monk, 1989), which also relied on the ingenious selection of nested primer DNA sequences to improve the sensitivity and specificity of amplification.

It is now entirely feasible that all the DNA markers which have been successfully applied to chorionic villus biopsy specimens, including linked DNA polymorphisms such as applied for the predictive testing of Huntington's disease (Brock et al, 1989), will be applicable to preimplantation embryo diagnosis. However, whilst PCR is clearly a very powerful tool in diagnostic genetics, a number of identified problems, particularly its ability to amplify any contaminant DNA, require caution about its use at this stage. Detection of gene sequences in individual sperm cells is now also possible using a PCR approach (Li et al, 1988), and this will probably also be used ultimately along with karyotyping approaches in prefertilization genetic screening.

Functional tests of embryo integrity

The above diagnostic procedures all carry relevance to implantation in the specific instance of known genetic carrier states and certain high-risk situations, e.g. for Down's syndrome. However, it is only the chromosome assessment of preimplantation embryos which is likely to be rewarding in preselecting embryos for transfer on a routine basis with the view to improving the chance of successful implantation. Even then, at best one might expect one-third of embryos to be discarded on the basis of chromosomal defects, yet, in the best hands, less than one-third of embryos can be successfully cultured through to morphologically normal blastocysts and less than one-fifth can implant with normal outcomes. Therefore, it appears likely that a proportion of embryos (perhaps 25–30%) may lack the functional capacity for implantation and full development. Some degree of laboratory limitation can be conceded, although this appears minor for IVF and embryo culture to the 4- and 8-cell stages, given tight adherence to the aforementioned principles. It is more likely that certain degrees of oocyte immaturity or dysmaturity may be reflected by deficient metabolic or other functional processes, and perhaps this might be measured in vitro for embryo preselection. A number of tests have been explored in research models: e.g. seeking the presence of β-hCG, platelet aggregating factor (PAF) (O'Neill and Spinks, 1988) or other early pregnancy factor (EPF) (Morton, 1984) within supernatants of the culture environment of the developing embryo; and metabolic uptake studies using agents such as fluoroscein diacetate, radiolabelled glucose (Wales et al, 1987) and both glucose and pyruvate in non-isotopic studies using a non-invasive technique (Hardy et al, 1989). Other studies have examined the follicle fluid of the relevant oocytes, e.g. for steroid hormones, pregnancy associated placental protein A (PAPP-A) (Stanger et al, 1985) and insulin-like growth factor (IGF-1)-binding protein. It suffices to summarize that the limitations of toxicity, development of appropriate microassay techniques and the relevance of any given marker or measurement for human embryos are inadequate at this stage to consider introducing such a test into clinical practice. For example, the PAF studies, which proved to be significantly relevant for mouse embryos, have so far not demonstrated the same relevance for human embryos. This might reflect assay limitations, and the development of a commercial radioimmunoassay that is sensitive in the range of 10–1000 pg (Baldo et al, 1990) is welcome.

UTERINE RECEPTIVITY

Given optimal embryo quality, the chance of implantation is dependent upon two further factors: uterine receptivity and mechanical factors (concerning embryo placement and transport within the genital tract). The question of uterine receptivity focuses upon the endometrium: its functional integrity and physiological considerations concerning the implantation window which influences the timing of embryo transfer procedures. These are extensively discussed in other sections of this book, hence the clinical considerations presented here will address the application of current

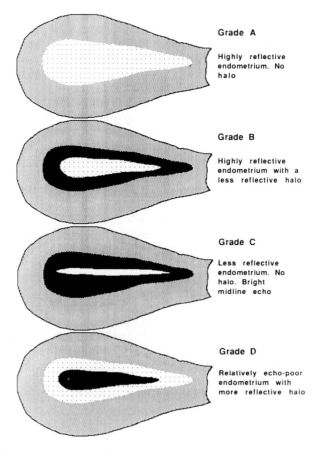

Grade A

Highly reflective endometrium. No halo

Grade B

Highly reflective endometrium with a less reflective halo

Grade C

Less reflective endometrium. No halo. Bright midline echo

Grade D

Relatively echo-poor endometrium with more reflective halo

Figure 6. Schematic diagram showing the four endometrial patterns recognized on real-time transvaginal ultrasound scans.

knowledge. This covers two areas: determining the optimum biophysical characteristics for successful implantation, and treatment to enhance endometrial receptiveness.

Seeking optimal characteristics

At PIVET a prospective study examining endometrial characteristics has been conducted using real-time transvaginal ultrasound. Over a 6-month period, scans were routinely performed in women attending for treatment of infertility during the follicular phase, and also in the luteal phase on days 10, 13 and 16 after hCG trigger or LH surge in the case of unstimulated, monitored cycles. Endometrial grades, based on earlier descriptions of the pattern of reflectivity seen at transvesical ultrasound scans (Smith et al, 1984), are depicted in Figure 6. The thickness of the inner and outer endometrial layers were recorded in each case.

Preliminary analysis of the results of 57 scans performed within 24 h of the hCG trigger in 39 women, and 54 scans performed in 31 women between days 12 and 16 after trigger, are shown in Figure 7. The data were analysed separately for scans performed around the time of trigger or during the luteal phase. There was no difference between the endometrial grade ascribed in scans in those women who failed to conceive and those who conceived either ongoing pregnancies or pregnancies which resulted in early pregnancy loss. We also failed to confirm earlier reports that endometrial thickness (Figure 8) is of predictive value in identifying those cycles in which conception is likely to occur (Gonen et al, 1989).

Measurement of the level of the placental protein PP14, the major secretory protein of the human endometrium, has been suggested as a marker of endometrial maturity (Joshi et al, 1986; Bell and Drife, 1989). Initial optimism has been confounded for a number of reasons: in particular, the wide variation among individuals and the close relation to β-hCG and progesterone levels. We measured PP14 levels in blood samples taken at the time of ultrasound scan in the above patients. Again, no significant correlation was demonstrated between PP14 level and endometrial thickness, and although PP14 is known to rise more rapidly in the late luteal phase of conception cycles, the wide individual variability precluded its use in a predictive capacity (Figure 8).

Other attempts to assess luteal phase characteristics include the measurement of E_2 and progesterone : E_2 ratios, with excessive E_2 indicating a diminished chance of implantation (Gidley-Baird et al, 1986; Forman et al, 1988). However, these measurements can reflect vagaries in stimulation regimens and appear to have no influence over outcomes when luteal support therapy is used (see below). At this stage a reliable and useful marker of endometrial quality has yet to be identified.

Luteal support therapy

Luteal support therapy, using progesterone, progestogenic compounds and/or hCG, has become a common component of infertility treatments involving ovarian stimulation, particularly where this is combined with assisted reproduction. There appears to be a reasonable rationale for luteal support in anovulatory women treated by hMG, as non-conception treatment cycles often display a markedly shortened luteal phase (Brown et al, 1980). This has also been observed among cycling women treated by hMG for assisted reproduction, particularly those with a high oestrogen output during the follicular phase (Edwards et al, 1980; Yovich, 1988b), hence luteal support is likely to be beneficial in hMG stimulated cycles. This

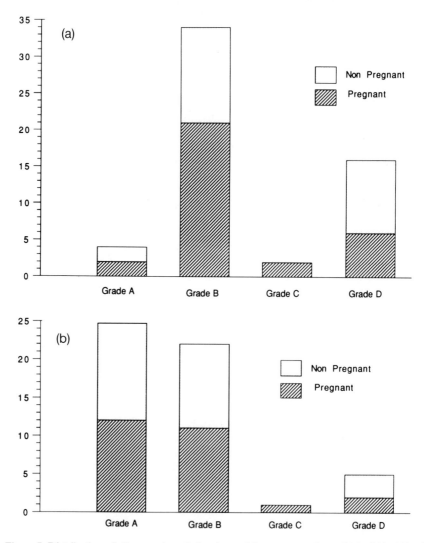

Figure 7. Distribution of ultrasound-graded endometrial patterns performed **(a)** within 24 h of the hCG trigger, and **(b)** during the luteal phase, categorized with respect to the achievement of pregnancy. (No significant relationship recognized.)

view is supported by a recently reported randomized matched study, which examined hormonal and pregnancy data in a small series (Hutchinson-Williams et al, 1990).

However, cycles stimulated by CC, with or without additional hMG, do not display shortened luteal phases (Yovich, 1988b). Furthermore, the early published reports of randomized controlled trials assessing luteal phase treatments using progesterone (Leeton et al, 1985; Yovich et al, 1985a; Trounson et al, 1986) or hCG support (Yovich et al, 1984; Mahadevan et al, 1985; Buvat et al, 1990) failed to show significant improvements in pregnancy rates, although there was usually a trend implying a benefit. However, despite the careful methodology in these studies, they have all been far too small to enable the significant detection of even a 10% variation in the pregnancy rate. Furthermore, they comprised a heterogeneous population of subjects within IVF programmes, which have usually been evolving through constant internal changes and which are generally reflected by inexplicable periods of poor pregnancy rates. One group attempting to study

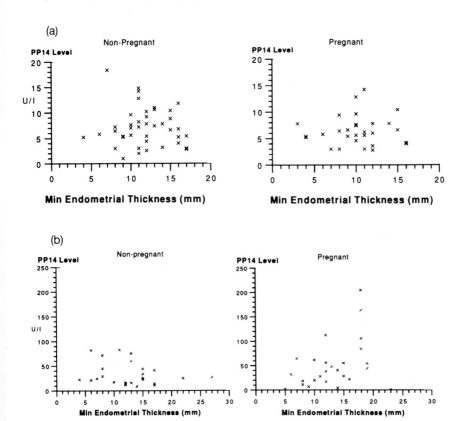

Figure 8. Scattergrams showing serum PP14 levels and endometrial thickness measured (**a**) within 24 h of the hCG trigger, and (**b**) during the luteal phase, categorized with respect to the achievement of pregnancy. (No significant relationship recognized.)

the effects of a progestagenic compound given during the luteal phase of IVF treatment cycles calculated that it would require two groups of 1500 subjects in each category to significantly detect a 5% improvement in the pregnancy rate, e.g. from 15% to 20% (Belaisch-Allart et al, 1987).

To minimize the inherent problems in luteal phase supplementation studies, a relatively large randomized controlled trial was performed at PIVET within a GIFT programme (Yovich et al, 1991), beginning around 9 months after it was established and shown to be characterized by stable pregnancy rates. Subjects were carefully screened to include a single infertility subcategory and exclude all known factors which might adversely affect the chance of pregnancy. Over a 12 month period (1986–1987), 280 couples were recruited after screening out all cases comprising any pre-existing factors deemed to be likely to influence the chance of pregnancy (e.g. age, ovulation disorders, presence of ASABs, endometriosis, male factors, previous IVF-related procedures) or any adverse factors in the treatment cycle (i.e. both poor and excessive responders excluded).

Couples fulfilling these criteria and providing informed consent were randomly selected by sequential allocation at the commencement of a treatment cycle into one of four groups:

1. Nil support.
2. hCG support: 1000 IU hCG (Profasi; Laboratoires Serono SA, Aubonne, Switzerland) given i.m.i. on days 4, 7, 10 and 13 of the luteal phase, where the day of oocyte retrieval is nominated as day 0.
3. Progesterone support: 50 mg progesterone in oil (Proluton; Schering AG, Berlin, Germany) given i.m.i. on days 0, 1, 2, 3 and 4 (i.e. 5 days), beginning in theatre immediately after oocyte retrieval. This regimen follows an implied benefit reported in a previous study (Yovich et al, 1985a).
4. Combined hCG/progesterone support: combines regimens (2) and (3), i.e. progesterone 50 mg i.m.i. on days 0–4 inclusive, followed by hCG 1000 IU i.m.i. on days 4, 7, 10 and 13 of the luteal phase.

The 280 cases selected into this trial had completely normal investigations, mild pelvic endometriosis only (American Fertility Society grades 1 or 2 only) or unexplained poor sperm–mucus interaction. They were therefore categorized as unexplained infertility. Such cases were usually treated by four cycles of ovarian stimulation therapy and, if postcoital tests were persistently negative, by additional intrauterine insemination of husband's washed, precapacitated spermatozoa (Yovich and Matson, 1988b) prior to inclusion in the GIFT programme. This was seen to be an ideal group for study as the patients had a good prognosis for pregnancy without luteal support therapy, hence any benefits of therapy which might be demonstrated would be likely to be of greater benefit in cases of repetitive unexplained failures.

The GIFT protocol applied a standard CC/hMG stimulation schedule to all cases, followed by laparoscopic oocyte recovery (the trial predated our introduction of the routine use of the transvaginal technique), followed by the selection of the highest graded oocytes for transfer. During the trial period the routine was for two oocytes into each tube with occasional patients having up to six oocytes in total (current protocols set a maximum limit of three oocytes per patient, usually all into one tube). Only clinical pregnancies were recorded in the trial, i.e. those demonstrating a rising β-hCG after day 16 of the luteal phase and the subsequent demonstration of a pregnancy sac(s) on ultrasound performed routinely in the 7th week, or histologically if an ectopic occurred. Pregnancy losses were diagnosed as

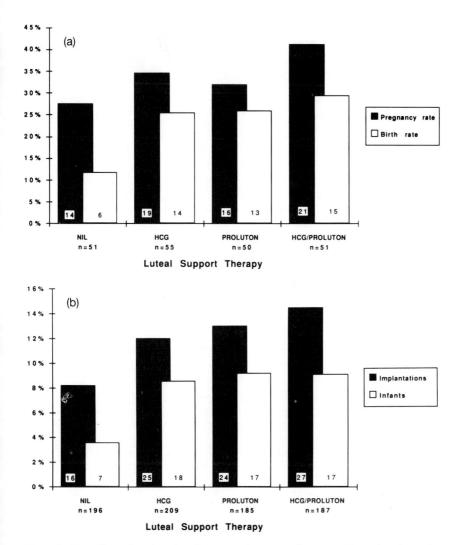

Figure 9. The effect of various luteal support therapy regimens on **(a)** total and ongoing pregnancy rates, and **(b)** total and ongoing implantation rates. Ongoing pregnancy rate ($P < 0.05$) and ongoing implantation rate ($P < 0.02$) significantly higher with luteal support. Courtesy of *Fertility and Sterility*.

blighted ovum if a viable fetus was not shown within the sac, or *spontaneous miscarriage* if a viable fetus was subsequently lost before the 20th week. All first trimester, pregnancy losses were classified as having single sacs. Those pregnancies progressing beyond 20 weeks were classified as ongoing or births.

The results are summarized in Figure 9 and indicate a significant benefit for luteal support therapy. The benefit is clearly shown with respect to

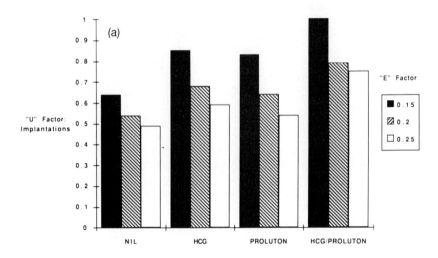

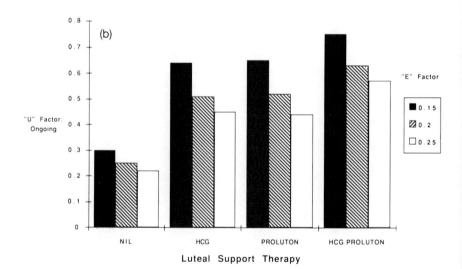

Figure 10. Statistical modelling of luteal support data showing that the uterine receptivity factor 'U' is improved most by luteal support therapy when embryo quality 'E' is lower. The improvement is apparent for all implantations **(a)** but highly significant for ongoing implantations **(b)**. Courtesy of *Fertility and Sterility*.

ongoing pregnancies and is apparent for individual implantations, particularly those which proceed to births. By applying a modelling technique on the data (using iterative procedures based on the binomial formula to derive uterine receptivity ('U' factors) for both implantation and ongoing pregnancy sacs, given various likely values for the proportion of optimum quality embryos ('E' factor); Figure 10), two interesting extrapolations could be made from the observed data. Firstly, it demonstrates the relationship between embryo quality and uterine receptivity in a manner which enables the relevance of luteal support to be seen in perspective. That is, the poorer the quality of the embryo, the greater the benefit of improvements in uterine receptivity. Secondly, there appears to be an interdependence of uterine receptivity to embryo quality. The optimum 'U' and 'E' factors both tended to be high where the outcome was best, and both were low where the outcome was poorest. This latter observation assumes the mean embryo quality was similar in all groups prior to the embryos reaching the uterus. It was not possible to measure embryo quality in this trial but it was designed to exclude every known bias. The observations are therefore considered to be real and support the concept of preimplantation embryo–endometrial interactions, whereby quality factors in one can benefit the other, and vice versa.

The study does not enable conclusions to be drawn regarding the best regimen of luteal support but the hCG/Proluton regimen is now incorporated as a routine at PIVET and is believed to be a significant contributing factor to the higher pregnancy and livebirth rates recorded overall during 1988 and 1989, as shown in Figures 3 and 4. Of 212 GIFT transfers during that period, 88 pregnancies arose (41.5%) and 57 (26.9%) proceeded through to birth. It is also now applied routinely in all other IVF related treatments, and during the same period 166 pregnancies arose after 566 embryo transfer procedures (29.3%) with 108 (19.1%) proceeding to births. These results are a significant improvement on our own data from the years preceding this trial (Webb, 1988) and from those reported nationally in Australia (Lancaster, 1990). Although other beneficial factors have been identified (Yovich et al, 1989d), luteal support therapy is believed to be a major contributor to the improvement.

MECHANICAL, TECHNICAL AND OTHER FACTORS

This section will consider the technical aspect of embryo transfer in so far as it relates to the chance and location of embryo implantation; the consideration of tubal as opposed to uterine transfers, as well as the relevance of transferring at different stages of oocyte to embryo development; and the relevance of certain underlying infertility disorders which appear to influence the chance of implantation.

Embryo transfer technique

A variety of techniques are applied with the aim of depositing embryos in the upper uterine cavity with the least degree of disturbance to the cervix, the uterine body and the endometrium. At PIVET a double cannulation technique is used. The external catheter is a soft polyurethane material which negotiates the cervical canal to a distance of 4 cm from the cervical os. Thereafter, an embryo-laden Teflon catheter is introduced through the outer sheath to a distance of 55–70 mm (as determined by prior evaluation by sounding and hysteroscopy during the investigatory work-up), to deposit the embryos a few millimetres short of the fundus. Prior to the process of embryo deposition, the outer catheter is withdrawn from the cervix and a settling period observed. Ultrasound control can be useful but is not usually required and the process should be totally atraumatic, i.e. instrumentation to grasp the cervix or dilate the canal should be avoided and both catheters should be blood-free on withdrawal. Best results are achieved by placing the patient in the Trendelenburg position with around 10° head-down tilt (knee–chest position is not required, regardless of the uterine position) and, after the transfer, the patient should maintain head-down tilt in bed for a minimum period of 4 h. A maximum of three embryos are transferred in 15–20 μl of culture medium containing 50% deactivated maternal serum.

The principles of the embryo transfer technique are simplicity of method, minimal disturbance to the mental and physical senses of the patient, atraumatic technique of catheter placement, slow entry and withdrawal of catheters, small transfer volumes, and minimum exposure of the embryos to the external environment between incubator and uterine cavity. Failure to adhere to any one of these principles reduces the chance of successful implantation. For example, rapid withdrawal of the transfer catheter can lead to a suction effect and up to 20% of embryo transfers may fail due to embryos exiting the uterine cavity via the cervix.

Once embryos have been deposited in the uterine cavity, it is clear that even with the best technique and confirmation of satisfactory uterine placement (Kovacs et al, 1987), embryos find their way into the fallopian tubes. This leads to ectopic pregnancies occurring in around 5% of IVF pregnancies as a universal experience. However, it is almost invariably tubal factor patients who are at risk from ectopics and the rate can be significantly raised if embryos are deliberately transferred to the fallopian tubes (e.g. by TEST (Yovich, 1990)) or inadvertently transferred by faulty techniques (Yovich et al, 1985c). In the latter situation, direct cannulation of the fallopian tube or rapid forced ejection of embryos in excessive fluid volumes may cause embryos to be pushed into the fallopian tube in cases with narrowed interstitial segments. Such embryos may be unable to return because of the narrowing or additional disorders of the distal intratubal lumen, as combined proximal/distal fallopian tube disorders often coexist.

Tubal versus uterine transfer

Since January 1988, the policy at PIVET for IVF related procedures has been to treat all tubal factor cases by IVF-ET; cases caused by endometriosis, unexplained infertility, poor sperm–mucus interaction or failed donor sperm therapy, by GIFT; and male factor cases, those with ASABs, those for donor oocytes or postcryopreservation and GIFT failures, by either

PROST or TEST. The last two techniques are still under comparative evaluation and include a laparoscopic or transcervical approach (TC-TEST) (Yovich et al, 1990). The results of oocyte and embryo transfers from these procedures over the 2-year period 1988–1989 are shown in Figures 3 and 4.

There were 253 pregnancies diagnosed following 776 transfer procedures (32.6%) and 165 pregnancies proceeded to livebirth deliveries (21.3% of transferred cases). The pregnancy rates were significantly higher following GIFT (3 d.f., $P < 0.01$), although pregnancy wastage was higher. None the less, the GIFT procedure still had a significantly higher chance of livebirth delivery per transfer procedure (3 d.f., $P < 0.05$). Conversely, the pregnancy rate and 'take-home-baby' rate for IVFET was significantly lower than the combined tubal transfer groups (1 d.f., $P < 0.02$ and $P < 0.005$ respectively).

With respect to individual implantations, 313 pregnancy sacs were diagnosed in the 7–8th week following the transfer of 2621 oocytes or embryos (failing pregnancies were diagnosed as single sacs). This indicated the overall implantation rate was 11.9%, and the rates ranged from a low of 8.7% for IVFET embryos to a high of 14.1% of GIFT oocytes or 18.8% of estimated GIFT 'embryos' (if one assumes that 75% of transferred oocytes will fertilize in vivo). The findings were highly significant (3 d.f., $P < 0.001$), mainly due to the lower implantation rate of embryos transferred to the uterus compared with the combined groups of oocyte and embryo transfers to the fallopian tubes (1 d.f., $P < 0.001$). Of further interest is the comparison of implantation rates for GIFT, PROST and TEST. It appears that in vivo generated embryos may (if the fertilization rate assumption holds) have an improved chance of implantation as GIFT 'E' rates are higher than combined PROST–TEST (1 d.f., $P < 0.005$).

Overall, 215 live infants were born providing an 'efficiency' level of 8.2% of oocytes or embryos transferred. The 'take-home-baby' rate ranged from 5.8% of IVF-ET embryos to 11.8% of PN oocytes transferred in the PROST procedure. The differences were highly significant (3 d.f., $P < 0.002$), virtually entirely due to the relatively low rate for uterine transfers compared with all tubal transfers (1 d.f., $P < 0.002$). Applying the aforementioned assumption to estimate GIFT 'embryos', an efficiency rate of 12.8% ongoing implantations was significantly higher than other tubal transfer procedures (1 d.f., $P < 0.05$). Again, the data indicates that tubal transfers are significantly better than uterine transfers and the improvement is greater the earlier the stage of transfer.

The above data confirms previous reports from PIVET (Yovich et al, 1988a, 1989b) but the precise reason for the benefit of tubal transfer remains uncertain. It is likely that oocytes and embryos transferred to the fallopian tube are more securely housed than with uterine placement, but the main reason is more likely to relate to the relatively unfavourable milieu within the uterine cavity in the early postovulatory phase, and this may be more marked after CC has been used for stimulation (Nelson et al, 1990). It is also possible that the fallopian tube contains factors of special benefit to the developing embryo, but one would expect greater differences if some crucial factor was not present in the uterus. The variation in implantation rates of tubal procedures with respect to the day of transfer implies that in vitro culture techniques are still not ideal and that further research is warranted in this area.

Underlying infertility disorder

It appears that factors in the female, associated with the underlying infertility disorder, may influence the likelihood of implantation. However, the differentiation between embryo factor and uterine receptivity is not always clear and specific studies in this area are required. The following conditions show variations from the general results in IVF.

Polycystic ovary disease and associated syndromes

The polycystic ovary (PCO) syndrome remains a contentious subject, with wide variations in its definition and management. In a decade of experience with subfertile couples treated by a broad range of methods, including IVF related procedures and GIFT, such patients have generally performed poorly when the stimulation regimen involved $CC \pm hMG$. The characteristics of the group included women with clinical PCO disease (i.e. infertility, oligomenorrhoea, obesity, hirsutism); those with histologically diagnosed polycystic ovaries; those with multifollicular ovaries diagnosed on ultrasound scans performed early in a non-treatment menstrual cycle; those with high basal LH:FSH ratio; and those women with raised serum androgens. Both reduced fertilization of oocytes when LH levels are raised (Stanger and Yovich, 1985) and reduced implantation of embryos when serum androgens are raised (Yovich, 1988b) have been described.

During 1988–1989, an alternative stimulation regimen was applied to the above group; this involved pituitary downregulation with GnRHa (Lucrin) followed by hMG stimulation as described earlier. The outcome was significantly improved in all the subcategories of the PCO syndrome. For example, 14 women with clinical PCO disease had 20 IVF related treatment cycles, resulting in the retrieval of 305 oocytes (15/patient). Following the transfer of up to four oocytes in GIFT or three embryos in IVF, nine pregnancies ensued with eight livebirths (57% of women). However, OHSS occurred in five treatment cycles (25%), and one patient required paracentesis. Three of the pregnancies were twin gestations (38%), and each had a successful outcome.

It appears the prognosis of women with PCO disease and PCO syndrome is markedly improved in assisted reproduction by avoiding CC and creating pituitary downregulation prior to stimulation; however, this group appears particularly predisposed to OHSS and multiple pregnancies.

Endometriosis

A wide range of abnormalities have been described in attempting to explain the cause of infertility in women with endometriosis, including hormonal anomalies, disordered ovarian function, peritoneal factors and immunological disturbances. A study from PIVET compared the outcome of 30 women with grade IV (i.e. most severe) pelvic endometriosis with a similar group of non-endometriotic tubal factor causes treated by IVF-ET. No differences were found in the stimulated hormone profiles but the endometriosis cases had a significantly reduced pregnancy rate (Yovich et al, 1988b). Significantly fewer oocytes were obtained from the endometriosis cases but the fertilization rate was normal, unlike the findings in another study (Wardle et al, 1985). The PIVET study also indicated no morphological differences in embryo quality but the implantation rate was significantly reduced, implying the presence of an implantation inhibitory factor. However, the subsequent experience of treating endometriosis patients by tubal transfer procedures, particularly GIFT, showed no limitations in the chance of pregnancy or implantation (Figure 11), regardless of the grade (Figure 12) or whether the women had been treated previously by either hormonal or surgical therapy (Yovich et al, unpublished data). There are some apparent differences related to the stimulation regimen, with the best results obtained after GnRHa downregulation. This further data appears not to support the presence of an implantation inhibitory factor but implies that embryos generated from women with endometriosis may be more susceptible to damage in utero, possibly when this follows CC stimulation. It is current policy at PIVET to downregulate women with grades III and IV (i.e. moderate and severe) pelvic endometriosis for 6 weeks prior to hMG stimulation for IVF related procedures, GIFT being preferred where applicable.

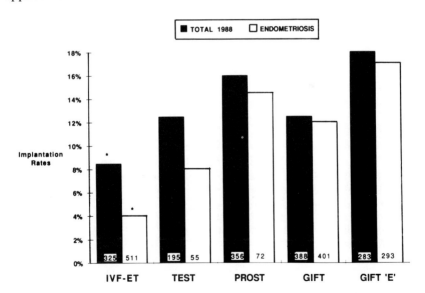

Figure 11. A comparison of implantation rates of embryos and oocytes for cases with endometriosis (1986–1988) compared with total cases treated from mixed causes during 1988 by various IVF related procedures. *IVF-ET had significantly lower implantation rates generally than tubal transfer procedures (combined data $P < 0.001$) and endometriosis cases were further reduced from other IVF-ET cases ($P < 0.05$). GIFT 'E' refers to estimated embryos (as Figure 4).

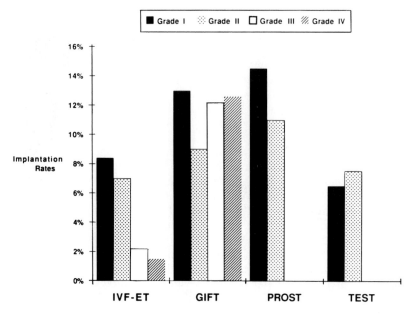

Figure 12. The implantation rates for oocytes and embryos transferred in various IVF related procedures according to the grade of endometriosis of the cases in Figure 11. (Total transferred = 1039; $*\chi^2$ 3 d.f., $P < 0.001$.)

EARLY PREGNANCY FAILURE

The clinician's interest in the phenomenon of implantation does not cease when pregnancy is diagnosed as there is a high proportion of wastage, mostly within the first 6 weeks after ovulation or embryo transfer. The pattern of wastage identified clinically at PIVET has been reported (Yovich and Matson, 1988a) and is shown in Figure 13. From a series of 1657 pregnancies diagnosed after infertility treatments to May 1989, 30.9% did not reach 20 weeks. The remaining 1145 pregnancies progressed to births, with the delivery of 1613 infants. These data are now incorporated into the routine counselling of patients seeking infertility treatments.

The clinical categories of pregnancy wastage were:

1. *Preclinical (biochemical) pregnancies* ($n = 98$; 5.9%): where loss occurred before the ultrasound diagnosis around week 7.
2. *Blighted ovum (anembryonic) pregnancy* ($n = 211$; 12.7%): early ultrasound examination revealed an empty intrauterine gestation sac associated with static or falling β-hCG levels.
3. *Spontaneous fetal death (spontaneous abortion or miscarriage)* ($n = 98$; 5.9%): absent fetal heart activity and failure in growth of the gestation sac, when positive fetal heart activity had previously been demonstrated at ultrasound scan.
4. *Ectopic pregnancy* ($n = 100$; 6.0%): an extrauterine implantation

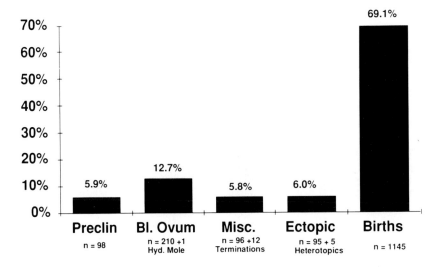

Figure 13. Outcome of 1657 monitored pregnancies conceived following infertility treatments at PIVET (July 1982–May 1989). Preclin., preclinical; Bl. Ovum, blighted ovum; Misc., miscarriage; Hyd. Mole, hydatidiform mole.

(usually tubal) with diagnosis made at laparoscopy if ultrasound examination failed to confirm the presence of an intrauterine gestation sac in association with raised serum β-hCG.

5. *Heterotopic pregnancy* ($n = 5$): a multiple pregnancy with both intrauterine and extrauterine gestational sacs.
6. *Hydatidiform mole* ($n = 1$): characteristic snowstorm appearance on ultrasound and hydropic chorionic villus vesicles at curettage.
7. *Therapeutic terminations* ($n = 12$): mostly for genetic reasons following amniocentesis or CVS diagnosis.
8. *Late pregnancy outcomes* ($n = 1145$): high incidence of multiple pregnancies (1.4 infants per birth) and preterm deliveries, even among singletons (13%). Fetal abnormalities ($n = 33$; 3.0%) are not increased over that reported in the local population (Bower et al, 1989), nor were recurring abnormalities a feature. An early study on the followup of children indicated normal development (Yovich et al, 1986a).

Patterns of early wastage

The patterns of early pregnancy wastage revealed some variations due to the underlying infertility disorder and the treatment method applied (Yovich and Matson, 1988a). For example, preclinical pregnancies were more common after GIFT and IVF-ET; blighted ovum pregnancies were more common after AIH or GIFT treatment for male factor infertility; and ectopic pregnancies were almost invariably found in women with known or suspected fallopian tube disease but were less common in male factor treatment groups, e.g. DI and PROST.

Monitoring early pregnancies

In some studies at PIVET and elsewhere early pregnancies have been monitored by hormonal and certain pregnancy associated protein estimations each week until a definitive diagnosis could be made, usually by ultrasound scan in the 7th to 8th week (Yovich et al, 1985b, 1986b, 1986c; Yamashita et al, 1989). Recently, an analysis on 675 monitored treatment cycles in women conceiving a singleton pregnancy, either following spontaneous ovulation ($n = 384$) or ovarian stimulation with CC/hMG ($n = 291$) between 1985 and 1989, has been completed (Lower et al, unpublished data). The prospective serum collection has been analysed to establish the value of early postimplantation hormonal estimations in the prediction of early pregnancy loss (Lower et al, unpublished data).

As expected, in the early weeks of pregnancy the levels of E_2 and progesterone are considerably higher in pregnancies conceived after ovarian stimulation with CC/hMG when compared with unstimulated cases. However, somewhat surprisingly, β-hCG levels were found to be significantly higher up to week 7 in unstimulated conceptions than in those following stimulation ($P < 0.005$). Frequency distribution curves plotting multiples of the median value (MoM, e.g. Figure 14) enabled comparisons of single and several hormone estimations for ongoing pregnancies and early pregnancy losses to be calculated as an odds ratio (i.e. true positives/false positives) (Wald and Cuckle, 1989). Significantly lower and falling β-hCG

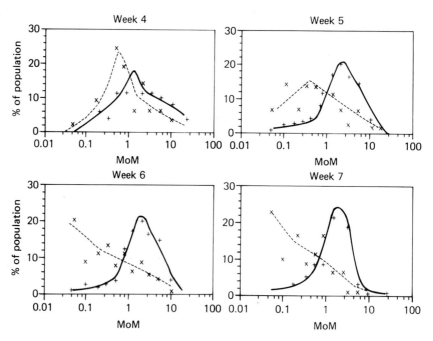

Figure 14. Multiples of the median value (MoM) curves for β-hCG in weeks 4–7 of ongoing (+——+) and failing (×---×) singleton pregnancies arising in unstimulated cycles.

levels discriminated the failing pregnancy group from ongoing pregnancies as early as the 5th week but the predictive value of any given result could often pose a clinical dilemma. Figure 15 considers the sensitivity and specificity of β-hCG estimations with receiver operating characteristic (ROC) (Vinatier and Monnier, 1988) curves for each week of gestation. For example, choosing a cut-off level of β-hCG below 0.5 MoM of the ongoing pregnancy range gives a sensitivity of 75% with an odds ratio of 8.61 at 7 weeks in unstimulated cycles. Similarly, a cut-off of 0.5 MoM for progesterone gives a sensitivity of only 41% and an odds ratio of 20. Such frequency

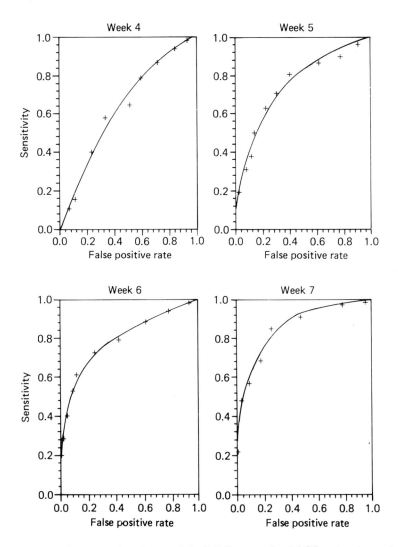

Figure 15. Receiver operating characteristic (ROC) curves for β-hCG estimations using a cut-off of 0.5 MoM for weeks 4–7 of singleton pregnancies.

distribution and ROC curves are currently being evaluated in prospective studies to determine their value in clinical practice.

Therapeutic strategies for early pregnancy wastage

In considering a therapeutic approach for high-risk pregnancies and those threatening to abort, the nature and causes of pregnancy wastage bear consideration. These can be broadly considered in three areas: general maternal conditions, intrinsic embryo abnormalities, and local uterine-endometrial factors.

General maternal disorders

Underlying maternal conditions may cause recurrent pregnancy losses, and comprehensive investigations with a view to specific counselling and treatments where applicable, should screen for the following.

Genetic causes. Detailed banded chromosome analysis is checked from both partners.

Anatomical causes. Detection of fibroids, cervical incompetence, active pelvic endometriosis, genital tract infections and uterine anomalies, including those from diethylstilboestrol exposure and intrauterine synaechiae, requires careful clinical evaluation, along with hysterography, laparoscopy and hysteroscopy.

Infective causes. Serological tests are performed for relevant antibodies in the detection of syphilis, brucellosis, toxoplasmosis and rubella immunological status. Endocervical swabs are cultured for aerobic and anaerobic bacteria and specific investigations are performed to exclude infection with cytomegalovirus, *Chlamydia trachomatis*, herpesvirus, *Listeria monocytogenes* and *Mycoplasma hominis. Mycobacterium tuberculosis* also requires consideration, depending upon clinical features and the patient's demographic background.

Maternal diseases. Tests are performed for systemic lupus erythematosis (Bresnihan et al, 1977), i.e. lupus anticoagulant and/or cardiolipin antibody (Exner, 1989), antinuclear factor and complement proteins C3 and C4, and fasting blood sugar for diabetes, as well as screening for cardiovascular, renal and thyroid diseases. Other considerations, such as exposure to anaesthetic gases, industrial chemicals and pesticides, the ingestion of antimetabolites and anticoagulants, and smoking/alcohol history, may be relevant in individual cases. The investigation of fertility parameters including ASABs (Junk et al, 1986; Haas, 1987) and luteal phase evaluation should be included.

Immunological factors. It has been suggested that the absence of an essential maternal immunoregulatory response to the genetically foreign fetus is the cause of at least some cases of recurrent miscarriages (Taylor and Faulk, 1981). It was therefore speculated that immunizing such women with their husbands' prepared lymphocytes would stimulate the appropriate maternal response, and one controlled study indicated the approach was valid (Mowbray et al, 1985). Certainly, women who recurrently miscarry often have negative mixed lymphocyte reactivity (MLR), whereas most women who have successfully completed at least one pregnancy have a positive MLR. This test, combined with the aforementioned screening protocol, forms the basis of an international multicentre study of paternal lymphocyte immunotherapy, and in which PIVET is a member (Moloney et al, 1989). So far a clear benefit for immunotherapy has not been demonstrated.

Embryo factors

Workers in the field of human reproduction have long been concerned that their efforts should not cause congenital abnormalities. The birth of Louise Brown in July 1978 was the climax of many years of painstaking research. She was one of four pregnancies achieved in that period, two of which resulted in normal children and two which failed to proceed. One of the latter was a first trimester abortion and tests on the fetus demonstrated a karyotype of 69XXX (Steptoe et al, 1980). Interestingly, the other was a midtrimester loss several weeks after amniocentesis had revealed pleiomorphism of 15D and a large Y chromosome, paternally derived anomalies which were not thought to have contributed to the loss.

As previously discussed, studies of preimplantation embryos generated following IVF have demonstrated a high rate of chromosomal abnormalities (23–40%) (Plachot et al, 1987; Papadopoulos et al, 1989). This may be compared with the historic findings of Hertig and Rock (Hertig et al, 1952), who described that only four of the eight preimplantation embryos they identified were morphologically normal. Of those embryos which do implant, by far the most common identifiable defect in early pregnancy losses is chromosomal abnormality in the conceptus. Abnormalities were detected in 60% of spontaneous abortions when the products of conception were analysed after the diagnosis had been made at a relatively late stage on clinical grounds (Boué et al, 1975). One might speculate that a number of other aetiological factors peculiar to pregnancies conceived following IVF could have an adverse effect. However, in a study conducted by postal questionnaire of more than 200 European IVF centres, 21 out of 34 (62%) abortuses karyotyped demonstrated a chromosomal abnormality (Plachot, 1989), suggesting no increase in the rate.

Pregnancies monitored at PIVET, and which have been diagnosed as blighted ovum, fetal deaths or ectopics, have undergone CVS and subsequent culture for chromosome identification using GTG banding (Lower et al, unpublished data). Fifty pregnancies were examined in this fashion over a 2 year period. Four have been excluded because of failed culture. Of the remaining 46 pregnancies, there were 29 blighted ova, nine spontaneous fetal deaths and eight ectopic pregnancies. In ten of 29 blighted ovum pregnancies and one of nine spontaneous fetal death pregnancies, readily identifiable villi

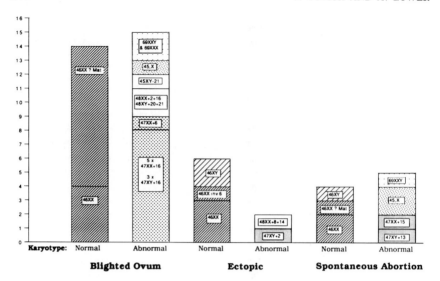

Figure 16. Distribution and type of chromosome abnormalities identified after chorionic villus sampling among 46 early failing pregnancies in a subfertile population.

could not be unequivocally separated and the culture specimen, consisting of membranous tissue, was classified as products of conception (POC). These 11 cases, mostly obtained early in the series when the initial assessment was less rigorous, all gave normal 46XX karyotypes. Whilst it is our belief that the majority of these karyotypes are of fetal origin, it was not possible to confirm conclusively that some were not of maternal origin.

Figure 16 summarizes the number and types of chromosomal abnormalities obtained in conceptions, both with and without gamete manipulation. The proportion of abnormalities in early pregnancy losses following gamete manipulation (14/26) was not significantly different from those following spontaneous conception (9/20). Anembryonic pregnancies and spontaneous abortions showed a higher proportion of chromosomal abnormalities than ectopic pregnancies. Maternal ages were not significantly different from those experiencing a loss showing a normal karyotype (32.2 ± 4.4 years) from those with an abnormal karyotype (32.8 ± 4.7 years).

These results from a subfertile population are in agreement with the findings of others in the general population. Data pooled from several series reveals an overall incidence of chromosomal abnormality in 46% of spontaneous abortions recognized in the first trimester (Simpson, 1989). The most common anomaly was autosomal trisomy, accounting for 50% of all abnormalities detected and 22% of all abortions for which karyotypes were available.

The imbalance between sexes in our data is interesting. Only 11 of 46 conceptuses karyotyped bore a Y chromosome, and of the 23 conceptuses with normal karyotypes only three were male. Even if the 11 pregnancies in which definite villi were not identified are excluded, only 25% of the karyotypically normal early pregnancy losses were male. This may represent a sampling error, although it appears that female conceptuses are more likely to abort in early pregnancy than males, as the finding has been reported in several series of spontaneous abortions (Boué et al, 1975; Creasy et al, 1976; Hassold et al, 1980). Of interest, the overall sex ratio in singleton births following IVF procedures was 1.03 (M:F) in Australia and New Zealand in 1988 (Lancaster, 1990).

Chromosomal abnormalities were seen in only two of our eight cases of ectopic pregnancy. A third case was identified with inversion of chromosome 6 of maternal origin, which was not considered to have contributed to the pregnancy loss. The ratio of male to female karyotypes was 0.6 for ectopic gestation. Clearly, larger numbers are required before any firm conclusions can be drawn from this data, however it is interesting to speculate that chromosomal anomalies do not appear to predispose to ectopic gestation, nor does there appear to be any gross imbalance between the sexes.

There is a clear and well-documented correlation between maternal age and aneuploidy, in particular trisomy 21 (Penrose, 1933). However, in our data there was no significant difference in maternal age between women losing normal and abnormal conceptuses.

Two of the three cases of triploidy are of particular interest. These occurred in consecutive pregnancies in the same patient following spontaneous conception. Whether these lesions were the result of polyspermic fertilization or caused by a defect of cell division is unknown. Controlled fertilization in vitro is proposed as a diagnostic test for this couple. If polyspermic fertilization is demonstrated at the pronuclear stage then the condition may be amenable to specific treatment by microinjection of a single spermatozoon. The importance of careful examination of the fertilized oocytes at the pronuclear stage has been stressed (Yovich and Grudzinskas, 1990). In particular this will enable oocytes with odd numbers of pronuclei to be discarded. There were no cases of polyploidy amongst those pregnancies conceived following fertilization in vitro in the present series.

Early diagnosis of pregnancy failure has therefore enabled accurate karyotyping of the abortus in a high proportion of the early pregnancy losses arising after infertility treatment. It indicates that around half the losses related to chromosomal abnormalities, similar to that observed after spontaneous abortions diagnosed on clinical grounds at a later stage of gestation in the general community. The study is currently being extended to determine the impact, if any, on the pattern of chromosome related wastage to luteal and obstetric support therapy.

Endometrial factors

The concept of potentially treatable hormonal deficiencies causing an inadequate endometrial bed for successful nidation remains an appealing but unproven hypothesis. Studies reported during the 1960s indicated that hormone support therapy was probably not effective (Shearman and Garrett, 1963; Goldzieher, 1964; Klopper and MacNaughton, 1965).

Furthermore, as shown in the preceding section, 50–60% of implantations and miscarriages demonstrate chromosomal abnormalities. However, in subfertile cases, pregnancy wastage appears to be more common than in the fertile population, and the demonstrated benefits of luteal support therapy in assisting implantation, as well as the finding that pregnancies will establish and be maintained in women without ovaries by simply providing exogenous oestradiol valerate and progesterone during the conception cycle and through the first trimester, lend support to the concept that implantation may be supported by hormonal therapy. The following regimens are undergoing trials at PIVET.

Threatened abortion. Women who present with vaginal bleeding in the first trimester are offered oral medroxyprogesterone acetate (MPA; Provera, Upjohn Pharmaceuticals). Early data from this study suggests a beneficial effect without causing the retention of abnormal fetuses or creating fetal abnormalities (Yovich, 1988a). The regimen commences with 4-hourly oral tablets to 120 mg/day, reducing to 6-hourly (80 mg/day) when bleeding ceases. Cases are monitored by hormonal and ultrasound investigations each week (see earlier) until the diagnosis is clear. If a viable fetus is demonstrated, hormonal support is continued until the 16th week, when it is ceased following a weaning regimen.

Recurrent abortion. In the belief that such cases may have a corpus luteal defect, hCG is used to maintain luteal activity and this is supported by MPA, which is thought to contribute further by maintaining uterine quiescence (i.e. dampening contractility). The regimen commences at the time of pregnancy diagnosis as follows:

hCG: 5000 IU i.m. twice each week to 10 weeks.
MPA: 80 mg/day by four divided doses to 16 weeks, thereafter weaning over the ensuing fortnight.

In selecting MPA as the support progestagen we were influenced by previous observations that the drug did not cause significant congenital abnormalities (Burstein and Wassermann, 1964). MPA is a substituted progesterone and therefore differs from the derivatives of the 19-nortestosterone group, which have been used in the past and have been clearly shown to have appreciable androgenic effects on the developing female fetus (Wilkins, 1960). The oral preparation of MPA appears satisfactory as it is well absorbed and stable plasma concentrations around 27 nmol/litre are established and maintained on the described regimens (Yovich et al, 1985d). That study also examined the profile of steroid metabolites in the maternal urine during the first trimester of pregnancy and showed no abnormal peaks on gas–liquid chromatography and mass spectrometry in a matched series.

CONCLUSIONS

A large number of factors are known or suspected to influence the chance of successful embryo implantation and these have been considered with a view to enhancing the process, where possible and appropriate. In clinical practice this falls into three broad areas: assisted reproduction for infertility disorders; enhancing the luteal phase and early weeks of pregnancy to minimize embryo wastage; and exploring management protocols to identify and treat pregnancies which threaten to abort or where women are at high risk for recurrent abortion.

Although the various techniques involved in assisted reproduction have developed rapidly over the past 15 years, the main limitation to their success relates to poor embryo quality. The numerous factors bearing on this have been considered and current research is being directed to improving the quality of embryos developed in vitro, and the identification of those embryos which have the full developmental potential to implant and proceed through to become healthy infants. Currently only around 10% of embryos have this potential. Certainly, a large part of the problem relates to underlying chromosomal abnormalities (up to 40% of preimplantation embryos and around 50% of both implanted gestational sacs and early developing fetuses). The rapidly evolving potential for preimplantation embryo diagnosis makes routine embryo selection seem a highly feasible proposition for the not-too-distant future, and one which can already be considered where there are known chromosome related disorders. However, other assessments of embryo quality are also important in order to improve the efficiency of assisted reproduction procedures for the management of both infertility and genetic disorders.

Treatments to enhance uterine receptivity appear to improve the chance of implantation and do significantly improve the chance of implantations proceeding to successful outcomes. This is most noticeable when embryos are of poorer quality. Luteal phase and early pregnancy treatments are currently given on an empirical basis and require further evaluation in relationship to the specific circumstances where benefits might be obtained. Although the treatments described here do not appear to cause maternal or fetal complications, caution must be expressed, in that numbers treated are still relatively small. Furthermore, the results obtained in studies on sub-fertile populations may not necessarily be relevant for fertile women.

Acknowledgements

We wish to acknowledge the support of staff members at PIVET Medical Centre who contributed in various ways to this work; in particular Jim Cummins, Rohini Edirisinghe, Jeanne Yovich, Jason Spittle and Ceinwin Gearon; also Marie Mulcahy of the cytogenetics department at the State Health Laboratories.

REFERENCES

Angell RR, Templeton AA & Aitken RJ (1986) Chromosome studies in human in vitro fertilization. *Human Genetics* **72:** 333–339.
Bahadori R (1986) Tuberculosis and infertility in Azerbaijan, Iran. In Ludwig H & Thomsen K (eds) *Gynecology and Obstetrics. Proceedings of the 11th World Congress of Gynecology and Obstetrics 1985, Berlin*, pp 675–676. Berlin: Springer-Verlag.

Baldo B, Smal M & McCaskill A (1990) Radioimmunoassay for platelet activating factor (PAF). *Life Sciences* **2:** 66.
Belaisch-Allart J, Testart J, Fries N et al (1987) The effect of dydrogesterone supplementation in an IVF programme. *Human Reproduction* **2:** 183–185.
Bell S & Drife J (1989) Secretory proteins of the endometrium—potential markers for endometrial dysfunction. *Clinical Obstetrics and Gynaecology* **3:** 271–291.
Boué J, Boué A & Lazar P (1975) Retrospective and prospective epidemiological studies of 1500 karyotyped spontaneous human abortions. *Teratology* **12:** 11–26.
Bower C, Forbes R, Rudy E et al (1989) Report of the Congenital Malformations Registry of Western Australia 1980–1988. Health Department of Western Australia.
Bresnihan B, Grigor R, Oliver M et al (1977) Immunological mechanism for spontaneous abortion in systemic lupus erythematosis. *Lancet* **ii:** 1205–1207.
Brock DJH, Mennie M, Curtis A et al (1989) Predictive testing for Huntington's disease with linked DNA markers. *Lancet* **ii:** 463–466.
Brown JR, Pepperell RJ & Evans JH (1980) Disorders of ovulation. In Pepperell RJ, Hudson B & Wood C (eds) *The Infertile Couple*, pp 7–42. Edinburgh: Churchill Livingstone.
Burstein R & Wasserman H (1964) The effect of Provera on the fetus. *Obstetrics and Gynecology* **23:** 931–934.
Buvat J, Herbaut J-C, Marcolin G et al (1990) Luteal support after luteinizing hormone-releasing hormone agonist for in vitro fertilization: superiority of human chorionic gonadotropin over oral progesterone. *Fertility and Sterility* **53:** 490–494.
Coutelle C, Williams C, Handyside A et al (1989) Genetic analysis of DNA from single human oocytes: a model for preimplantation diagnosis of cystic fibrosis. *British Medical Journal* **299:** 22–24.
Cox LW (1975) Infertility, a comprehensive programme. *British Journal of Obstetrics and Gynaecology* **82:** 2–6.
Creasy M, Crolla J & Alberman ED (1976) A cytogenic and histological analysis of spontaneous abortions. *Human Genetics* **45:** 239–251.
Cummins J, Breen T, Harrison K et al (1986) A formula for scoring human embryo growth rates in in vitro fertilization: its value in predicting pregnancy and in comparison with visual estimates of embryo quality. *Journal of In Vitro Fertilization and Embryo Transfer* **3:** 284–295.
Cummins JM, Yovich JM, Edirisinghe WR et al (1989) Pituitary down-regulation using leuprolide for the intensive ovulation management of poor prognosis patients having IVF-related treatments. *Journal of In Vitro Fertilization and Embryo Transfer* **6:** 345–352.
Edwards RG, Steptoe PC & Purdy JM (1980) Establishing full-term human pregnancies using cleaving embryos grown in vitro. *British Journal of Obstetrics and Gynaecology* **87:** 737–756.
Exner T (1989) Lupus anticoagulants. *Today's Life Science* **1:** 40–46.
Forman R, Fries N, Testart J et al (1988) Evidence for an adverse effect of elevated serum estradiol concentrations on embryo implantation. *Fertility and Sterility* **49:** 118–122.
Foulot H, Ranoux C, Dubuisson JB et al (1989) In vitro fertilization without ovarian stimulation: a simplified protocol applied in 80 cycles. *Fertility and Sterility* **52:** 617–621.
Garcia J (1989) Return to the natural cycle for in vitro fertilization (Alleluia! Alleluia!). *Journal of In Vitro Fertilization and Embryo Transfer* **6:** 67–68.
Gidley-Baird AA, O'Neill C, Sinosich MJ et al (1986) Failure of implantation in human in vitro fertilization and embryo transfer patients: the effects of altered progesterone/estrogen ratios in humans and mice. *Fertility and Sterility* **45:** 69–74.
Goldzieher J (1964) Double-blind trial of a progestin in habitual abortion. *Journal of the American Medical Association* **188:** 651–654.
Gonen Y, Casper R, Jacobson W et al (1989) Endometrial thickness and growth during ovarian stimulation: a possible predictor of implantation in in vitro fertilization. *Fertility and Sterility* **52:** 446–450.
Grillo J, Gamerre M, Noizet A et al (1991) Influence of the morphological aspect of embryos obtained by in vitro fertilization on their implantation rate. *Journal of In Vitro Fertilization and Embryo Transfer* (in press).
Haas GJ (1987) Immunologic infertility. *Obstetric and Gynecology Clinics of North America* **14:** 1069–1085.
Haines C, O'Shea R & Emes A (1989) The relationship between follicular diameter,

fertilization rates and embryo quality. *Proceedings of the VIth World Congress on IVF and Alternate Assisted Reproduction, Jerusalem*. Jerusalem: Plenum Press.

Handyside A, Penketh R, Winston R et al (1989) Biopsy of human preimplantation embryos and sexing by DNA amplification. *Lancet* **i:** 347–349.

Handyside AH, Kontogianni EH, Hardy K et al (1990) Pregnancies from biopsied preimplantation embryo sexed by Y-specific DNA amplification. *Nature* **344:** 768–770.

Hardy K, Hooper M, Handyside A et al (1989) Non-invasive measurement of glucose and pyruvate uptake by individual human oocytes and preimplantation embryos. *Human Reproduction* **4:** 188–191.

Hassold T, Chen N, Funkhouser J et al (1980) A cytogenetics study of 1000 spontaneous abortions. *Annals of Human Genetics* **44:** 151–178.

Hertig A, Rock J, Adams E et al (1952) Thirty-four fertilized human ova, good, bad and indifferent, recovered from 210 women of known fertility. *Pediatrics* **23:** 202–211.

Holding C & Monk M (1989) Diagnosis of beta-thalassaemia by DNA amplification in single blastomeres from mouse preimplantation embryos. *Lancet* **ii:** 532–535.

Homburg R, Eshel A, Abdalla HI et al (1988) Growth hormone facilitates ovulation induction by gonadotropins. *Clinical Endocrinology* **29:** 113–117.

Homburg R, West C, Torresani T et al (1990) Cotreatment with human growth hormone and gonadotropins for induction of ovulation: a controlled clinical trial. *Fertility and Sterility* **53:** 254–260.

Hutchinson-Williams KA, Diamond MP, DeCherney AH et al (1990) Luteal rescue in in vitro fertilization-embryo transfer. *Fertility and Sterility* **53:** 495–501.

Joshi S, Rao R, Henriques E et al (1986) Luteal phase concentrations of a progestagen-associated endometrial protein (PEP) in the serum of cycling women with adequate or inadequate endometrium. *Journal of Clinical Endocrinology and Metabolism* **63:** 1247–1249.

Junk S, Matson PL, O'Halloran F et al (1986) Use of immunobeads to detect human anti-spermatozoal antibodies. *Clinical Reproduction and Fertility* **4:** 199–206.

Kerem B-S, Rommens JM, Buchanan JA et al (1989) Identification of the cystic fibrosis gene: genetic analysis. *Science* **245:** 1073–1080.

Klopper A & MacNaughton M (1965) Hormones in recurrent abortion. *Journal of Obstetrics and Gynaecology of the British Commonwealth* **72:** 1022–1028.

Kovacs GT, Shekleton P, Leeton J et al (1987) Ectopic tubal pregnancy following in vitro fertilization and transfer under ultrasonic control. *Journal of In Vitro Fertilization and Embryo Transfer* **4:** 124–0740.

Lancaster P (1990) IVF and GIFT pregnancies Australia and New Zealand 1988. National Perinatal Statistics Unit.

Leeton J, Trounson A & Jessup D (1985) Support of the luteal phase in in vitro fertilization programs: result of a controlled trial with intramuscular Proluton. *Journal of In Vitro Fertilization and Embryo Transfer* **2:** 166–169.

Lenz S, Lauritsen JG & Kjellow M (1981) Collection of human oocytes for in vitro fertilization by ultrasonically guided follicular puncture. *Lancet* **i:** 1163–1164.

Li H, Gyllesten U & Cui X (1988) Amplification and analysis of DNA sequences in single human sperm and diploid cells. *Nature* **335:** 414–417.

Macnamee MC, Taylor PJ, Howles CM et al (1989) Short-term luteinizing hormone-releasing hormone agonist treatment: prospective trial of a novel ovarian stimulation regimen for in vitro fertilization. *Fertility and Sterility* **52:** 264–269.

Mahadevan MM, Leader A & Taylor PJ (1985) Effects of low-dose human chorionic gonadotrophin on corpus luteum function after embryo transfer. *Journal of In Vitro Fertilization and Embryo Transfer* **2:** 190–194.

Marrs R, Saito H, Yee B et al (1984) Effect of variation of in vitro culture techniques upon oocyte fertilization and embryo development in human in vitro fertilization procedures. *Fertility and Sterility* **41:** 519–523.

Martin RH (1988) Human sperm karyotyping: a tool for the study of aneuploidy. In Vig BK & Sandberg AA (eds) *Aneuploidy, Part B: Induction and Test Systems*, pp 297–316. New York: Alan R Liss.

Maudlin I & Fraser L (1977) The effect of PMSG dose on the incidence of chromosomal anomalies in mouse embryos fertilized in vitro. *Journal of Reproduction and Fertility* **50:** 275–280.

Moloney M, Bulmer J, Scott J et al (1989) Maternal immune responses and recurrent miscarriage. *Lancet* **i:** 45–46.

Monk M (1989) Preimplantation diagnosis. In Edwards RG (ed.) *Establishing a Successful Human Pregnancy*, Serono Symposia Publications, Vol. 66, pp 185–197. New York: Raven Press.

Morton H (1984) Early pregnancy factor, a link between fertilisation and immunomodulation. *Australian Journal of Biological Sciences* **37:** 393–407.

Mowbray J, Gibbings C, Liddell H et al (1985) Controlled trial of treatment of recurrent spontaneous abortion by immunisation with paternal cells. *Lancet* **i:** 941–943.

Nelson LM, Herslag A, Kuri RS et al (1990) Clomiphene citrate directly impairs endometrial receptivity in the mouse. *Fertility and Sterility* **53:** 727–731.

O'Neill C & Spinks N (1988) Embryo-derived platelet activating factor. In Chapman M, Grudzinskas G & Chard T (eds) *Implantation: Biological and Clinical Aspects*, pp 83–91. London: Springer-Verlag.

Papadopoulos G, Templeton A, Fisk N et al (1989) The frequency of chromosome anomalies in human preimplantation embryos after in-vitro fertilization. *Human Reproduction* **4:** 91–98.

Penrose L (1933) The relative effects of paternal and maternal age in mongolism. *Journal of Genetics* **27:** 219.

Pickering S, Braude P, Johnson M et al (1990) Transient cooling to room temperature can cause irreversible disruption of the meiotic spindle in the human oocyte. *Fertility and Sterility* **54:** 102–108.

Pickering SJ & Johnson MH (1987) The influence of cooling on the organisation of the meiotic spindle of the mouse oocyte. *Human Reproduction* **2:** 207–216.

Plachot M (1989) Chromosome analysis of spontaneous abortions after IVF. A European survey. *Human Reproduction* **4:** 425–429.

Plachot M, Junca A-M, Mandelbaum J et al (1987) Chromosome investigations in early life. II. Human preimplantation embryos. *Human Reproduction* **2:** 29–35.

Plachot M, Veiga A, Montagut J et al (1988) Are clinical and biological IVF parameters correlated with chromosomal disorders in early life: a multicentric study. *Human Reproduction* **3:** 627–635.

Puissant F, Van Rysselberge M, Barlow P et al (1987) Embryo scoring as a prognostic tool in IVF. *Human Reproduction* **2:** 705–708.

Purdy J (1982) Methods for fertilization and embryo culture in vitro. In Edwards R & Purdy J (eds) *Human Conception In Vitro*, pp 135–156. London: Academic Press.

Riordan JR, Rommens JM, Kerem BS et al (1989) Identification of the cystic fibrosis gene: cloning and characterization of complementary DNA. *Science* **245:** 1066–1073.

Roberts CG & O'Neill C (1988) A simplified method for fixation of human and mouse preimplantation embryos which facilitates G-banding and karyotypic analysis. *Human Reproduction* **3:** 990–992.

Rommens JM, Iannuzzi MC, Kerem B-S et al (1989) Identification of the cystic fibrosis gene: chromosome walking and jumping. *Science* **245:** 1059–1065.

Rudak E, Jacobs PA & Yanagimachi R (1978) Direct analysis of the chromosome constitution of human spermatozoa. *Nature* **274:** 911–913.

Saiki R, Gelfand D, Stoffel S et al (1988) Primer-directed enzymatic amplification of DNA with a thermostable DNA polymerase. *Science* **239:** 487–491.

Saiki RK, Scharf S, Faloona F et al (1985) Enzymatic amplification of beta-globin genomic sequences and restriction site analysis for diagnosis of sickle cell anemia. *Science* **230:** 1350–1354.

Shearman R & Garrett W (1963) Double-blind study of the effect of 17-hydroxyprogesterone caproate on abortion rate. *British Medical Journal (Clinical Research)* **1:** 292–295.

Simpson JL (1989) Aetiology of pregnancy failure. In Chapman M, Grudzinskas J, Chard T & Maxwell D (eds) *The Embryo: Normal and Abnormal Development and Growth*. London: Springer-Verlag (in press).

Smith B, Porter R, Ahuja K et al (1984) Ultrasonic assessment of endometrial changes in stimulated cycles in an in vitro fertilization and embryo transfer program. *Journal of In Vitro Fertilization and Embryo Transfer* **1:** 233–238.

Stanger JD & Yovich JL (1985) Reduced in-vitro fertilization of human oocytes from patients with raised basal luteinizing hormone levels during the follicular phase. *British Journal of Obstetrics and Gynaecology* **92:** 385–393.

Stanger JD, Yovich JL & Grudzinskas JG (1985) Relationship between pregnancy-associated plasma protein A (PAPP-A) in human peri-ovulatory follicle fluid and the collection and fertilization of human ova in vitro. *British Journal of Obstetrics and Gynaecology* **92:** 786–792.

Steptoe PC, Edwards RG & Purdy JM (1980) Clinical aspects of pregnancies established with cleaving embryos grown in vitro. *British Journal of Obstetrics and Gynaecology* **87:** 757–768.

Taylor C & Faulk W (1981) Prevention of recurrent abortion with leucocyte transfusion. *Lancet* **ii:** 68–70.

Trounson A, Howlett D, Rogers P et al (1986) The effect of progesterone supplementation around the time of oocyte recovery in patients superovulated for in vitro fertilization. *Fertility and Sterility* **45:** 532–535.

Veiga A, Calderón G, Santaló J et al (1987) Chromosome studies in oocytes and zygotes from an IVF program. *Human Reproduction* **2:** 425–430.

Vinatier D & Monnier J-C (1988) La courbe R.O.C. (receiver operating curve), une aide à la décision. Principes et applications à travers quelques exemples. *Journal de Gynecologie, Obstetrique Biologie de la Reproduction* **17:** 981–989.

Wald N & Cuckle H (1989) Reporting the assessment of screening and diagnostic tests. *British Journal of Obstetrics and Gynaecology* **96:** 389–396.

Wales R, Whittingham D, Hardy K et al (1987) Metabolism of glucose by human embryos. *Journal of Reproduction and Fertility* **79:** 289–297.

Walters DE (1985) An assessment of two mathematical models of embryo implantation. In Edwards RG, Purdy JM & Steptoe PC (eds) *Implantation of the Human Embryo*, pp 219–232. London: Academic Press.

Wardle P, McLaughlin E, McDermott A et al (1985) Endometriosis and ovulatory disorder: reduced fertilization in vitro compared with tubal and unexplained infertility. *Lancet* **ii:** 236–239.

Webb S (1988) In Vitro Fertilization and Related Procedures in Western Australia 1983–1987. A Demographic, Clinical and Economic Evaluation of Participants and Procedures. Health Department of Western Australia.

West JD, Gosden JR, Angell RR et al (1988) Sexing whole human preimplantation embryos by in-situ hybridization with a Y-chromosome specific DNA probe. *Human Reproduction* **3:** 1010–1019.

Wikland M, Hamberger L, Enk L et al (1989) Technical and clinical aspects of ultra-sound guided oocyte recovery. *Human Reproduction* **4**(supplement): 79–82.

Wilkins L (1960) Masculinization of female fetus due to use of orally given progestins. *Journal of the American Medical Association* **118:** 1028–1032.

Yamashita T, Okamoto S, Thomas A et al (1989) Predicting pregnancy outcome after in vitro fertilization and embryo transfer using estradiol, progesterone, and human chorionic gonadotropin beta-subunit. *Fertility and Sterility* **51:** 304–309.

Yovich JL (1985) Embryo quality and pregnancy rates in in vitro fertilization. *Lancet* **i:** 283–284.

Yovich JL (1988a) Medroxyprogesterone acetate therapy in early pregnancy has no apparent fetal effects. *Teratology* **38:** 135–144.

Yovich JL (1988b) Treatments to enhance implantation. In Chapman M, Grudzinskas G & Chard T (eds) *Implantation: Biological and Clinical Aspects*, pp 239–254. Berlin: Springer-Verlag.

Yovich JL (1990) Tubal transfers: PROST & TEST. In Asch RH, Balmaceda JP & Johnston I (eds) *Gamete Physiology*, pp 305–317. Norwell, Massachusetts: Serono Symposia USA.

Yovich JL & Grudzinskas JG (1990) *The Management of Infertility: A Practical Guide to Gamete Handling Procedures*. London: Heinemann.

Yovich JL & Matson PL (1988a) Early pregnancy wastage after gamete manipulation. *British Journal of Obstetrics and Gynaecology* **95:** 1120–1127.

Yovich JL & Matson PL (1988b) The treatment of infertility by the high intrauterine insemination of husband's washed spermatozoa. *Human Reproduction* **3:** 939–943.

Yovich JL, Stanger JD, Yovich JM et al (1984) Assessment and hormonal treatment of the luteal phase of in vitro fertilization cycles. *Australian and New Zealand Journal of Obstetrics and Gynaecology* **24:** 125–130.

Yovich JL, McColm SC & Yovich JM (1985a) Early luteal serum progesterone concentrations are higher in conception cycles. *Fertility and Sterility* **44:** 185–189.

Yovich JL, Stanger JD, Yovich JM et al (1985b) Hormonal profiles in the follicular phase, luteal phase and first trimester of pregnancies arising from in-vitro fertilization. *British Journal of Obstetrics and Gynaecology* **92**: 374–384.

Yovich JL, Turner SR & Murphy AJ (1985c) Embryo transfer technique as a cause of ectopic pregnancies in in vitro fertilization. *Fertility and Sterility* **44**: 318–321.

Yovich JL, Willcox DL, Wilkinson SP et al (1985d) Medroxyprogesterone acetate does not perturb the profile of steroid metabolites in urine during pregnancy. *Journal of Endocrinology* **104**: 453–459.

Yovich JL, Parry TS, French NP et al (1986a) Developmental assessment of twenty IVF infants at their first birthday. *Journal of In Vitro Fertilization and Embryo Transfer* **3**: 253–257.

Yovich JL, Willcox DL, Grudzinskas JG et al (1986b) Placental hormone and protein measurements during conception cycles and early pregnancy. In Thomsen K & Ludwig H (eds) *Proceedings of XIth World Congress of Gynecology and Obstetrics*, pp 854–857. Berlin: Springer-Verlag.

Yovich J, McColm S, Willcox D et al (1986c) The prognostic value of β-hCG, PAPP-A, oestradiol and progesterone in early human pregnancy and the effect of medroxyprogesterone. *Australian and New Zealand Journal of Obstetrics and Gynecology* **26**: 59–64.

Yovich J, Draper R & Edirisinghe W (1988a) The relative chance of pregnancy following tubal or uterine transfer procedures. *Fertility and Sterility* **49**: 858–864.

Yovich JL, Matson PL, Richardson PA et al (1988b) Hormonal profiles and embryo quality in women with severe endometriosis treated by in vitro fertilization and embryo transfer. *Fertility and Sterility* **50**: 308–313.

Yovich JL, Cummins JM, Bootsma B et al (1989a) The usefulness of simultaneous IVF and GIFT in predicting fertilization and pregnancy. In Capitanio GL, Asch RH, De Cecco L & Croce S (eds) *GIFT: From Basics to Clinics*, pp 321–332. New York: Raven Press.

Yovich JL, Draper RR, Turner SR et al (1989b) The benefits of tubal transfer procedures. *Proceedings of the VIth World Congress on IVF and Alternate Assisted Reproduction, Jerusalem.* Jerusalem: Plenum Press (in press).

Yovich JL, Matson PL & Yovich JM (1989c) The optimization of laparoscopic oocyte recovery. *International Journal of Fertility* **34**: 390–400.

Yovich JL, Turner S, Yovich JM et al (1989d) In-vitro fertilization today. *Lancet* **ii**: 688–689.

Yovich J, Draper R, Turner S et al (1990) Transcervical tubal embryo-stage transfer (TC-TEST). *Journal of In Vitro Fertilization and Embryo Transfer* **7**: 137–140.

Yovich J, Edirisinghe W & Cummins J (1991) Evaluation of luteal support therapy in a randomized controlled study within a GIFT program. *Fertility and Sterility* (in press).

Index

Note: Page numbers of article titles are in **bold** type.